Primary Care of Adolescent Girls

Edited by

Susan M. Coupey, M.D.

Professor of Pediatrics
Albert Einstein College of Medicine
Associate Director, Division of Adolescent Medicine
Montefiore Medical Center
Bronx, New York

Philadelphia / HANLEY & BELFUS, INC.

Publisher: HANLEY & BELFUS, INC.
Medical Publishers
210 South 13th Street
Philadelphia, PA 19107
(215) 546-7293; 800-962-1892
FAX (215) 790-9330
Web site: http://www.hanleyandbelfus.com

Note to the reader: Although the information in this book has been carefully reviewed for correctness of dosage and indications, neither the authors nor the editor nor the publisher can accept any legal responsibility for any errors or omissions that may be made. Neither the publisher nor the editor makes any warranty, expressed or implied, with respect to the material contained herein. Before prescribing any drug, the reader must review the manufacturer's current product information (package inserts) for accepted indications, absolute dosage recommendations, and other information pertinent to the safe and effective use of the product described.

Library of Congress Cataloging-in-Publication Data

Primary care of adolescent girls / edited by Susan M. Coupey.
p. / cm.
Includes bibliographical references and index.
ISBN 1-56053-369-2 (alk. paper)
1. Adolescent medicine. 2. Teenage girls—Diseases. 3. Primary care (Medicine). I. Coupey, Susan M.
[DNLM: 1. Adolescent Medicine. 2. Primary Health Care. 3. Women's Health. WS 460 P952 2000]
RJ550.P75 2000
616'00835'2—dc21

99-047482

Primary Care of Adolescent Girls ISBN 1-56053-369-2

Last digit is the print number: 9 8 7 6 5 4 3 2 1

Contents

Contributors

Elizabeth M. Alderman, M.D.
Associate Professor of Clinical Pediatrics, Department of Pediatrics, Albert Einstein College of Medicine, Division of Adolescent Medicine, Montefiore Medical Center, Bronx, New York

Sharon Rose Beier, M.D.
Assistant Professor, Department of Pediatrics, Albert Einstein College of Medicine, Beth Israel Medical Center, Bronx, New York

Frank M. Biro, M.D.
Associate Professor, Department of Pediatrics, University of Cincinnati College of Medicine, Division of Adolescent Medicine, Children's Hospital Medical Center, Cincinnati, Ohio

Robert T. Brown, M.D.
Clinical Professor, Department of Pediatrics, Ohio State University College of Medicine and Public Health, Chief, Section of Adolescent Medicine, Children's Hospital, Columbus, Ohio

Peter G. Burk, M.D.
Clinical Associate Professor, Department of Medicine, Albert Einstein College of Medicine, Division of Dermatology, Montefiore Medical Center, Bronx, New York

Susan M. Coupey, M.D.
Professor, Department of Pediatrics, Albert Einstein College of Medicine, Associate Director, Division of Adolescent Medicine, Montefiore Medical Center, Bronx, New York

Ron Davis, Ph.D.
Associate Professor, Department of Psychology, Lakehead University, Consulting Psychologist, Eating Disorders Program, St. Joseph's Care Group, Thunder Bay, Ontario, Canada

Nancy Neveloff Dubler, L.L.B.
Professor, Department of Epidemiology and Social Medicine, Albert Einstein College of Medicine, Director, Division of Bioethics, Montefiore Medical Center, Bronx, New York

Ann L. Engelland, M.D.
Private Practice of Pediatrics, Westchester County, New York Presbyterian Hospital, New York, White Plains Hospital, White Plains, New York

Donna Futterman, M.D.
Associate Professor, Department of Pediatrics, Albert Einstein College of Medicine, Director, Adolescent AIDS Program, Montefiore Medical Center, Bronx, New York

Melanie A. Gold, D.O.
Assistant Professor, Department of Pediatrics, University of Pittsburgh School of Medicine, Division of Adolescent Medicine, Children's Hospital of Pittsburgh, Pittsburgh, Pennsylvania

Alvin F. Goldfarb, M.D.
Professor, Department of Obstetrics and Gynecology, Jefferson Medical College of Thomas Jefferson University, Philadelphia, Pennsylvania

Estherann Grace, M.D.
Associate Clinical Professor, Department of Pediatrics, Harvard Medical School, Division of Adolescent/Young Adult Medicine, Children's Hospital, Boston, Massachusetts

Richard B. Heyman, M.D.
Clinical Professor, Department of Pediatrics, University of Cincinnati College of Medicine, Children's Hospital Medical Center, Cincinnati, Ohio

Debra K. Katzman, M.D.
Associate Professor, Department of Pediatrics, University of Toronto Faculty of Medicine, Medical Director, Eating Disorder Program, Hospital for Sick Children, Toronto, Ontario, Canada

Paritosh Kaul, M.D.
Postdoctoral fellow, Department of Pediatrics, Albert Einstein College of Medicine, Division of Adolescent Medicine, Montefiore Medical Center, Bronx, New York

Lisa M. Lewis, Ph.D.
Assistant Professor, Department of Pediatrics, University of Cincinnati College of Medicine, Division of Adolescent Medicine, Children's Hospital Medical Center, Cincinnati, Ohio

Alec L. Miller, Psy.D.
Assistant Professor, Department of Psychiatry and Behavioral Sciences, Albert Einstein College of Medicine, Division of Adolescent Psychiatry, Montefiore Medical Center, Bronx, New York

Catherine Monk, Ph.D.
Research Fellow, Department of Psychiatry, Columbia University, Developmental Psychobiology Department, The New York State Psychiatric Institute, New York, New York

David Muram, M.D.
Professor, Department of Obstetrics and Gynecology, State University of New York Health Sciences Center at Brooklyn, University Hospital at Brooklyn, Brooklyn, New York

Wendy Neal, M.D.
Assistant Professor, Department of Pediatrics, Mount Sinai School of Medicine, Mount Sinai Adolescent Health Center, New York, New York

Kim O'Connor, M.S.W.
Social Worker, Teenage Pregnancy and Parenting Program, New York Presbyterian Hospital, Cornell Medical Center, New York, New York

Margaret Polaneczky, M.D.
Assistant Professor, Department of Obstetrics and Gynecology, New York Presbyterian Hospital, Cornell Medical Center, New York, New York

M. Max Quinn, J.D.
Fellow in Pediatric Bioethics, Department of Epidemiology and Social Medicine, Albert Einstein College of Medicine, Montefiore Medical Center, Bronx, New York

Walter D. Rosenfeld, M.D.
Associate Professor, Department of Pediatrics, University of Medicine and Dentistry of New Jersey, Director, Adolescent/Young Adult Center for Health, Morristown Memorial Hospital, Morristown, New Jersey

Susan L. Rosenthal, Ph.D.
Associate Professor, Department of Pediatrics, University of Cincinnati College of Medicine, Division of Adolescent Medicine, Children's Hospital Medical Center, Cincinnati, Ohio

Caitlin C. Ryan, M.S.W., A.C.S.W.
Senior Research Fellow, Human Sexuality Studies Program, San Francisco State University, San Francisco, California

Kathy Silverman, D.O.
Postdoctoral Fellow, Department of Pediatrics, Division of Adolescent Medicine, Albert Einstein College of Medicine, Montefiore Medical Center, Bronx, New York

Eric Small, M.D., F.A.A.P.
Clinical Instructor, Department of Pediatrics, Mount Sinai School of Medicine, New York, Founder and Director, The Sports Medicine Center for Young Athletes, Blythedale Children's Hospital, Valhalla, New York

Elaine E. Yordan, M.D.
Clinical Professor, Department of Pediatrics, University of Connecticut School of Medicine, Farmington, Associate Director, Section of Adolescent Medicine, Saint Francis Hospital and Medical Center, Hartford, Connecticut

Preface

The substantial changes in the role of women in society that took place in the second half of the 20th century have had a profound effect on the lives of adolescent girls. Girls have many more career options and lifestyle choices than in the past, but also are exposed to more stress and health risks. Primary care provided in clinicians' offices encompasses preventive screening as well as diagnosis and management of acute and chronic, biomedical and psychosocial conditions. Primary care clinicians require a broad-based knowledge of all aspects of health in order to deliver the high-quality care that young women need and deserve. This book gathers the medical, gynecological, developmental, psychological, and bioethical information needed to provide comprehensive primary health care to girls ages 10 through 22 years. It focuses on the unique biopsychosocial developmental needs of girls and their impact on the delivery of health care. Throughout the book there is an emphasis on the differences between the care of adolescent girls and that of boys, younger children, or adult women.

This text is not intended as a complete reference but as a concise resource that will be useful in a clinical setting. It is divided into three sections. The first section, entitled *The Adolescent Girl as a Patient,* contains three chapters outlining physical and psychosocial development of early, middle, and late adolescent girls and special considerations for the health care visit at each of these three stages of adolescence. Two additional chapters focus on body image and sexual development, important areas in the diagnosis and treatment of many different health problems of girls in this age group. The second section, *The Patient–Provider–Parent Relationship*, contains two thoughtful chapters by experienced practitioners addressing the special issues faced by male versus female clinicians caring for adolescent girls. Also in this section are important chapters addressing the management of confidentiality and legal and ethical considerations for providing health care to adolescents. The third and final section entitled *Primary Care* contains 17 chapters covering common conditions encountered in the clinical or office setting, including the preparticipation sports examination, contraceptive counseling, depression and suicide, breast and menstrual disorders, eating disorders, abdominal pain, sexual assault, and others.

This book is addressed to the broad range of clinicians who currently provide health care to adolescent girls. I hope it will be useful to gynecologists, pediatricians, family physicians, nurse practitioners, mental health professionals, health educators, and other health care professionals. Because residents in pediatrics, internal medicine, and family medicine require training in adolescent medicine and residents in obstetrics and gynecology must become competent in primary care of young women, the book also should be of interest to trainees in these disciplines. Adolescent girls are best served by clinicians who understand their needs, communicate effectively with them and their parents, and deliver comprehensive primary care services. I hope this book will provide much of the information needed to accomplish these goals.

Susan M. Coupey, M.D.

Dedication

This book is dedicated to my daughter, Ariane, and to the many adolescent girls who allowed me to participate in their health care and who taught me so much.

Susan M. Coupey, M.D.

Acknowledgment

Many wonderful people helped with the planning, writing, and production of this book and I would like to thank a few of them personally. First and foremost, I want to express my gratitude and admiration to the authors for their patience, faith in the book, and the many nights and weekends they spent writing the chapters. Without the organizational skills and editing help of Mary Sharkey and Paritosh Kaul, M.D., this project would have been much more difficult to accomplish—thank you both. The sage advice of my two dear friends, esteemed colleagues, and mentors, Stanford B. Friedman, M.D., and Alvin F. Goldfarb, M.D., has helped me immeasurably in planning the book and seeing it through to publication. Thank you, Stan and Alvin. Last but certainly not least, I thank my husband, James R. English, and my son, Marc, for their support and understanding, and Linda Belfus, extraordinary editor and publisher, for making this publishing experience a pleasure.

Susan M. Coupey, M.D.

CHAPTER 1

The Early Adolescent Girl: Ages 10–13 Years

Elaine E. Yordan, M.D.

Although the developmental process of adolescence has been described as a time of storm and stress, most adolescents are not overwhelmed by turmoil and inner conflict. Early adolescence is a time of growth, change, and expanding horizons. Most early adolescents emerge from childhood feeling happy with their lives and having positive perceptions about the changes taking place in their bodies and their minds. Notwithstanding an eventual transfer of orientation away from the family and newly directed toward independence and autonomy, most early adolescents live at home and depend on the material support, emotional security, and boundaries provided by the family. Most early adolescents feel optimistic about their future.

Human development is influenced on multiple levels by biologic and psychologic characteristics, society and culture, historical developments, and the ecological environment. For early adolescents there are the normative, age-graded influences of puberty, linear growth, and entrance into middle school or junior high school. However, early adolescent development also is affected by historical and societal variables such as periods of national economic depression or prosperity and changes in societal sex-role expectations, child-rearing practices, and the educational system.

Entering early adolescence, girls must address several issues simultaneously. The burgeoning capacity for sexual reproduction is the most notable. The early adolescent girl also must come to accept the outward physical changes brought about by growth and pubertal development. The events that take place in intrauterine life and early infancy can be compared in magnitude only with those that transpire in early adolescence. The degree of biological development and the pace with which it occurs in early adolescence are truly dramatic. Furthermore, the early adolescent girl must integrate these changes into an increasingly complicated social environment.

Who is the early adolescent girl? She is between 10 and 13 years old and entering puberty. She has breast development, pubic hair development, and may have had menarche (Table 1). Her brain has achieved 95% of its adult weight. She is accumulating subcutaneous fat on the lower portion of her trunk and

TABLE 1. Mean Ages for Appearance of Pubertal Characteristics in United States' Girls

Characteristic	White Girls	African-American Girls
Breasts	10 years	8.9 years
Pubic hair	10.5 years	8.8 years
Menarche	12.9 years	12.2 years

Adapted from Herman-Giddens ME, Slora EJ, Wasserman RC, et al: Secondary sexual characteristics and menses in young girls seen in office practice: A study from the pediatric research in office settings network. Pediatrics 99:505–512, 1997.

extremities. She may have acne and apocrine gland secretion causing axillary odor. She functions in three environments: family, school, and peer group.

This chapter reviews the physical and psychosocial development of early adolescent girls as well as important aspects of the medical history and the general physical and gynecologic examination. In addition, common problems encountered in the primary medical care of early adolescent girls are discussed.

PHYSICAL AND PSYCHOSOCIAL DEVELOPMENT

Physical Development

Shortly after birth the hypothalamic–pituitary–ovarian axis enters a state of dormancy. The production of the gonadotropins, follicle-stimulating hormone (FSH), and luteinizing hormone (LH) from the anterior pituitary gland and gonadotropin-releasing hormone (GnRH) from the hypothalamus is suppressed by an intrinsic central nervous system inhibitor and negative feedback caused by a hypersensitivity to minute amounts of circulating ovarian estrogen. Ovarian hormones and pituitary gonadotropins are produced only in small amounts and remain suppressed until the age of 8 or 9 years.

At the initiation of puberty the intrinsic suppression of endogenous GnRH gradually disappears; there is decreased sensitivity to the negative feedback of estrogen; and the pulsatile secretion of GnRH is initiated. At first, the GnRH pulses occur during sleep. The increasing amplitude and frequency of the GnRH pulses lead to the sleep-associated secretion of detectable serum levels of LH, which is the biochemical sign that marks the beginning of puberty. As a consequence of continuing increases in gonadotropin secretion, the ovaries enlarge and begin to produce estrogen. For adolescent girls, the first clinical sign of puberty is the appearance of breast budding (thelarche) at age 9 or 10 years. See Figure 1 for the Tanner classification of adolescent breast stages. Serum estradiol levels are about 2 ng/dl in girls just before breast development begins. The peak growth spurt in girls occurs later at Tanner breast stage 3–4, but it begins at about age 11 or 12 years, which is 2 years earlier than in boys.

Following the appearance of breast budding, pubic hair (Fig. 2) and axillary hair begin to grow under the influence of several androgens (dehydroepiandrosterone, dehydroepiandrosterone sulfate, and androstenedione) secreted from the adrenal cortex. Estrogen production continues and menarche follows at about age 12½ years (range 9–15 years). The timing of menarche is associated with inherited family patterns shared by mothers and daughters as well as

Breast Stage 1 (B_1)
The infantile stage, which persists from the postnatal period until the onset of puberty.

Breast Stage 2 (B_2)
The "bud" stage. The breast and papilla are elevated as a small mound. The diameter of the areola is increased.

Breast Stage 3 (B_3)
The breast and areola are further enlarged with a continuous rounded contour.

Breast Stage 4 (B_4)
The areola and papilla continue to expand and form a secondary mound projecting above the contour of the breast.

Breast Stage 5 (B_5)
The adult form with a smooth rounded contour. The secondary mound present in Stage 4 is gone.

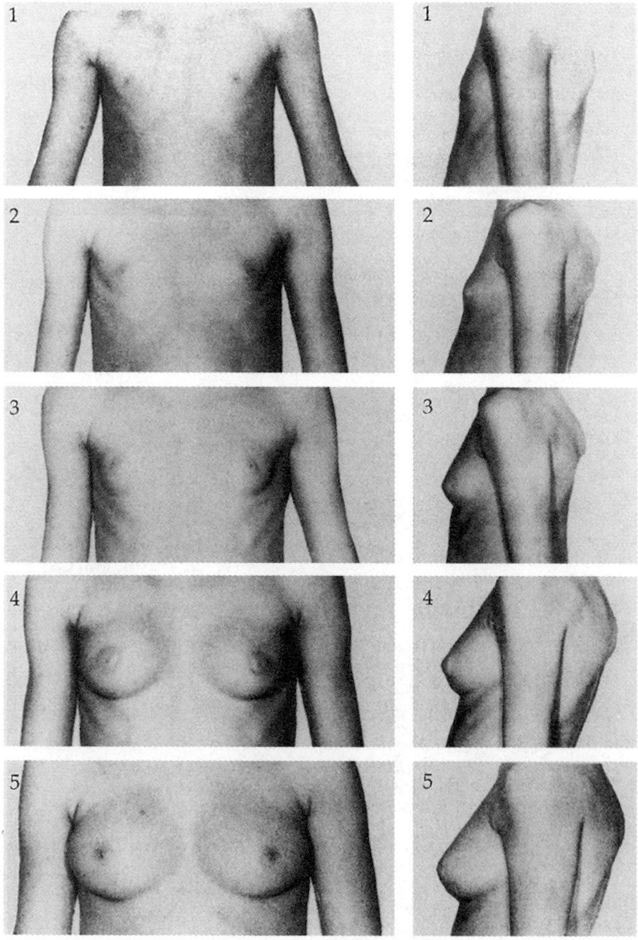

FIGURE 1. Tanner breast stages. (From Herman-Giddens ME, Bourdony CJ: Assessment of Sexual Maturity Stages in Girls. Elk Grove Village, IL, American Academy of Pediatrics, 1995, with permission. Photographs originally printed in Tanner JM: Foetus into Man. Cambridge, MA, Harvard University Press, 1978, p 197.)

by environmental factors. Although the average age at menarche for white girls in the United States is currently 12.9 years, ethnic differences have been noted, with African-American girls having earlier menarche (Table 1). Chronic illnesses and vigorous athletic training may be responsible for a delay in onset of menstruation. Eating disorders can disrupt normal growth and cause a delay of pubertal development. Among girls with Tanner stage 2 breasts, there is a 10% incidence of menarche. Thirty percent of girls with Tanner stage 3 breasts have had menarche, whereas 90% will have menarche by the time their breast development has reached Tanner stage 4.

The first several menstrual periods are usually anovulatory. It may be as long as a year after menarche that the last milestone of puberty is reached. Ovulation and regular, predictable ovulatory menstrual cycles may not be established until a few years after menarche.

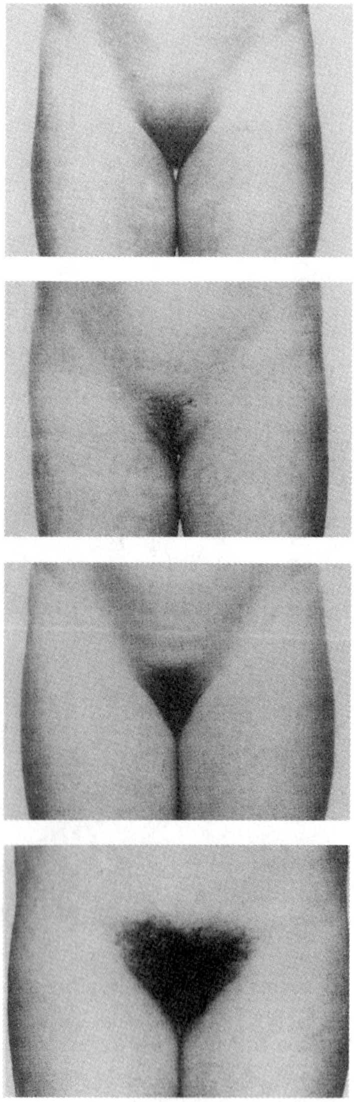

Pubic Hair Stage 1 (PH_1)
None.

2

Pubic Hair Stage 2 (PH_2)
Small amount of long, downy hair along the labia majora.*

3

Pubic Hair Stage 3 (PH_3)
Moderate amount of more curly, pigmented, and coarser hair. The hair also begins to extend laterally.

4

Pubic Hair Stage 4 (PH_4)
Hair that resembles adult hair in coarseness and curliness but area covered is smaller and there is no extension to the medial surface of thighs.

5

Pubic Hair Stage 5 (PH_5)
Adult type and quantity, sometimes extending to medial surface of thighs.

* The shadow in this photograph obscures the detail of this stage.

FIGURE 2. Tanner pubic hair stages. (From Herman-Giddens ME, Bourdony CJ: Assessment of Sexual Maturity Stages in Girls. Elk Grove Village, IL, American Academy of Pediatrics, 1995, with permission. Photographs originally printed in Tanner JM: Foetus into Man. Cambridge, MA, Harvard University Press, 1978, p 199.)

Psychosocial Development

As the early adolescent girl begins to experience the physical changes of puberty, she also must begin to integrate these changes into her self-concept. Her perception of her body image may lead her to worry that she is abnormal in some way. She may focus on and worry excessively about minor aches and pains, body shape, weight, and acne. The early adolescent struggles with the inner question, "Am I normal?" This increased body awareness is also expressed by a greater interest in privacy and increased shyness and modesty. Self-esteem commonly declines in early adolescence. Self-esteem is the positive or negative way in which one evaluates one's values, feelings, attitudes and beliefs, fears and desires, and strengths and weaknesses. Early adolescents begin to evaluate themselves more on inner thoughts and emotions, thinking that they know themselves better than others know them.

The Changing Parent–Child Relationship

The vast majority of adolescents love and appreciate their parents. However, a major imperative of adolescent psychological development is to individuate and develop a separate identity from parents. Girls at this age begin to form new relationships outside of the family with peers. Conflict may be a feature in the reorganization process of the parent–adolescent relationship. A conflict develops between dependency needs and the need to detach from parents. However, if both parents and children can compromise and adapt during this period of change, it can be a positive time of exploration for both.

Adolescent behavior is affected by parenting styles. Adolescents with authoritarian parents tend to be withdrawn and moody and to have low self-esteem. Those with permissive parents may be impulsive and aggressive and have trouble dealing with limits. Adolescent girls with neglectful parents are in the most danger of deviant behavior because of lack of supervision and emotional support. Adolescents with authoritative parents are likely to be in a situation that fosters positive development.

The Peer Group

The formation of close relationships outside of the immediate family with peers assumes a new importance in early adolescence. Although the family is the primary means of socialization for the individual, during early adolescence peer groups become powerful modifiers of girls' thoughts and activities. A peer group is a small group of similarly aged, fairly close friends who share the same activities. In early adolescence a peer group is often comprised of same-sex friends.

During early adolescence girls begin to develop a sense of independence and autonomy. Early adolescents are old enough that they do not need constant supervision, and they enjoy their new sense of freedom. Early adolescent activities are more peer-focused and independent of adults. To be part of a group is a powerful need in adolescence, and it coincides with the adolescent tendency to experiment with novel experiences and risk-taking behavior. It is from such experiences that close friendships gain importance. Often, best friends become intensely close, and a best friend's parent may actually be regarded by some early adolescent girls as a surrogate parent.

The peer group usually provides a social environment that is safe and secure. Within the protective context of same-sex friendships and group activities, the early adolescent girl has the opportunity to interact socially and to experiment. Peer groups provide support for the adolescent while she defines her identity, abilities, and personality. Popularity depends on a youngster's social skills. Besides providing the adolescent with the opportunity to learn how to interact with others, peer groups are central influences on her general interests, musical tastes, and clothing styles. Within the secure framework of idealized friendships, the girls dress alike, have the same makeup, hair styles, outfits, and backpacks; they even employ the same slang vocabulary.

Although peer groups may provide positive influences such as scholastic and extracurricular achievement, they also may be the source of negative influences such as drug and alcohol use. High self-esteem and self-confidence are two personal attributes that enable adolescent girls to avoid succumbing to peer pressure that promotes undesirable activities. To influence risk-taking behaviors (such as the use of cigarettes, marijuana, and alcohol), the peer group may use verbal methods, including daring and provoking a girl until she feels uncomfortable and then engages in the behavior, or nonverbal methods such as excluding the girl from social activities until she complies with the behavior.

Ideally, within the supportive structure of the peer group, the early adolescent will initiate experimentation and begin to test rules and limits, build and maintain friendships, and learn about autonomous function while still protected by adults and parents. For example, an adolescent girl may want to start dating at age 12 years, but her parents may feel that she is not ready. In this situation, one acceptable compromise is a "get together" with a group of friends.

Although peer relationships are an important part of early adolescence, the early adolescent girl still turns to the family for support in times of crisis. The combination of a supportive family and healthy peer relationships is associated with higher levels of social skills that empower the early adolescent girl to feel competent.

Emerging Sexuality

Paradoxically, while puberty may occur at the time of early adolescence, it imparts the capacity to engage in adult sexual and reproductive behaviors. A number of factors contribute to the initiation of sexual activity. Social influences have a great impact upon sexual behavior. Simply the occurrence of pubertal development is associated with peer pressure encouraging sexual behavior as part of the standards of the peer group. Having sexually permissive friends is a major factor contributing to adolescent sexual behavior. Adolescents with early pubertal development are more likely to engage in sexual behaviors at an early age than adolescents with late pubertal development. As early adolescent girls begin the process of sexual socialization, their sexual orientation and interest start to become manifest.

The appropriate age for adolescent dating varies with the individual, but certain factors contribute to the onset of dating. As youngsters progress beyond early adolescence, the same-sex peer groups that characterize that period begin to dissolve. Adolescent peer group relationships modify into couples, and dating activities begin. Currently, many adolescent girls begin to date at age 12 or 13, and early dating may lead to early sexual activity. Girls who mature early tend to have older friends. This may predispose some early adolescent girls with low self-esteem and emotional difficulties to engage in problem behaviors, including sexual intercourse. Early adolescents with a history of sexual abuse are also at risk of initiating sexual intercourse at an earlier age. The chief reasons why early adolescent girls engage in sexual intercourse are peer pressure, pressure from boys, curiosity, and the perception that everyone does it.

Cognitive Development

Early adolescents are concrete thinkers, have limited ability to understand abstract concepts, and best appreciate things that they can recognize with one of the five senses. However, it is during adolescence that the ability to think more abstractly, employ logic, consider hypothetical situations, and view issues from multiple perspectives develops. It is important to remember that early adolescents are only beginning to acquire these abilities; adults must be supportive and understand that while girls may look physically mature, their thought processes may remain quite concrete and childlike.

THE HEALTH CARE VISIT

The Medical Interview

The medical interview with the early adolescent should include a discussion of nutritional habits, bowel function, sleep pattern, school situation, after-school activities, social relations (i.e., friends and family), emotional well-being, and any risk-taking behaviors (e.g., smoking, drinking, illicit drugs). For girls, questions about menarche, menstrual pattern, dysmenorrhea, and menstrual hygiene are appropriate.

The early adolescent girl may exhibit difficulties, however, in providing the salient information. It can be a challenging task to motivate young adolescents to respond to questioning with a detailed and complete reply. The difficulty can be made worse when a parent, usually the mother, is present during the medical interview and dominates the situation. The best way to avoid this set of circumstances is to make a deliberate effort to develop rapport with the patient over an extended period. Ideally, this takes the form of a longstanding doctor–patient relationship. Over a period of years a clinician can gradually promote a comfortable and trusting atmosphere that facilitates easy communication with the early adolescent. However, not every relationship is longstanding, and it is important to develop rapport with new patients quickly.

When the early adolescent girl is new to your practice and schedules a routine annual examination, it is useful to send an introductory letter or pamphlet to the parents that describes the scope of the visit, including information on confidentiality and about genital examination. It is worthwhile to communicate to parents that early adolescence is an ideal time to help girls begin to learn how to have more responsibility for their own health care. It is also appropriate to raise the issue of confidentiality as part of the routine approach to providing medical care to adolescents. As such, although interaction with the parents continues to be important, a private confidential conversation with the early adolescent girl begins to lay the foundation for trusting and candid exchanges between clinician and patient over the years to come.

Managing Privacy and Confidentiality

Depending on the circumstances, the clinician should begin by speaking with the accompanying parent and the patient together. This meeting provides a way for the clinician to observe the dynamics of the relationship between the parent and the adolescent. Occasionally, a parent who has a specific concern or question may request to speak to the clinician privately. A private interview is helpful because it gives the clinician an additional opportunity to assess the parent's concerns and attitudes. Sometimes it is helpful to take advantage of the time during which the adolescent girl is changing her clothing and spend a minute or two asking the parents if there are any special concerns that they may have. They may reveal some important information or simply be grateful that their input is included in your evaluation. Having had the opportunity to discuss issues with the parent, either privately or with the girl present, the clinician should speak privately with the early adolescent girl in the consultation office.

Speaking with the early adolescent girl alone provides an appropriate opportunity to introduce the concept of confidentiality in concrete, easy-to-understand terms. During the private conversation the clinician should be open, honest, interested, concerned, and supportive; he or she should attempt to communicate at the patient's developmental level. The conversation should be nonjudgmental, with careful attention to tone of voice, content of discussion, and body language.

Ample time needs to be set aside for a careful and thoughtful dialogue. Remember that this interview influences the adolescent's attitude (positively or negatively) toward medical care and other health care professionals with whom she will interact in the future. Initially, the conversation with an early adolescent may be frustratingly one-sided, with the clinician asking questions to which the response is a nod or a short, barely audible, mumbled phrase. Although this can be discouraging, the clinician's persistence and patience usually helps the patient to feel comfortable.

How Concrete Thought May Affect the Medical Interview

Although adolescence is the time during which abstract thinking develops, interaction with the early adolescent girl needs to be conducted in concrete terms. The physical changes that are taking place in the early adolescents girl's body are the focus of her constant attention. This heightened emphasis on physical characteristics is reflected by frequently expressed concerns. It will have an effect on the way in which an early adolescent girl responds to a review of systems. She may conceivably report having every possible symptom. Headaches, nausea, chest pain, and abdominal pain are all symptoms that the girl may acknowledge. Usually, thorough questioning as a follow-up to a positive response reveals that these symptoms are minor issues. At this point the adolescent needs reassurance that everything is normal. It is a mistake for the clinician to trivialize these concerns. Also, the fact that these complaints have been addressed and resolved should be communicated to the parent, who likely has heard all these complaints endlessly from the teenager.

Occasionally, a physical symptom that may be the early adolescent's chief complaint is not related to organic pathology but instead is the result of narcissism and intense self-scrutiny. Early adolescents are filled with questions and the desire to ascertain whether the new developments they are noticing about themselves are normal or deviant. It may be extremely difficult for the early adolescent to express these concerns and worries because of concrete thinking processes. Success in uncovering these underlying concerns and working with early adolescents to help them understand the changes that are taking place in their lives and bodies depend on how the medical interview is structured and paced.

The Psychosocial History

Equal in importance to a thorough review of systems is a thorough psychosocial history. Although it may be time-consuming, asking appropriate questions may lead to an understanding of the underlying cause of a somatic complaint. It may not be until the final segments of the psychosocial interview that a key piece of information comes to light. For example, after a lengthy talk with a girl complaining of headaches, it eventually may become clear that the headaches are linked to issues uncovered in the psychosocial history. In one case, careful discussion of the girl's home life and parents' occupations revealed that the headaches were related to anxiety over the dangers that her father encountered as part of his job as a policeman.

The Home

The home environment is a key area that should be considered in the medical interview. It is important to identify the composition of the family, the size of the house or apartment, and its occupants. Does the girl have her own room and privacy at home? Because complex family characteristics often exist, the clinician should ascertain if the mother and father live together at home and the nature of their relationship to each other. The presence of a step-parent, a parent's unmarried sexual partner, siblings, and other relatives may be a significant factor affecting the early adolescent's physical and mental health. All of these relationships need to be explored.

If the adolescent girl has a problem, does she turn to one of her parents? If not to a parent, then to whom does she turn for help and why? The safety of the neighborhood, the prevalence of local gang violence, and the presence of weapons in the home are all issues that have an impact on the early adolescent's psychosocial well-being.

School

School is another area that demands careful consideration. Simply asking the early adolescent girl what school she attends and about her favorite subject, worst subject, her grades, and if she has had to repeat a grade can lead to many revealing facts. Participation in school clubs, extracurricular activities, and sports should be noted. Although your patient may not have formulated specific goals, a discussion of future plans may be fruitful. One way to facilitate this discussion is to ask, "If you could be anything in the whole wide world, what would you like to be?" It is also quite normal for the early adolescent to express a set of future goals that may appear to be totally unrealistic. In addition, a problem of truancy, detention, suspension, or expulsion for an early adolescent is always of great concern and needs to be explored carefully.

Leisure Time and Friends

Leisure time activities are an important component of the lives of early adolescent girls. It is helpful to review what she does together with her family.

After-school activities, weekend time, summer vacation, local "hang-outs," peers, and television are all influences that affect the early adolescent.

It is important to inquire about the early adolescent girl's friendships. Does she have a best friend? Who? What is the best friend's age; what habits does she have, and what do they do together? For example, if the best friend smokes cigarettes, it is likely that the patient will feel pressure to smoke. If the patient is 12 years old and the best friend is 16 years old, the patient possibly will be pressured to engage in other risky behaviors such as drinking and sexual activity. Does the early adolescent girl have friends who are boys? What are the boys' involvement in the peer group? Does she have a "crush" on one of the boys? Has she been on an individual date with him or dated within the context of the peer group? It is important to know the exact nature of her involvement with the boyfriend.

When watching television, movies, listening to music, and sleeping are the primary leisure activities for early adolescent girls, boredom is often the result. Attempts to relieve the boredom may lead to engaging in risky behaviors such as unprotected sexual intercourse, the use of illicit substances, or delinquent behaviors. Affirmative responses to these issues merit concerns of possible depression and need to be further assessed.

Risk-taking Behaviors and Sexual History

Risk-taking behavior in an early adolescent may be a sign of depression. A discussion of the early adolescent's friends is a nonthreatening way of initiating a conversation about the issues of sexual activity and substance abuse. Questions about the peer group's involvement in dating, sexual activity, cigarette smoking, alcohol consumption, and the use of illicit substances may help to uncover problems that the patient herself is having in these areas. In addition, it may be difficult for an early adolescent to divulge the fact that she is voluntarily sexually active with an older teenage boyfriend, but a general discussion of sexual activity may help her to become comfortable with discussion of her own sexual activity. For example, if an early adolescent girl is sexually active with her 17-year-old boyfriend, it is important to know if the activity is truly voluntary. The circumstances may be consistent with "date rape," in which the early adolescent has been subjected to coercion to have sex. In addition, it is possible that the early adolescent in this situation may also be a victim of physical abuse.

As part of taking a history from a sexually active early adolescent, the standard questions of age at first intercourse, number of lifetime partners, contraception and condom use apply. Early onset of sexual activity may be associated with a history of sexual abuse. Questions about a possible history of sexual abuse should be addressed to the early adolescent who is sexually active. It is also appropriate to begin a discussion about sexually transmitted diseases, human immunodeficiency virus (HIV), and contraception. The diagnosis of a sexually transmitted disease in an early adolescent aged 12 years and under may be a reportable occurrence to child-protective services in some jurisdictions.

Depression

Specific questions relating to symptoms of depression should be asked. It is not helpful to ask, "Do you feel depressed?" It is better to bring up the subject of emotions and feelings casually while conducting the physical examination. It is a good way to keep the conversation going, and by now the patient may be somewhat more relaxed. Start by asking her to describe what kind of person she is most of the time. Ask her how she balances out on a scale of 1 to 10 (sad to happy). Ask her to describe situations that make her feel "sad, down or blue." Replies like "grandmother dying" are appropriate and should not heighten concern. Conversely, if she says that she feels sad "a lot of the time," she should be evaluated for a significant clinical depression. If she admits to current or past thoughts of suicide or previous suicide attempts, it is vital to ask if she has a plan. In this circumstance immediate intervention is required.

Suicidal ideas and thoughts are serious problems. Careful questioning is always important. Sometimes suicidal thoughts and attempts are obvious, and sometimes they are subtle. Consider the case of a girl who at bedtime swallows a handful of acetaminophen tablets expecting to die, but who merely falls asleep and wakes up the next morning, never telling anyone. Such an incident, clearly indicative of some degree of depression, may never come to light unless the physician creates an atmosphere that is conducive to such a revelation. A suicide attempt in the history puts the patient at risk for a repeat act.

A history of runaway behavior needs to be thoroughly explored because it often may be rooted in the turmoil of physical or sexual abuse. Runaway behavior also may be linked to ambivalence over sexual orientation or to issues of parental substance abuse. Life on the street is commonly associated with drug and alcohol abuse, depression, low self-esteem, sexually transmitted diseases, survival sex, and sex in exchange for drugs.

The General Physical Examination

Guidelines for health supervision from the American Academy of Pediatrics address the scope of the annual visit for 10- and 11-year-old girls. Depending on the desires of the patient, the physical examination may be done with or without the mother present. Routine records of height, weight, pulse, and blood pressure should be recorded. For girls, expect a growth spurt between ages 11 and 13½ years. The complete physical examination should include assessment for hearing and vision, acne, scoliosis (Fig. 3), Tanner staging of the breasts and pubic hair (Figs. 1 and 2), and examination of the external genitalia. Discussion of breast self-examination is appropriate.

Routine testing for hematocrit, urinalysis, and a tuberculosis skin test are indicated. Also indicated are a tetanus-diphtheria booster and, if not already done, the sequence of hepatitis B immunization. Lipid screening may be indicated by family history. Between the ages of 12 and 13 years, a second dose of mumps, measles, and rubella vaccination should be given if not already done. If an adolescent has not acquired immunity to chickenpox or had the varicella vaccine, the vaccine sequence should be administered. Keep in mind that these vaccines are contraindicated in an early adolescent who is pregnant or having unprotected intercourse.

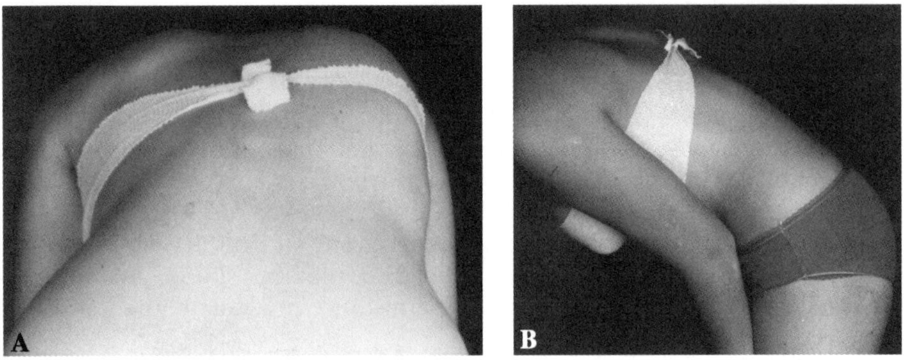

FIGURE 3. Adam's forward bend test, the primary screening physical examination for scoliosis. A, Frontal view. B, Sagittal view. (From Stanitski CL: Conditions of the spine. Adolesc Med 9:520, 1998, with permission.)

The Gynecologic Examination

The scope of the gynecologic examination of the early adolescent as part of a routine annual physical examination varies and depends on the clinical circumstances. It always is helpful to first discuss the character of the examination with the patient. Anatomic models and illustrations facilitate the dialogue. The examiner should familiarize the patient with the instrumentation for the examination and describe the sounds (i.e., metallic) and physical sensations (i.e., speculum temperature, pressure) that she will experience (see chapter 2, Table 3).

For a patient who has had a longstanding relationship with the same health care provider, an external genital examination is a customary component of the visit. There is nothing unusual about proceeding to assess all organ systems in an orderly manner, including the reproductive system. As a clinician may inquire about any respiratory symptoms during the examination of the patient's chest, it is appropriate to discuss issues pertinent to reproductive health as part of a genital examination.

When performing a gynecologic examination on an early adolescent girl, the clinician should use a chaperone as an assistant who helps to make the patient feel at ease. Although there may be instances in which the presence of a longstanding doctor–patient relationship precludes the need for a chaperone, having a chaperone to corroborate a clinician's professionalism during a gynecologic examination of an early adolescent is always prudent and beneficial. In addition, a chaperone should always be present for the medical evaluation of sexual abuse. This presence should be documented on the clinical chart.

It is appropriate to introduce the patient to the dorsal lithotomy position. Placement of a cloth drape folded around her legs and directed inward to lie flat on her abdomen makes it easier for her to look down and observe. Offer her a mirror that she can hold to watch as you examine the vulva. Describe to her what you are doing. Inspection of the vulva should be performed with adequate direct lighting. Gentle lateral separation of the labia majora is usually sufficient to allow visual examination of the vestibule of the vagina. The hymen should be observed to verify its patency.

The decision to perform a speculum examination should be tailored specifically to each early adolescent girl and the history given. If the early adolescent girl is sexually active or has been sexually assaulted (penile penetration of the vagina), examination of the vagina and cervix with an appropriately sized vaginal speculum is indicated. In this age group, a Huffman or Pederson vaginal speculum is comfortable for the patient and allows the examiner to see the vagina and cervix clearly. The exam should be as gentle as possible because it may have a lasting influence on the patient's attitude toward gynecologic health care. You should put her in control and assure her that if she has discomfort during the examination, she should tell you immediately and you will stop.

A pregnancy test should be done if there is any question of pregnancy. A Papanicolaou smear and testing for *Neisseria gonorrhoeae* and *Chlamydia trachomatis* should be obtained (culture media are necessary for cases of sexual abuse). A wet mount should be performed on any vaginal discharge. Testing for syphilis also should be done on a routine basis in all sexually active adolescents. Consider a discussion of HIV testing when appropriate. Papanicolaou smears should be performed annually, and testing for *Neisseria gonorrhoeae* and *Chlamydia trachomatis* should be obtained at the time of each pelvic examination in sexually active girls.

A bimanual pelvic examination also should be performed. When the patient is an early adolescent, a single examining finger can be placed in the vagina with the examiner's other hand placed on the patient's lower abdomen. With the availability of ultrasound, questionable or abnormal findings on physical examination can be further evaluated. For the early adolescent patient who is not sexually active, a routine speculum examination is not indicated.

Encourage the early adolescent patient who is not sexually active to continue to remain abstinent and the early adolescent patient who has been sexually active to reestablish abstinence. Other subjects to consider discussing with the patient include signs and symptoms of sexually transmitted diseases, contraceptive options, and condoms.

COMMON PROBLEMS ENCOUNTERED IN PRIMARY CARE

Common issues encountered in primary care of early adolescent girls include the timing of menarche, use of tampons, misconceptions about physiologic leukorrhea, and patient concerns about increase in body weight and fat distribution.

The Timing of Menarche

An early adolescent girl and her mother often seek an estimate of when the girl's menarche will occur. The timing of the first period depends on multiple factors. Menarche usually occurs on the downslope of the height velocity curve when the girl has at least Tanner stage 3 breast development. The first period also tends to coincide with the peak of the weight velocity curve, and 90% of normal girls who have developed Tanner stage 4 breasts have had menarche.

Tampons

Whether to use vaginal tampons for menstrual hygiene is a frequently encountered question in reproductive health in this age group. Tampons are popular, convenient, and widely advertised, and early adolescent girls often specifically request information about their use. Tampons are convenient for use during athletic activity, a day at the beach, summer camp, or simply any time. It is necessary to remind the patient that tampons should be changed during the day as often as one changes a sanitary napkin and not worn to bed at night.

The early adolescent's desire to use tampons provides the clinician with an excellent opportunity to discuss the basics of pelvic anatomy and menstruation. During these discussions the clinician should refer to illustrations depicting the relationship of the internal and external reproductive organs. It is helpful to use a plastic model of female pelvic anatomy to demonstrate the correct application of a tampon. Occasionally, it is necessary to actually assist a patient as she inserts a tampon in the vagina so that her method of application is successful and comfortable.

The tampon manufacturers have sizes designed for use by early adolescent girls ("Slimfits," "Junior," and "Slender Regular"). The tampon manufacturers also have literature available that clearly explains to the early adolescent girl puberty, menstruation, and correct tampon use; it is worthwhile to have these materials handy in your office.

Physiologic Leukorrhea

A white vaginal discharge is a common complaint in this age group. Although such discharges can be associated with vulvovaginitis, physiologic leukorrhea is perfectly normal. A normal vaginal discharge is white, nonhomogeneous, and odorless. Microscopically, a normal discharge is characterized by superficial epithelial cells, flora composed of lactobacilli (long, stringlike bacteria), and occasional leukocytes. The addition of 10% potassium hydroxide to the discharge does not change the odor as it would for bacterial vaginosis.

Patient Concerns about Increase in Body Weight and Fat Distribution

Early adolescent girls frequently are alarmed about the normal weight gain associated with the developmental changes and the deposition, location, and distribution (lower trunk, lower extremities, and posterior thighs) of adipose tissue that occur during puberty. One hazard of this occurrence is an attempt by the girl to lose weight through dieting. Such diets often subject the patient to a significant reduction of calcium and iron intake. Another consequence of dieting is the risk of a caloric deficiency that may potentially compromise her longitudinal growth and final height.

As part of the regular anticipatory guidance given to early adolescent female patients, it is important to explain the normal physical changes that will be taking place in her body and how her body's appearance will change.

CONCLUSION

Early adolescence is a period of profound physical changes, including rapid skeletal growth, weight gain, and maturation of the reproductive system. Cognitive and psychological adaptation to these physical changes begins at this time, as does a focus outward from the family toward peer group. Health concerns include those related to abnormal growth, such as scoliosis, and those related to hormonal changes such as leukorrhea, menstrual irregularity, and acne. Emotional problems, depression, and risk-taking behaviors also may affect the health of some early adolescent girls.

SUGGESTED READING

1. American Academy of Pediatrics: Guidelines for Health Supervision III. Elk Grove Village, IL, American Academy of Pediatrics, 1997.
2. Goldenring J, Cohen E: Getting into adolescent heads. Contemp Pediatr 5:75–90, 1988.
3. Lerner RM: A life span perspective for early adolescence. In Lerner RM, Foch TT (eds): Biological-Psychological Interactions in Early Adolescence. Hillsdale, NJ, Lawrence Erlbaum, 1987, pp 9–29.
4. Offer D, Boxer AM: Normal adolescent development: Empirical research findings. In Lewis M (ed): Child and Adolescent Psychiatry. Baltimore, Williams & Wilkins, 1991, pp 266–278.
5. Speroff L, Glass RH, Kase NG: Abnormal puberty and growth problems. In Speroff L, Glass RH, Kase NG (eds): Clinical Gynecologic Endocrinology and Infertility, 5th ed. Baltimore, Williams & Wilkins, 1994, pp 361–399.
6. Vaughan VC, Litt IE (eds): Child and Adolescent Development. Philadelphia, W.B. Saunders, 1990.
7. Yordan EE: Tips, tricks, and tests for the gynecologic exam of young females. In Goldfarb AF (ed): Clinical Problems in Pediatric and Adolescent Gynecology. New York, Chapman and Hall, 1996, pp 3–18.

CHAPTER 2

The Middle Adolescent Girl: Ages 14–17 Years

Susan M. Coupey, M.D.

For girls, middle adolescence between the ages of 14 and 17 years is the riskiest period in the adolescent decade. Physical changes of puberty are complete, but the psychological and behavioral changes necessary to ensure a healthy and happy young adulthood are rapidly progressing. Whenever such a process of rapid developmental maturation occurs, health risk increases because of experimentation and the inevitable errors in judgment that are made. Middle adolescence roughly correlates with the high school years. Nearly 1 out of every 5 high school girls describes her health as fair or poor, despite the relative health of this age group by objective measures.[1] In contrast, younger girls in grades 5–8 are more likely to describe their health as good to excellent. Thus, among girls there is a deterioration in the perception of health during middle adolescence.

Appropriate counseling and screening for health problems require an awareness of the developmental and environmental stressors affecting middle adolescent girls and the associated health risks (Table 1). Girls in this age range are at the peak of body consciousness, having recently completed pubertal maturation, and many are unhappy with the way their bodies have grown. Disordered eating and dieting are prevalent as are poor nutrition, iron deficiency, and constipation. In addition, girls are under developmental pressure to achieve a degree of autonomy and independence from their families, which often results in conflict at home. Middle adolescence is a particularly difficult time for the mother–daughter relationship, so mothers may need support and parenting advice at this time. Many girls initiate sexual activity during the high school years, and many also begin experimenting with alcohol and illicit drugs. Just over one-third of 9th-grade girls (average age 14.5 years) and nearly two-thirds of 12th-grade girls (average age 17.5 years) report having had sexual intercourse at least once, and 48% of 12th-grade girls have tried marijuana.[2] Therefore, providers must screen for health risks related to sex and drugs in all 14–17-year-old girls. Middle adolescent girls are at higher risk of mental health problems, particularly depression, than are boys. Many more girls than boys in this age range report feeling stressed, lacking in self-confidence, and experiencing depressive symptoms.[1] Of 10th-grade girls in the United States, 14%

TABLE 1. Prevalence of Selected Health Risk Behaviors in High School Girls—United States 1997*

Behavior	Grade 10 (%)	Grade 12 (%)
Dieted to lose weight (past 30 days)	47	46
Took laxatives/vomited to lose weight (past 30 days)	9	6
Did not participate in 20 minutes of vigorous physical activity in 3 of the past 7 days	44	56
Made a suicide plan (past 12 months)	24	15
Made one or more suicide attempts (past 12 months)	14	12
Frequent cigarette use (smoked on > 20 of past 30 days)	14	19
Episodic heavy drinking (≥ 5 drinks/episode in past 30 days)	26	34
Current marijuana use (past 30 days)	21	22
Currently sexually active (past 3 months)	31	50
Four or more lifetime sex partners	12	21
Have been pregnant	9	11

* Data from Kann L, Kinchen SA, Williams BI, et al: Youth risk behavior surveillance—United States, 1997. MMWR 47(SS-33):1–89, 1998.

attempted suicide in 1997 compared with only 4% of boys in the same grade.[2] Talking to middle adolescent girls about their emotional health and identifying risk of suicide are a priority for primary care providers.

This chapter reviews physical and psychosocial development of middle adolescent girls, important aspects of the medical history and physical examination in this age group, and some common problems encountered in primary care.

PHYSICAL AND PSYCHOSOCIAL DEVELOPMENT

Pubertal Development

In general, by the end of their 14th year, most girls have completed their growth in height and are fully mature reproductively. The average girl has her first menstrual period in her 12th year; linear growth is completed within 2 years of the menarche by age 14. However, girls who mature later than average experience menarche in their 13th or 14th year; thus some middle adolescent girls entering high school are still pubertal. For girls early pubertal development is associated with more difficult psychosocial adjustment, including more depression, disruptive behavior, and eating disorder symptoms, than on-time development.[3] However, late pubertal development in girls does not show any consistent pattern of adjustment problems, and, in fact, late developers are more likely than their earlier developing peers to have high academic goals.[3,4] Indeed, later puberty in girls may be protective in terms of risk-taking behavior because the physical appearance of late-maturing girls is more childlike than that of their peers; thus they are less likely to be invited to participate in risky behaviors by physically mature peers and adults. When late-maturing girls do complete puberty at age 15 or 16 years, they are more educated and experienced and make better judgments about risk behaviors than do early-maturing girls who may complete puberty before high school by age 12 or 13 years.

Weight and Body Image

For the majority of girls with early or average pubertal maturation, middle adolescence is associated with weight gain. As linear growth decelerates after menarche, the proportion of body fat increases. Girls gain on average about 6.5 kg (14.3 lb.) in the 5 years following menarche and, even with normal weight gain, have a greater potential for fat deposition centrally than boys.[5] By late adolescence, girls accumulate approximately 23% body fat, whereas in boys of this age, body fat decreases to approximately 12%. Excessive weight gain in middle adolescent girls may lead to large gains in central fat, thus increasing long-term risk for metabolic and cardiovascular diseases. Unfortunately, middle adolescent girls are less likely to exercise regularly than younger girls, increasing their risk for obesity (see Table 1). Approximately 25% of middle adolescent girls are obese, and about half of these are very obese.

Postpubertal body and behavioral changes also contribute to the development of eating disorders in some girls. Our culture idealizes thinness for women, and this message is certainly heard by adolescent girls. More advanced pubertal development is associated with increasing weight preoccupation, more negative body image, and elevated levels of eating disturbance in girls.[6] Early-maturing girls tend to be fatter and shorter than late-maturing girls, and they have been shown consistently to be at higher risk for developing eating disorders.[6,7] The mean age at onset of anorexia nervosa is 14 years. Weight and dieting concerns are prevalent among middle adolescents, and there is a strong association between these concerns and depressive mood and emotional distress.[8] For girls, satisfaction with their body shape and size is an important determinant of self-esteem and psychological health. A large study assessed the prevalence of other health-compromising behaviors in high school students who engaged in unhealthy weight loss methods tht included vomiting and use of laxatives and diet pills. Compared with girls who did not engage in unhealthy weight loss methods, girls using such methods were more likely to use tobacco, alcohol, and marijuana; to have made a suicide attempt, to have unprotected sex; and to engage in delinquent behaviors. Thus disordered eating and poor body image are markers for other risk behaviors in girls.

Psychological, Social, and Cognitive Development

Middle adolescent girls are preoccupied with exploring their identities and discovering what kind of an adult they will ultimately become. Girls spend less time with their families, and, along with a group of friends, they experiment with different clothing, hairdos, music, and vocabulary. As they acquire more independence, they test rules, develop strong opinions, and often challenge parental authority. Parents may become frustrated and angry, and family communication may be strained. Many girls feel a particular need to reject the values and opinions of their mothers in their efforts to differentiate themselves from the parent they most closely resemble. A daughter may adopt a style of dress, for example, that is diametrically opposite to her mother's style, or she may choose a boyfriend of whom her mother disapproves and flaunt her new-found sexual power. Such behaviors tend to annoy even the most understanding of mothers. Some mothers experience sadness and grief over the loss of a close relationship with their daughters. Clinicians can provide support and encourage mothers to keep the lines of communication open and trust that their daughters will eventually pass through this developmental stage.

Although many middle adolescents remain primarily concrete thinkers, some begin to make the transition to formal operational thinking. They become more future-oriented, able to understand and discuss abstract concepts, and begin to appreciate the perspectives of others. Middle adolescent girls often become engaged with community and societal issues such as care of the elderly, racism, homelessness, or violence. Girls may begin part-time employment at this developmental stage and have significant amounts of discretionary income. However, jobs may interfere with school achievement and lead to fatigue and stress, and money may be spent on fast foods, cigarettes, alcohol, or drugs. School achievement and future career goals become very important at this age and can be a source of anxiety, but they also can allow girls to excel and receive praise and respect for their competence.

Mental Health

Although most middle adolescents are well adjusted and happy, a significant minority are depressed. Girls are more likely than boys to have low self-esteem, to exhibit more depressive symptoms, and to attempt suicide. Peterson and colleagues studied depression longitudinally in adolescents from 6th–12th grade and at a young adult follow-up at age 21 years.[9] The investigators found that emotional tone, an index of psychological well-being, improved in girls from 6th–8th grade, then declined steadily through high school and into young adulthood, whereas for boys, emotional tone increased each year. In addition, girls reported significantly more depressive episodes on a diagnostic interview than boys. The gender difference in depression was explained in this study, because the investigators found that adolescent girls were more likely than boys to experience a convergence of simultaneous stressors during early and middle adolescence.[9] Stressors included changing schools from elementary to junior high school while in the midst of puberty (boys' puberty occurs later, after they have changed schools, whereas girls experience both stresses simultaneously) and experiencing more major life events such as parental divorce, which is more likely among parents of girls.[9] An analysis of data from the Commonwealth Fund survey of a nationally representative sample of adolescents in grades 5–12 found that 10% of girls were depressed.[10] Girls were more likely than boys to report high levels of stress, and stress level was a stronger predictor of depression for girls than for boys. Abuse was significantly associated with depression, and girls were significantly more likely than boys to have experienced both physical abuse (14% vs. 11%) and sexual abuse (10% vs. 4%). Thus, data from different sources indicate that middle adolescence is a vulnerable period for girls' mental health.

THE HEALTH CARE VISIT

The American Medical Association's *Guidelines for Adolescent Preventive Services* (GAPS) and the National Center for Education in Maternal and Child Health's *Bright Futures: Guidelines for the Health Supervision of Infants, Children, and Adolescents* recommend annual preventive services visits for adolescents.[11,12] The first few minutes of the health care visit consist of a review of the structure of the visit and a brief medical history with both the parent(s) and adolescent girl together, after which the clinician should request that the parent(s) leave the consulting room. For middle adolescent girls, most of the medical interview should take place with the adolescent alone. At the end of the visit, the adolescent and the clinician can briefly review the findings and treatment plan with the parent(s). Generally, 30 minutes is sufficient time for an initial health maintenance visit. The first 5 minutes can be spent with the adolescent and parent(s) together, followed by 10 minutes for a private interview with the adolescent, 10 minutes for the physical examination during which the interview and anticipatory guidance can continue, and 5 minutes for discussion of findings and treatment with the girl and her parent(s). Follow-up visits may require only 15 minutes and no parental contact because many girls at this age are able to travel to the medical office alone. The GAPS materials, available from the American Medical Association, include written questionnaires for both parents and adolescents to screen for health problems. Such questionnaires are helpful and can save time; however, they must be reviewed by the clinician at the time of the visit, and any problems identified should be acknowledged and addressed.

The Medical Interview

The medical interview with the middle adolescent girl is most efficient and effective in identifying salient health problems if the clinician uses open-ended questions to explore specific areas known to be problems for many girls in this age group, including body image, weight, and nutrition; sexual behavior; health habits; family interactions; emotional health; and exposure to violence and abuse.[13] Suggested trigger questions are listed in Table 2. Because many health problems in middle adolescent girls result from private, embarrassing behaviors, explicit assurance of confidentiality should be given by the clinician along with an explanation of the limits of that confidentiality (see chapter 6). Parents should be educated by the clinician about the need to provide private confidential care to their daughter, but they also should be reassured that they will be informed if a major health problem is uncovered. The clinician should take the opportunity to encourage and facilitate mother–daughter communication about health risk whenever the occasion presents itself, because such communication has been shown to decrease risk behaviors.

A review of systems for middle adolescent girls is a systematic screening for common problems and should include inquiry about frequency of headaches; glasses, contact lens, or vision problems; last dental examination; breathing problems or history of asthma; abdominal pain; bowel habits; dysuria or urinary frequency; menstrual history; history of sexually transmitted diseases and pregnancy; fractures, joint, or muscle problems, and/or sports injuries.

TABLE 2. Suggested Trigger Questions for Girls Aged 14–17 Years

1. Body image, weight, and nutrition
   a. How do you feel about the way you look?
   b. Are you trying to change your weight ?
   c. Are you on any special diet?
2. Sexual behavior
   a. Are you involved in a romantic relationship now? In the past?
   b. Is (was) sex a part of that relationship?
   c. How do you feel about the decisions you have made about your sexual life?
3. Health habits
   a. Do you smoke cigarettes?
   b. How often do you drink alcohol?
   c. What drugs do kids in your school use most often? Have you tried any?
4. Family interactions
   a. Who do you get along with best in your family?
   b. Is there anyone in your family with whom you do not get along so well?
   c. Are you worried about any family members and how much they drink or take drugs?
   d. What would you like to change about your family if you could?
5. Emotional health
   a. Have you ever felt so upset or stressed that you wanted to speak to a counselor or therapist? Have you seen a therapist for one or more visits?
   b. Tell me about the last time you felt really down and depressed. Did you ever feel so depressed that you didn't want to live anymore?
   c. Tell me about the last time you felt really happy.
6. Violence and abuse
   a. Are you concerned about your personal safety at home? At school? In your neighborhood?
   b. Has anyone ever touched you in a way you didn't like? Forced you to have sex?

The General Physical Examination

Important procedures to include in the general physical examination of a middle adolescent girl are related to assessment of growth and development, the skin, and the skeletal examination. Because both over- and underweight are common, height and weight should be carefully measured and body mass index (BMI) plotted (see chapter 14).[11] A body mass index of 23 kg/m^2 is at the 85th percentile for a 16-year-old girl, and a BMI of 29 kg/m^2 is at the 95th percentile and indicates overweight. As part of the assessment of growth and development, sex maturity rating (SMR) or Tanner staging of both breasts and pubic hair should be noted (see chapter 1). Blood pressure should be measured yearly using the appropriate-size cuff. Multiple recordings (at least 3) should be done if the blood pressure is elevated. The 95th percentile for systolic and diastolic blood pressure in 16-year-old girls is 131/85 mmHg (see chapter 10).[11] Skin problems, including acne, eczema, infections, and trauma, are common in girls, and a careful assessment of the skin should be done (see chapter 18). In addition, for thin girls, a visual assessment of the amount of subcutaneous fat can be made. In order to accomplish these examinations, the clinician should ask the girl to remove her clothes, except her underwear, and put on a gown. A complete examination cannot be achieved when the adolescent is clothed. A teaching breast examination should be done to evaluate for masses (see chapter 17). Finally, because skeletal problems and trauma or sports injuries are common in girls, the spine should be carefully examined for scoliosis (see chapter 1), and joints, especially knees, should be examined (see chapter 11).

The Pelvic Examination

All middle adolescent girls who have had sexual intercourse should have a complete pelvic examination; this includes approximately one-third of 16-year-old and one-half of all 17-year-old girls in the United States (see Table 1). The examination is required to screen for sexually transmitted diseases such as genital warts, genital herpes, vaginitis, cervicitis, and others (see chapter 21). In addition, Papanicolaou (Pap) smear screening should be done yearly. Pelvic examination also is indicated in girls with certain symptoms regardless of whether or not they have been sexually active. Such indications include acute abdominal pain, dysmenorrhea, dysfunctional uterine bleeding, and abnormal vaginal discharge.

For virginal girls, a speculum examination may not be necessary because Pap smears and cervical cultures usually are not indicated. It may be sufficient to inspect the external genitalia, take samples of vaginal discharge with a swab, and perform a rectoabdominal bimanual examination to assess the pelvic contents. Assessment of the size and tenderness of the cervix and uterus or any pelvic mass can be accomplished by a rectoabdominal bimanual examination. This examination is better tolerated by virginal girls than is a vaginal bimanual examination. Occasionally, a speculum examination is necessary in a virginal girl, and, most often, the clinician can do it in the office with proper preparation of the patient and use of a small speculum. It is important to reassure the girl and her mother that this examination will not damage her in any way and will not rupture the hymen.

In preparation for the pelvic examination the patient should be instructed to empty her bladder, after which she should be gowned and draped. A brief explanation of the procedure should be given before she is placed in the lithotomy position with her feet in stirrups (Table 3). First, inspect the vulva, assessing the degree of estrogenization of the tissues, the size of the clitoris, and the type of hymenal opening, as well as looking for any abnormal lesions. The speculum should be inserted while putting pressure posteriorly and aiming towards the small of the patient's back. The cervix should be inspected, and the presence and characteristics of any discharge should be noted. A sample of the discharge may be taken for wet mount examination. Many girls have an ectropion or eversion of the endocervical columnar epithelium onto the portio of the cervix. This ectropion appears as a symmetrical reddish ring around the os, contrasting with the lighter pink, stratified, squamous epithelium covering the rest of the cervix. The ectropion does not represent an abnormality and will eventually be replaced with squamous epithelium through the process of metaplasia. However, the columnar cells are more readily infected with sexually transmitted pathogens, and the presence of an ectropion is a feature that increases risk of sexually transmitted diseases (STDs). An endocervical sample should be taken for a Pap smear using a cytobrush or a cotton swab; then the exocervix should be sampled by rotating an Ayer spatula

TABLE 3. Tips for Conducting a First Pelvic Examination

1. Take 2 minutes while the patient is sitting on the examining table to conduct a "show and tell" explanation of the exam before positioning her in the lithotomy position.
   a. Hand her the speculum to hold.
   b. While she is holding the speculum, explain that the instrument is used to separate the walls of her vagina so that you can see her cervix and touch it with a cotton swab to test for sexually transmitted diseases and take a Pap smear.
   c. Allow her to try to open the blades of the speculum so she can see how it works and hear any noise it might make.
   d. Take the speculum from her and ask her to make a circle with her thumb and index finger.
   e. Insert the speculum into the circle of her fingers. Ask her if she can feel the speculum in her hand; then ask her if it hurts.
   f. She will have to acknowledge the difference between feeling something and having something hurt.
   g. Explain that she will feel the speculum in her vagina but it will not hurt.
2. As you are positioning her, acknowledge that this exam is different and may be embarrassing, but express your hope that she will feel reassured to know that she is getting the health care she needs.
3. Raise the head of the examination table to a 45° angle, and arrange the drape over the patient's knees and abdomen so that she can see you during the examination.
4. Ask her to assist you by holding the speculum and handing it to you when you ask.
5. Talk your way through the examination, telling her what you are doing and why.
6. Touch her first with your gloved hand, using firm pressure on the inner thigh as a desensitizing technique before moving to touch her vulva.
7. Insert the speculum quickly with one smooth fluid movement, pressing down and back; then stop and allow her to adjust to the feeling before opening the speculum to expose the cervix.

around the cervix. Testing for *Chlamydia trachomatis* and *Neisseria gonorrhoeae* should be done next and the speculum removed. The bimanual examination is accomplished by inserting two fingers into the vagina and the other hand on the abdomen and carefully palpating the uterus and adnexae. Normal ovaries are often difficult to palpate, but when an ovary is palpated, it is mildly tender.

COMMON PROBLEMS ENCOUNTERED IN PRIMARY CARE

The main problems that primary care clinicians encounter in middle adolescent girls include emotional and psychosomatic symptoms, gynecologic problems related to sexual behavior or menstruation, skin disorders, upper respiratory infections, and injuries or trauma. Most of these health problems are discussed in depth in other chapters in this book; however, it may be helpful to briefly discuss psychosomatic symptoms here.

Psychosomatic Symptoms

It is not surprising, given the multitude of stressors faced by middle adolescent girls today, that psychosomatic symptoms are prevalent. Such symptoms are defined as physical symptoms that have organic expression but that are caused primarily by psychosocial factors.[14] The most frequently reported symptom is recurrent or chronic abdominal pain (see chapter 19). Headache is also a frequent psychosomatic symptom reported by middle adolescent girls. It is important to approach the diagnosis initially from both a physical and psychosocial perspective, looking in particular for a positive history of stressful life events within the girl's family or environment. Clues that a symptom may be psychosomatic include a chronic symptom associated with little objective evidence of debility, asynchrony between the reported severity of the problem and the girl's reaction to it, and discovery of a role model for the symptom within the family.[14] The physical examination should be conspicuously thorough so that the clinician will have credibility when he or she reassures the adolescent and family that there are no abnormal findings. Laboratory testing and imaging studies should be kept to a minimum. Even if the clinician is not sure that the symptoms are psychosomatic in origin, it is helpful to request an assessment by a mental health professional as a way of helping the girl to cope with her pain during the time it takes to complete the evaluation. Often the therapist will uncover more clues to the cause of the girl's symptoms and may diagnose a significant psychiatric disorder such as depression that is amenable to treatment. Management begins by establishing a therapeutic relationship with the patient and her family, showing them that their concerns are taken seriously. It is important to offer symptomatic therapy such as nonsteroidal antiinflammatory drugs for pain, a regimen to relieve constipation, even suggesting vitamin pills to help counteract fatigue can be helpful. It is also important to initiate a program to restore normal activities. If, for example, the girl has been missing many school days because of the symptom, a program of gradual return to school should be developed.

CONCLUSION

Middle adolescence is a complex and exciting but risky developmental period for girls. Although most negotiate this 4-year period with only minimal health problems, a large number of girls experience one or more problems with body image, mental health, sexual health, violence, or trauma. Clinicians should screen for health risk behaviors and provide appropriate referral and management when they are diagnosed. These tasks of the clinician demand excellent interpersonal communication skills as well as the relevant medical, gynecologic, and psychiatric knowledge.

REFERENCES

1. Schoen C, Davis K, DesRoches C, Abrams M: The Commonwealth Fund survey of the health of adolescent girls. New York, The Commonwealth Fund, 1997.
2. Kann L, Kinchen SA, Williams BI, et al: Youth risk behavior surveillance—United States, 1997. MMWR 47(SS-3):1–89, 1998.
3. Brooks-Gunn J: Antecedents and consequences of variations in girls' maturational timing. J Adolesc Health 9:365–373, 1988.
4. Graber JA, Lewinshon PM, Seeley JR, Brooks-Gunn J: Is psychopathology associated with the timing of pubertal development? J Am Acad Child Adolesc Psychiatry 36:1768–1776, 1997.
5. Hediger ML, O'Scholl TO, Schall JI, Cronk CE: One-year changes in weight and fatness in girls during late adolescence. Pediatrics 96:253–258, 1995.

6. Koff E, Rierdan J: Advanced pubertal development and eating disturbance in early adolescent girls. J Adolesc Health 14:433–439, 1993.
7. Killen JD, Hayward C, Litt I, et al: Is puberty a risk factor for eating disorders? Am J Dis Child 146:323–325, 1992.
8. Casper RC, Offer D: Weight and dieting concerns in adolescents, fashion or symptom? Pediatrics 86:384–390, 1990.
9. Petersen AC, Leffert N, Graham B, et al: Depression and body image disorders in adolescence. Women's Health Issues 4:98–108, 1994.
10. Schraedley PK, Gotllib IH, Hayward C: Gender differences in correlates of depressive symptoms in adolescents. J Adolesc Health 25:98–108, 1999.
11. Elster AB, Kuzsets NJ: AMA Guidelines for Adolescent Preventive Services (GAPS). Baltimore, Williams & Wilkins, 1994.
12. Bright Futures: Guidelines for Health Supervision of Infants, Children, and Adolescents. Arlington, VA, National Center for Education in Maternal and Child Health, 1994.
13. Coupey SM: Interviewing adolescents. Pediatr Clin North Am 44:1349–1364, 1997.
14. Brown RT: Psychosomatic problems in adolescents. Adolesc Med 3:87–96, 1992.

CHAPTER 3

The Young Adult Woman: Ages 18–22 Years

Melanie A. Gold, D.O.

The physical and psychosocial development of the late adolescent and young adult woman, aged 18–22 years, marks the end of adolescence and the beginning of adulthood. The history-taking approach is closer to that used with adult women, as are the general physical and gynecologic examinations. Although many of the health issues of the young adult woman may begin in early and middle adolescence, there is a unique quality to health problems that occur in this final stage of adolescent development.

PHYSICAL AND PSYCHOSOCIAL DEVELOPMENT

Physical Development

In the young woman between the ages of 18 and 22 years, physical development is complete so long as there have not been any underlying chronic illnesses or nutritional deficiencies to delay normal growth. Secondary sex characteristics are fully developed, with breasts reaching Tanner stage 5 sexual maturity rating and pubic hair development reaching Tanner stage 4 or 5, depending on ethnicity. Skin can vary, but often acne, which is prominent during early and middle adolescence, clears at this time. Skin, particularly if exposed to the sun, may develop increased freckling or areas of hyper- or hypopigmentation during young adulthood.

Although linear growth has ceased by late adolescence, the young woman continues to accrue skeletal mass. During this time, adequate nutrition, especially calcium and vitamin C, is crucial to adequate mineralization of bone. Dietary calcium requirements are high (1200 mg/day) and are attained by few young women. From age 18–22 years, weight distributes into adultlike patterns with fat pads developing on the hips and abdomen. Subcutaneous fat also distributes around the breasts, upper arms, buttocks, and thighs. The majority of young adult women menstruate regularly with stable patterns of flow, duration, and dysmenorrhea by age 22 years.

Psychosocial Development

The transition from adolescence to adulthood is amorphous and lacks a clear-cut right of passage. The young adult woman may attain various privileges that seem to convey adultlike status, such as a driver's license and the right to vote, marry, join the armed services, or purchase tobacco and alcohol. Yet in American culture, there is no universal ritual marking the transition to adulthood for young women.

A major psychological task of young adulthood is to consolidate a realistic self-identity. In earlier adolescence, girls are awkward, uncomfortable, and frequently dissatisfied with their changing bodies. A stable, realistic body image and sense of comfort with her mature body characterize the well-adjusted, late adolescent woman. The young woman develops a sense of ownership and acceptance of her body as well as a realistic appraisal of its appearance, abilities, and limitations.

A second important developmental milestone of late adolescence is cognitive maturation. In early adulthood, the young woman attains the ability to employ higher levels of reasoning, which include formal operational thought and the ability to think in abstractions and metacognitions. She becomes introspective, develops insight, and can make complex and sophisticated judgments about human relationships and behavior. She has a fuller understanding of her own and others' motivations. She can see contradictions and fallacies in her own and others' arguments. As cognitive abilities mature, the young woman acquires the ability to assess fully the future consequences of her actions and can plan ahead for a career or future education.

As the young adult woman's identity solidifies, she achieves other tasks of adulthood such as developing autonomy from her family, forming enduring partner relationships, and developing work or career paths. She renegotiates her relationship with her parents and progresses towards attaining both emotional and financial autonomy. Emancipation from the family is often demonstrated by the young woman's moving away from home and living independently. Although emotional autonomy is frequently attained by young adulthood, financial independence in the United States may be deferred until completion of advanced education when the young woman is 22 years old or older. One-half of 18–22-year-old women attend college and remain financially dependent on their families.

An integral part of identity development includes sexual identity. Although adolescence is a time of exploring sexual orientation, attractions, and formation of intimate relationships, by early adulthood most young women know their sexual orientation. However, in contrast with men, some young women may remain unsure of their sexual orientation until their mid-20s to early 30s (see chapter 25). Development of sexual identity also includes the formation of intimate one-on-one relationships and physical intimacy. By the age of 19 years, three-quarters of all young women have had intercourse at least once, and many are regularly sexually active. Young adult women frequently contemplate forming a family and, depending on their academic and career aspirations, may plan marriage and childbearing.

THE HEALTH CARE VISIT

Young adults often present for medical care without their parents. Generally, the young woman should be interviewed alone. However, it is appropriate to collect information from the parents that may not be known to the young woman, such as family medical history, including history of mental illness or substance abuse, and the patient's early childhood development if relevant. More importantly, it is helpful to determine what concerns or questions the parents may have regarding their daughter's health and to communicate clearly that is it now their daughter's responsibility to interact with the health care provider as an adult. The patient should take primary responsibility for making and canceling appointments, taking medications, understanding treatment options, and making her own medical decisions, although certainly parents can be helpful in assisting their daughter in her decision making.

Confidentiality and consent-to-treatment issues are more clear-cut and less complex than they were for the younger adolescent. Once the patient is 18 years old or older, she can consent to her own medical care, and all of her care can be kept confidential from her parents if she wishes. It is important to remind the parents and their daughter that an adult patient–physician relationship includes confidential care and the ability to consent to medical treatment. However, the clinician can emphasize that parental involvement still is helpful in decision making. The issues of confidential care also may become entangled with the financial aspects of medical care. It is important to establish to whom the medical bills will be sent, who will be responsible for purchasing medication or other prescribed treatments, and whether the young adult woman is still eligible to be covered under her parents' health insurance. Some family insurance policies cover minors only up to the age of 18 years, whereas others cover children to the age of 21 years or through college graduation.

The Medical Interview

The interview should begin with an assessment of the primary purpose of the visit. If the visit is for a routine examination and the patient has no complaints or concerns, the history can proceed with the past medical history, including past medical and surgical problems; history of injuries, fractures, and burns; current medications; allergies; immunization history; and family medical history. The psychosocial assessment should follow. If the visit is for evaluation of a problem or complaint, a detailed exploration of the complaint should precede the past medical history. When inquiring about medication, the clinician should ask not only about prescription medication but also specifically about the use of over-the-counter medications, laxatives, vitamins, herbal remedies, and oral contraceptives, that frequently are not considered as "medications" by the patient. Immunization history should include questions about receipt of diphtheria-tetanus booster in the past 10 years and completion of three hepatitis B immunizations. It also should assess the need for varicella immunization and a second mumps, measles, and rubella (MMR) immunization, and determine whether a PPD tuberculosis screen was done in the past 2 years. Annual influenza vaccination is indicated for young adult women with

TABLE 1. Prevalence of Selected Health Risk Behaviors of College Women—United States, 1995*

Behavior	Age 18–24 Years (%)
Objectively overweight (BMI ≥ 27.3)	14
Perceive themselves as overweight	42
Made a suicide plan (past 12 months)	7.5
Made a suicide attempt (past 12 months)	1.6
Frequent cigarette use (smoked on > 20 of past 30 days)	15
Episodic heavy drinking (≥ 5 drinks/episode in past 30 days)	35
Current marijuana use (past 30 days)	15
Ever used cocaine (lifetime)	6.5
Currently sexually active (past 3 months)	67
Currently sexually active and used any method of contraception at last intercourse (includes withdrawal)	89
Currently sexually active and used birth control pills prior to last intercourse	48
Currently sexually active and used a condom during last intercourse	34
Six or more lifetime sex partners	24

* Data from Centers for Disease Control and Prevention: Youth Risk Behavior Surveillance: National College Health Risk Behavior Survey—United States, 1995. MMWR 46(SS-6):1–54, 1997.

certain chronic conditions and should be recommended for young women who live in college dormitories or who are enrolled in military services.

Because the major causes of morbidity and mortality in late adolescence are secondary to risk-taking behaviors, a careful psychosocial history is crucial (Table 1). The acronym "HEEADDSSS" helps clinicians remember to inquire about all the elements of the psychosocial history (Table 2). The stability of the young woman's environment should be assessed, for she may have lived in a variety of different group and individual environments that may have affected her health. Because disordered eating behaviors are common among young adult women, it is important to ascertain how she views her body shape and weight and whether she is satisfied with her appearance. It is particularly important to ask her how she regulates her weight and whether she tries to alter her weight with any special diets, exercise, laxatives, diuretics, or self-induced vomiting. Regularity and type of physical activity also should be assessed. Asking about hobbies or activities in which the young woman engages can be a good indicator of her mental health. Young women who are busy with many

TABLE 2. HEEADDSSS Acronym for Psychosocial History

Home
Education/**E**mployment
Eating/**E**xercise
Activities
Drugs
Depression
Suicidality
Sexuality
Safety

activities generally have higher self-esteem and are less likely to engage in unhealthy risk-taking behaviors than women who are inactive. Inactivity frequently is associated with overweight, substance use, and poor self-esteem.

A substance use evaluation is essential and should include questions about cigarette and alcohol use, as well as use of marijuana and other illicit substances. Clinicians should assess patterns of use such as amount, frequency, duration, situation in which drugs are used (e.g., alone or socially), and reason for substance use (e.g., likes to feel high, to reduce tension or stress, to deal with shyness or depression). In addition, because the most common causes of mortality are automobile accidents, suicide, and homicide, it is imperative to inquire about drinking and driving habits, seat belt use, protective gear for sports, and whether the young woman has a gun or is a victim of physical or sexual violence.

Mood disorders are common at this age, so every young woman should be asked about her current mood and about past and current suicidal ideation. It is also helpful to assess the young woman's general coping techniques by inquiring about what she does to help herself feel better when she feels upset or sad. Young women with active coping strategies such as talking to friends, writing poetry, or exercising are at lower risk for suicidal ideation and attempts than those who have no identifiable coping techniques or use less healthy coping strategies such as sleeping or substance use.

A natural way to introduce questions about sexuality is to begin with a gynecologic history, which includes age at menarche; menstrual regularity, flow, and duration; and history of dysmenorrhea. Then follow up with questions about sexual behavior. Asking about feminine hygiene practices such as use of tampons and douching can identify risk factors for toxic shock syndrome or bacterial vaginosis. Sexual orientation should be assessed by asking whether the young woman feels sexually or physically attracted to men, women, both, or neither. The clinician can then ask about specific sexual behaviors, including whether the young woman has ever experienced or performed oral–genital, penile–vaginal, or anal intercourse. This line of questioning allows the clinician to assess risk of sexually transmitted diseases (STDs) and to determine which screening physical and laboratory examinations to perform. Questions about sexual behavior should be asked of all young adult women, including those with chronic illness or physical and mental handicaps. It is also important to ask the young woman about history of sexual abuse. History of pregnancy should be elicited, including outcomes. Type and frequency of current and prior contraception use together with the number of lifetime sexual partners and duration of the current sexual relationship may help to identify young women at high risk for sexually transmitted diseases and pregnancy.

The General Physical Examination

The physical examination of the young adult woman is performed to diagnose illness; to provide clearance for participation in college/vocational training, sports, and employment; and for routine preventive health check-ups. It should be performed without the mother in the room. If a chaperone is needed for breast and genital examinations, a female member of the office staff should perform this function. Exceptions to this rule are for young adult women who are developmentally delayed or severely mentally handicapped, in which case a parent may be needed to interpret the patient's needs. When the young woman is severely physically handicapped, the parent can assist in positioning of the patient. The physical examination should be performed in an examination room with a door that can be locked so that the young woman is assured of privacy. Ideally, she should be completely undressed and wearing a hospital gown.

Height, weight, and body mass index are important to document, as is annual blood pressure screening, because 1–2% of all adolescents in the general population have hypertension. Standardized curves are used to evaluate whether a particular adolescent has elevated blood pressure for her age. For young adult women aged 18–22 years, a systolic blood pressure above 135 mmHg or a diastolic pressure above 85 mmHg is greater than the 95th percentile. Particular attention should be paid to teeth and gums, which should be examined for caries, malocclusions, and inflammation, because decayed, missing, or filled teeth and gingivitis increase with age. Every young adult woman should be referred for a biannual dental check-up. The thyroid gland should be palpated for thyromegaly or other masses because thyroid disorders are more common in women. The breast examination can be performed with the patient sitting up or lying supine. The arm should be raised above the head during the breast examination to fully examine the tail of the breast, which extends into the axilla. The breasts should be examined visually for any anatomic anomalies, skin discolorations, dimpling, or thickening, and the Tanner stage should be noted (see chapter 1). Then each breast should be palpated using the finger tips of the second, third, and fourth digits, beginning at the outer border of the breast and spiralling in concentric circles towards the nipple, including the areola (see chapter 17). The axilla should be palpated for adenopathy as well. Finally, the nipple should be gently squeezed to express any discharge. Although some controversy exists over teaching self-breast examination to younger adolescents, late adolescence is the optimal time to teach this technique to young women. They should be counseled to check their breasts monthly, about a week after menses so that they learn what is normal for them and can recognize any changes in texture or masses as they age.

Although it is no longer necessary to examine the back for scoliosis in the young adult woman, it is helpful to evaluate her musculoskeletal system, including range of motion of the spine and all joints. The skin of the back should be inspected for signs of fungal infections, acne, café-au-lait spots, and pilonidal cysts. Skin should be examined to look for sites of tattoos, body piercing, infections (both fungal and bacterial), acne, eczema, striae, and scars.

The Pelvic Examination

The American College of Obstetricians and Gynecologists recommends that the first gynecologic examination with a pelvic examination should be performed between the ages of 18 and 21 years even if the patient is not sexually active. A history of tampon use aids in the examination because tampons gradually stretch the vaginal introitus. If individual lubricant jelly packets are used for the bimanual examination, before beginning the exam, it is helpful to ask the patient to hold the packet in her palm to warm it in preparation for the examination. Feedback should be given to the patient continuously during the examination to verify what looks normal and what does not. The process of the examination is similar to that described for the middle adolescent in chapter 2. Screening tests for gonorrhea and chlamydia should be performed annually, regardless of signs or symptoms of sexually transmitted disease. Vaginal secretions can be applied to a PH strip to determine the acidity or alkalinity as an aid in the diagnosis of bacterial vaginosis and trichomonas. An extra swab of the vaginal secretions should be taken for wet mount evaluation for the presence of yeast, bacterial vaginosis, trichomonas, and abnormal leukocytosis (see chapter 21). After cultures and diagnostic samples are collected, the speculum should be removed and a bimanual examination should be performed. The rectal examination, which is conducted in adults to screen for colon cancer, can be deferred in the young adult woman because colon cancer is rare among young adults. However, a rectal examination is necessary if the patient has complaints of abdominal pain, tenesmus, rectal itching or bleeding, or has a retroverted uterus that cannot be palpated adequately on bimanual vaginal examination.

COMMON PROBLEMS ENCOUNTERED IN PRIMARY CARE

Despite their overall good health, young adult women have some distinctive health issues as compared with men, older women, or younger girls. Many of these health issues are the result of engaging in high-risk social activities such as unprotected sexual intercourse or substance use. The physical and mental health issues deemed most urgently in need of attention at a recent meeting of college health services directors are listed in Table 3. Most health information about 18–22-year-old women has been collected from college settings. Although such data are informative, they may not reflect the different health care issues of young women who work, are unemployed, or are in vocational schools or the military. Because national data on young adult women are collected and presented in age ranges of 15–19 years and 20–24 years, disaggregating the statistics for 18–22 year olds is difficult. Much of the health-related data on young adult women are either mixed with data on women of similar age who are in college or are mixed with data on men.

ACCESS TO HEALTH SERVICES

In a survey of coed university students, Smiley[2] found that only 65% of all participants reported they had used student health services and that 16% had

TABLE 3. Urgent Health Needs of U.S. College Students Endorsed by College Health Service Directors

• Preventive and self-care	• Mental health (stress, anxiety, depression, suicide)	• Self-esteem
• Sexually transmitted diseases	• Violence	• Body image
• Contraception	• Eating disorders	• Nutrition
• Substance use		

Adapted from The Commonwealth Fund, Commission on Women's Health, Notes on College Health Services Directors' Meeting. Personal communication, 1995.

no health insurance coverage. However, there was no breakdown by gender. Despite limitations of the data, much is known about young women's access to health services. Young adult women often have difficulty accessing health care and paying for medical services. In addition, they frequently have concerns about confidentiality of health care, lack knowledge about preventive health services, and have misconceptions about medical institutions and their own medical needs. As they grow older and become increasingly responsible for their own health care, young adult women often find themselves in jobs without health insurance. Young women also may have difficulty communicating with physicians, especially those who are older and male. This may result in poor utilization of acute and preventive health services, including failure to follow appropriate medical advice. Many young women lack information about common women's health conditions, particularly those associated with increasing age such as osteoporosis, cervical and breast cancer, and cardiovascular disease. Thus, young women often do not participate in health-screening and health-promoting activities to decrease the risks of these conditions.

Young adult women are most likely to receive their health care from pediatricians, family practitioners, obstetrician/gynecologists, and dermatologists. Sixty-six percent of all visits by young adult women are to these four specialists. In fact, older adolescents are more likely to receive their primary care from obstetrician/gynecologists than pediatricians as compared with younger adolescents, who are more likely to be seen by pediatricians. The most common reasons for office visits by young adult women are shown in Table 4.

Reproductive Health Issues: Unintended Pregnancy and Sexually Transmitted Disease

Among the most prevalent health care needs of 18–22-year-old women are those related to sexual behavior. More than 70% of 19-year-old women have engaged in sexual intercourse.[3] Among college populations, 67–75% of women have had sexual intercourse. In 1992, 112 pregnancies occurred per 100,000 U.S. women aged 15–19 years, and of these, 61 ended in birth, 36 in abortions, and 15 in miscarriages.[5] In 1996, women aged 20–24 years obtained 32% of all the abortions, and women aged 19 years or younger obtained 20% of abortions.[6] In one college study, 75% of sexually active men and women claimed to use contraception all the time, 58% reporting using condoms or avoiding intercourse; however, 12% experienced an unplanned pregnancy.[2] The high percentage of young women who are sexually active places them at increased risk for sexually transmitted diseases (STDs). In one study of college students, 9% of

TABLE 4. The Most Common Reasons for Health Care Visits by Young Adult Women in Order of Frequency

1. Prenatal care
2. General physical examination
3. Throat complaint
4. Evaluation of acne
5. Cough

Adapted from Nelson C: Office Visits by Adolescents. Vital and Health Statistics of the National Center for Health Statistics, Advance Data, 1991.

those who were sexually active had an STD, and 85% said that they never or seldom worried about STDs.[2] Studies indicate that age is the sociodemographic factor most associated with STDs caused by *Chlamydia trachomatis* infection, with adolescents having the highest prevalence of infection. Among 8,234 college women presenting for routine gynecologic care at a student health center in Florida, Herold[8] found a monthly variation in the chlamydia rate from 11% in August and September compared with 9% during the rest of the year. A review of over 1,000 medical records of University of South Florida students revealed that chlamydia was the most prevalent STD diagnosed. Among normal asymptomatic women students with no known history of STD contact, 7% had a positive chlamydia test. Women with vaginal symptoms were more likely to be positive for chlamydia, and almost one-half of those with a recent STD contact tested positive for chlamydia.[9] If undetected and untreated, many STDs, especially chlamydia, can progress to pelvic inflammatory disease (PID) (see chapter 19). Human papilloma virus (HPV) is a viral sexually transmitted infection prevalent among young adult women that is associated with increased risk for cervical cancer. Estimates of the prevalence of HPV range from 5–19% in women attending family planning clinics and university health centers to 27% among women attending STD clinics.[11] Some believe these rates still underestimate the actual prevalence, which may be as high as 30–40%.[12]

Substance Use: Tobacco Alcohol, and Illicit Drugs

A dramatic increase in women's mortality from lung cancer began in the 1960s, and now lung cancer is the number one cause of death among American women. Adult women's smoking behavior is generally initiated in middle-to-late adolescence (see chapter 16). Smoking is associated with early menopause and infertility, and environmental exposure to tobacco smoke causes lung cancer, lower respiratory tract infection, chronic middle ear infection, and exacerbation of asthma. According to the 1993 National Health Interview Survey, 23% of current smokers are 18–24 year olds; this represents a 50% decline from 1965.[14,15] However, the rate of decline in smoking prevalence was greater for men than for women. Primary care clinicians should ask about cigarette smoking and strongly advise young women who smoke to quit. Help with smoking cessation should be offered and may include prescription of medications such as bupropion (Wellbutrin, Zyban®) and referral to cessation programs.

The leading cause of death among young adult women is alcohol-related motor vehicle accidents. The prevalence of alcohol use among young adult women, particularly those in colleges, is high, ranging from 85–91%, and the prevalence of problem drinking among college students can be as high as 72%, depending on the college setting. Women are at greater physical risk from alcohol than men because of their smaller size as well as differences in alcohol metabolism.[17] In a national survey of college students from 140 campuses, Wechsler found that 16% of female students did not drink, whereas 45% drank alcohol but did not binge.[18] Thirty-nine percent of female students were classified as binge drinkers, defined as consuming more than 5 drinks per sitting at least once in the past 2 weeks, and 17% reported drinking binges 3 or more times in 2 weeks. Frequent binge drinkers were more likely to experience serious health and social consequences of their drinking behaviors; 47% reported injuries and engaging in unplanned sex.

Risk factors associated with problem drinking patterns include initiation of drinking before age 15 years and having a best friend who drinks heavily. Blackouts are reported by nearly one-half of female students during their freshman year. Alcohol is involved in more than 60% of college student suicides, in 90% of campus rapes, and in 95% of violent crimes on campus. Over one-third of young adult women engage in some form of sex that is influenced by drinking alcohol and may abandon safe-sex techniques because of alcohol use. The interaction between alcohol use and high-risk sexual activity suggests that intervention efforts should address the connection between the two risk factors as well as techniques for negotiating and avoiding these situations. Clinicians have a significant role to play in counseling young adult women, particularly college women, about the consequences of binge drinking.

Reliable data on the prevalence of illicit substance use are difficult to obtain from college students because of issues of confidentiality. Thirty-one percent of the women in the 1994 Fund for the Improvement of Post-Secondary Education (FIPSE) Core Drug and Alcohol Survey reported using marijuana in the past year, and 15% in the past month.[20] Seventeen percent used another illicit drug in the past year, and 7% were current users in the past month of illicit drugs other than marijuana. Marijuana and amphetamines are the two most frequently reported illegal drugs used. There are no reliable data about illicit drug use by young adult women who are not in college, but clinical evidence and evidence from testing of young pregnant women suggest that use is common.

Mental Health

Young adult women are more likely to seek health care for mental health problems than young men of similar age. Complaints include depression, anxiety, and somatic complaints related to stress, as well as distorted body image and eating disorders. Young women also suffer from the psychologic and physical ramifications of physical and sexual abuse, both recent and in childhood.

Stress is a by-product of college or working life that can adversely affect the health of young adult women. Perceived stress is higher for college students than for persons with only high school education or less and for persons who are college graduates. Stresses include financial obligations, parental expectations, and a change in living situation. Stress is often associated with other unhealthy behaviors.

Bulimia nervosa, an eating disorder characterized by recurrent episodes of binge eating often followed by self-induced vomiting or purging to maintain or lose weight, occurs predominantly in young adult women. Bulimia nervosa is 2–6 times more common than anorexia nervosa. Employing stringent DSM-IIIR psychiatric diagnostic criteria and a nationally representative sample of college students, Drewnowski found a prevalence of bulimia nervosa of 1.0% for college women and 0.2% for men.[21] In addition, bulimic behaviors that do not meet diagnostic criteria are widespread among college-aged women. Providing early diagnosis and treatment for bulimia can prevent significant morbidity and mortality.

Interpersonal violence is the leading cause of morbidity and mortality among adolescents and young adults, second only to motor vehicle accidents. Although males are at greatest risk of violent injury or death within the community, women are at greatest risk due to sexual assault and violence within the home. National data from the U.S. suggest one in four women experiences physical or sexual abuse by the time of adulthood (see chapter 26). Rape victimization rates are greatest for women aged 16–19 years (7.1 per 1,000), followed by women aged 20–24 years (3.0 per 1,000). Young women at greatest risk for rape are single, live in central cities, have recently moved, and have lower income.[22] Clinicians should always consider physical and sexual abuse as an underlying issue in young adult women with mental health and psychosomatic problems.

CONCLUSION

Young adult women are excellent targets for preventive health interventions. They have prevalent health concerns in reproductive health, substance use, and mental health that have the potential for significant reduction of morbidities and mortalities through health behavior changes. This age group also requires diagnosis and treatment for health consequences of risk behaviors, including contraceptive counseling, routine screening for STDs, routine Pap smear screening, identification of problem drinking patterns, and mental health problems stemming from violence. In addition, provision of health care to the young adult woman requires attention to preventive counseling and screening for adult diseases such as breast cancer, hypertension, and osteoporosis.

REFERENCES

1. The Commonwealth Fund, Commission on Women's Health, Notes on College Health Service Directors' Meeting. Personal communication, 1995.
2. Smiley K, Johannessen K, Marsh K, Collins C: Surveying University of Arizona students' health. J Am College Health 41:75–77, 1992.
3. Forrest JD, Singh S: The sexual and reproductive behavior of American women, 1982–1988. Fam Plann Perspect 22:206–214, 1990.
4. Nelson C: Office Visits by Adolescents. Vital and Health Statistics of the National Center for Health Statistics, Advance Data, 1991.
5. Henshaw SK: Teenage abortion and pregnancy statistics by state, 1992. Fam Plann Perspect 29:115–122, 1997.
6. Abortion surveillance—United States, 1996. MMWR 48:1–42, 1999.
7. U.S. Department of Health and Human Services: Healthy People 2000: National Health Promotion and Disease Prevention Objectives. DHHS Pub. No. (PHS) 91-50212. Washington, DC, Department of Health and Human Services, 1991.
8. Herold AH, Woodward LJ, Roetzheim RG, et al: Seasonality of *Chlamydia trachomatis* genital infections in university women. J Am College Health 42:117–120, 1993.
9. Lee H: Genital chlamydial infection in female and male college students. J Am College Health 37:288–291, 1989.
10. Washington AE, Arno PS, Brooks MA: The economic costs of pelvic inflammatory disease. JAMA 255:1735–1738, 1986.
11. Aral SO, Holmes KK: Epidemiology of sexual behavior and sexually transmitted disease. In Holmes KK, Mordh P, Sparling PF, et al (eds): Sexually Transmitted Disease, 2nd ed. New York, McGraw-Hill, 1990, pp 19–36.
12. Bauer HM, Ting Y, Greer CE, et al: Genital human papillomavirus infection in female university students as determined by a PCR-based method. JAMA 265:2809–2810, 1991.

13. Husten CG, Chrismon J, Reddy MN: Trends and effects of cigarette smoking among girls and women in the United States, 1965–1993. J Am Med Womens Assoc 51:11–18, 1996.
14. Centers for Disease Control and Prevention: Cigarette smoking among adults—United States, 1993. MMWR 43:925–930, 1994.
15. Centers for Disease Control and Prevention: Surveillance for selected tobacco-use behaviors—United States, 1900–1994. MMWR 43:43, 1994.
16. French SA, Perry CL: Smoking among adolescent girls: Prevalence and etiology. J Am Med Womens Assoc 51:25–28, 1996.
17. Frezza M, di Padova C, Pozzato G, et al: High blood alcohol levels in women: The role of deceased gastric alcohol dehydrogenase activity and first-pass metabolism. N Engl J Med 322:95–99, 1990.
18. Wechsler H, Davenport A, Dowdall G, et al: Health and behavioral consequences of binge drinking in college: A national survey of students at 140 campuses. JAMA 272:1672–1677, 1994.
19. Butcher AH, Manning DT, O'Neal EC: HIV-related sexual behaviors of college students. J Am College Health 40:115–118, 1991.
20. Fund for the Improvement of Post-Secondary Education (FIPSE), Core Drug and Alcohol Survey, Unpublished data, 2 June 1993 and 15 February 1994. UCCS/Office of Measurement Services, University of Minnesota, 2502 Broadway Drive, Room 130, St. Paul, MN 55113.
21. Drewnowski A, Hopkins SA, Kessler RC: The prevalence of bulimia nervosa in the US college student population. Am J Public Health 78:1322–1325, 1988.
22. Bureau of Justice Statistics: Criminal Victimization in the United States, 1991: A National Crime Victimization Survey Report. Washington, DC, Bureau of Justice Statistics, 1992.
23. Koss MP, Gidycz CA, Wisniewcski N: The scope of rape: Incidence and prevalence of sexual aggression and victimization in a national sample of higher education students. J Consult Clin Psychol 55:162–170, 1987.

CHAPTER 4

The Female Body Image

Debra K. Katzman, M.D.
Ron Davis, Ph.D.

Body image is a multidimensional construct[1] that girls and boys experience differently.[2,3] For adolescents, body image is the way they experience the body.[4] Body image has two basic dimensions: body satisfaction and body-size perception.[1] Body satisfaction refers to a person's affect, behaviors, and cognitions about his or her size and appearance. Body-size perception involves not only a person's estimation of his or her size, but also the distorted perception that the body is far from the idealized standard.[1] It is the way young persons see themselves and the way they think others perceive them. Evidence suggests that children and adolescents probably differ from adults in their perception of their body images.[5] This is understandable since body image is a concept that changes with physical and psychosocial growth and development and is affected by the young person's interaction with the social world.[6]

Dissatisfaction with body image and consequent dieting behavior are major concerns of adolescent girls. Interest in the issue of body-image dissatisfaction and dieting in adolescent girls has become particularly important because of its association with disordered eating and eating disorders such as anorexia nervosa and bulimia nervosa. Many young women commonly believe that they are overweight and have the concomitant desire to weigh less.[6] In fact, one study[7] looking at body image demonstrated that although 81% of the young adolescent girls were within or below the range for ideal weight, 78% preferred to weigh less. Only 14% of these girls were satisfied with their current weight.

These body-image concerns are not restricted to older adolescents. Koff and Rierdan[8] found that young girls between the ages of 11 and 12 years want to weigh less and date the emergence of such feeling to when they were between the ages of 9 and 11 years old. What more and more young girls would call a normal weight would actually be considered underweight by normal reference standards. In fact, although many girls are aware of appropriate weight norms, they nevertheless want to be underweight. The desire for extreme thinness seems to be occurring at younger ages now than in the past.[9]

Body shape and size are important criteria that children use to judge attractiveness. Evidence suggests that as early as age 7 years, children from Western societies have acquired adult cultural perceptions of attractiveness,[9] in particular, the idealization of thinness and the fear of fatness. Young girls believe that the worst consequences of being fat include being unattractive, feeling bad about themselves, getting teased, and being unpopular.[8] It is, therefore, not surprising that over 50% of these girls have a history of dieting.

This chapter reviews the concept of body image in the adolescent girl. It discusses the various influences that mold a young girl's body image, considers the concept of an unhealthy body image, reviews issues about assessing body image in the adolescent girl, and examines ways to help adolescents modify an unhealthy body image.

SOCIOCULTURAL INFLUENCES ON THE ADOLESCENT FEMALE BODY IMAGE

The cultural ideal for women's body size and shape has become considerably thinner and leaner over time. To understand the sociocultural factors that have an impact on the adolescent girl's body image, it is important to review the changing standards of the ideal body image for women over time (Table 1).

Historically, women of Western society have tried to adapt to the specific era's image of beauty. The trends of ideal beauty can be traced back to the fifteenth century, when beauty was depicted by the fleshy body shape and rounded stomachs of the reproductive figure. This figure was the ideal body image because of the social importance of fertility.[10] The rounded and heavy female habitus continued to be considered the ideal image throughout the eighteenth and nineteenth centuries: women had corseted waistlines, full breasts, and plump arms and necks. A plump shape was regarded as a sign of health.

The cultural ideal began to change in the early 1920s when women acquired a thinner, more boylike body shape. Women did away with corsets and padding their bodices and began to bind their breasts to flatten their silhouettes. This perception of the thin female beauty has evolved over the late twentieth century. In the 1960s, the boyish figure of Twiggy became the fashion. When Garner et al.[11] collected data on Miss America winners from 1959 through 1978, they found a significant decrease in their body weight and measurements over time. Over the same period of time, data collected about *Playboy* magazine centerfolds revealed a decrease in the average weight of a centerfold model from 91% of the standard body weight in 1960 to 83% in 1978.[11]

Studies continue to show that the cultural ideal for a young woman's body size has become thinner and lighter.[4] In the early 1980s, the female ideal body changed to a more muscular, slim physique. Women in the 1990s strive not

TABLE 1. Factors Affecting Body Image

• Sociocultural:	Twentieth century ideal is "thin and light"
• Gender:	Intense focus on physical appearance for girls
• Puberty:	Associated with increased body weight and fat
• Ethnicity:	Subcultural differences
• Socioeconomic status:	Desire for thinness correlated with higher SES

only to be lean, but also to cope with the added pressure to be healthy and physically fit. The thin and fit female physique symbolizes self-control, hard work, ambition, and success.[6] These cultural standards explain, in part, why many adolescent girls are preoccupied with their bodies and dissatisfied with their body image, and are willing to try a variety of dangerous weight-loss practices in their quest for the perfect body.

INFLUENCE OF GENDER ON THE ADOLESCENT FEMALE BODY IMAGE

From an early age, a child's body image is influenced by his or her adult caregivers and how they perceive and respond to the child. Evidence suggests that parents tend to focus on the body's physical appearance in girls and physical functioning and strength in boys.[12]

In general, girls are more dissatisfied with their weight and shape than boys.[2] Studies[13,14] have shown that body-image dissatisfaction among girls increases as puberty progresses. Girls are most dissatisfied with the fat-bearing areas of body, such as upper thighs, buttocks, and stomach. Adolescent boys, on the other hand, want to be bigger and taller; they are more interested in gaining or maintaining weight, so they place more emphasis on exercise than on diet for weight and shape manipulation.[4]

Studies have reported that between 50% and 69% of normal-weight adolescent girls are dissatisfied with their body weight and want to lose weight.[15] In addition, approximately 16% of the underweight girls studied wanted to lose weight, and 60% were extremely fearful of being overweight. On the other hand, 21% of normal-weight high school boys thought that they were underweight, and 10% thought that they were overweight. It is unusual for boys who are not overweight to want to lose weight.

Gender differences in body image are evident from an early age. Children as young as 7 years want to become slimmer and engage in weight-losing behaviors.[9] Hill et al.[3] investigated the self-perception and body-shape satisfaction of 9-year-old girls and boys in different weight categories. The heaviest children expressed the most discontent: they had a low body-esteem, a desire for thinness, and higher levels of dietary restraint. The desire for thinness and associated motivation to diet were apparent in some children in all weight categories.[3] Furthermore, this pattern was more characteristic of girls than boys. At the age of 9 years, girls and boys differed in their body-shape satisfaction and in their body-shape aspirations.

The most current data about unhealthy body images and dietary behaviors come from a report on the Youth Risk Behavior Surveillance Program.[16] The data from this program characterized a nationwide sample of 10,904 United States high school students. Approximately one-quarter of all students surveyed thought they were overweight. Female students from all racial and ethnic groups were much more likely to think of themselves as overweight than male students and were more likely to have tried to lose weight.

It seems that girls wish to lose weight even when they are of normal weight or are underweight; boys, however, are more often satisfied with their weight. They are more likely to see themselves as underweight and wish to gain weight. The most important body-image concern of both males and females, however, is the fear of becoming overweight.[4]

INFLUENCE OF PUBERTY ON THE ADOLESCENT FEMALE BODY IMAGE

Body-image disturbance, disordered eating, and a drive for thinness increase with pubertal development. This trend is particularly remarkable among adolescent girls. The relationships between the stage of pubertal development and body image, body satisfaction, and disordered eating have shown that postmenarchal girls have a poorer body image and higher levels of dieting behavior and eating disturbances related to weight control than premenarchal girls.[17] This relationship is independent of age. Davies and Furnham[14] found that body satisfaction declined among British adolescents during adolescence. Overall satisfaction with nine body features, particularly the upper thigh, buttocks, and stomach measurements, declined from age 12 to 18 years.

Increased body weight and percentage of body fat are normal and necessary parts of the pubertal process. This may account for higher rates of body dissatisfaction in pubertal girls.[17] This finding is in direct contrast with findings for adolescent boys, who show increased body satisfaction after puberty begins.[18]

INFLUENCE OF ETHNICITY ON THE ADOLESCENT FEMALE BODY IMAGE

The literature suggests that some racial differences exist in the attitudes that adolescents harbor about their body image. For the most part, adolescents from different ethnic backgrounds have perceptions and attitudes about body satisfaction similar to those of adolescents from developed countries and white backgrounds.

Studies[19–21] that have examined race or ethnic group differences consistently show that black adolescent girls are less likely to view themselves as overweight, are more satisfied with their body size and shape, and are less likely to diet than white adolescent girls. Schreiber et al.[22] found that even though black girls were taller and heavier and had earlier signs of puberty than white adolescent girls, the black girls were more satisfied with their weight, body shape, and body parts. In addition, the predictors for girls trying to gain weight were being black, having a low body-mass index, and having a mother telling the girl that she was too thin.[22] Another study[23] found that black female adolescents preferred a heavier ideal female body size than white adolescent girls. Black adolescent girls' body-size preferences were significantly more influenced by family members than were white subjects', whose preferences were significantly more influenced by their peer group.[23]

Some unhealthy weight-control behaviors, however, are more frequent in ethnic or racial subgroups than in white adolescent girls, independent of socioeconomic factors or body-mass index. One study[24] found that about twice as many Hispanic adolescent girls reported using laxatives or diuretics to lose weight than adolescent girls of other ethnicities. Binge eating was also reported more frequently by Asians and less frequently by black adolescent girls.

This study also revealed that black and Asian adolescent girls are the least likely to view themselves as overweight.

INFLUENCE OF SOCIOECONOMIC STATUS ON THE ADOLESCENT FEMALE BODY IMAGE

Weight concerns and body dissatisfaction were once thought to be largely confined to middle-to-upper socioeconomic-status (SES) girls. In a recent large, comprehensive health survey administered to 36,320 students in grades 7–12, Story and colleagues[24] found that adolescent girls of a higher SES may be more likely to diet and may view themselves as overweight; they may be less likely to engage in unhealthy weight-control behaviors and may be more likely to adopt healthy eating and exercise behaviors than lower-SES adolescents. Perhaps these behaviors are due to the higher-SES youth's greater resources and greater access to health information, weight-loss programs, health clubs, cosmetics, plastic surgery, and variety of foods, which may have an impact on their health behaviors and appearance.[25] The higher-SES females dieted more frequently than lower-SES females, and lower-SES females were less likely to perceive themselves to be overweight. Dornbusch et al.,[26] who reported on a national sample of American 12–17-year-olds for the National Health Examination Survey, demonstrated that a higher socioeconomic class and increasing sexual maturity were positively correlated with a desire to be thinner, regardless of weight. The thinner the female, the greater the impact of social class on the desire for thinness.

HEALTHY VERSUS UNHEALTHY BODY IMAGES

Understanding the concept of an unhealthy body image first requires understanding what it means for an adolescent girl to have a healthy body image. An adolescent girl's body image, as defined earlier, concerns the manner in which she experiences her body. If an adolescent's representation of her own body is accurate according to normative standards and if she feels positive and confident about her body, she probably has a healthy body image. Young people who care for their bodies and have developed positive self-esteem and confidence in themselves are likely to have a secure, healthy body image.

When, then, is a young girl's body image considered unhealthy? The concept of body image involves a perceptual component in which the physical manifestation of the body is judged. Many adolescent girls misperceive their size as being overweight when, in fact, they are normal or even underweight according to weight-for-height normative standards. Body image also involves an affective component in which personal meaning and feeling are associated with the body.[6] Many adolescent girls attribute negative evaluations to their bodies: for example, "I am inferior because I am fat." On both dimensions of body image, a normative discontent has been observed among adolescent girls within contemporary society.[6] The typical adolescent girl at some point in her life will either misperceive her actual size or attribute some negative feeling toward her body.

The effect that body image has on adolescent girls' lives must, therefore, be examined. The extent to which a person's body image has a negative impact on that person may be a measure of how unhealthy that image is. The following case of a 16-year-old teen named Ema, who consults her physician with a complaint about her weight, illustrates this issue:

Ema: I have to lose weight because I can't fit into my clothes anymore. I need a diet plan to help me lose 15 pounds.

Physician: According to your weight, you are well within the healthy range for your age and height. There are no medical reasons for you to lose weight. Tell me, why do you think you need to go on a diet?

Ema: Well, I don't like my body. I really feel fat and it depresses me. All my girlfriends are so much skinnier than me. Lately, I've avoided being around them because I'm so self-conscious about my weight. Guys won't even look at me. That's because I'm fat. Last week I skipped school for two days and stayed in my bedroom because I felt so fat. I starved myself, and I didn't even leave my house until I'd lost 5 pounds. All I've been living off is cigarettes and coffee. If I were just 15 pounds thinner, I'd be much happier.

This case reflects the unhealthy consequences of Ema's poor body image. She feels inferior to her peers and avoids them because of her negative feelings about her body size. Like many female adolescents, Ema truly believes herself to be fat and believes that others perceive her that way, too. Ema's body image also produces an affective experience: she feels depressed.

DISORDERED EATING

Numerous studies[27–29] have documented the association between psychological distress, low self-esteem, body dissatisfaction, and disordered eating symptoms in young people. In one cross-sectional study[27] of adolescent girls in grades 7–10, body dissatisfaction and emotional distress were the strongest predictors for such disordered eating behaviors as fasting, vomiting, and laxative misuse. Prospective studies[28,29] confirm the importance of self-esteem and body image in the development of disordered eating behaviors. Girls with low self-esteem at age 11 or 12 years are at significantly greater risk of developing more severe disordered eating symptoms and other psychological problems by the age of 15 or 16 years.[28] In another 4-year prospective study[29] of adolescent high school girls, those with the poorest body image at younger ages were most likely to develop disordered eating symptoms as they advanced through adolescence.

Ema's case illustrates how an unhealthy body image may compel some young people to behave in a manner that has biological consequences: she starved herself and increased her caffeine and cigarette consumption so that she might lose weight. With the achievement of puberty, it is not uncommon for females to experience body dissatisfaction and to begin to engage in methods of weight loss. In one study,[30] postpubertal girls ate only three-quarters of the recommended amount of food and nutrients for their age, and they had a more negative body image than a comparable sample of prepubertal girls.

Numerous studies have documented the frequency with which adolescents engage in weight-control practices and disordered eating behaviors. In two large-scale American surveys[31,32] of girls in grades 9–12, 41–44% were trying to lose weight, in spite of the majority being within a healthy weight range.

Methods of weight control ranged from the less pernicious practices of exercise, skipping meals, and reducing calories, to the more dangerous methods of forced vomiting, complete fasting, and the use of substances such as laxatives, emetics, diet pills, and cigarettes. Interestingly, female adolescents with such chronic medical illnesses as diabetes, asthma, and seizure disorders are more likely to experience a poor body image and to engage in dangerous weight-loss methods than girls without chronic medical conditions.[33]

The medical consequences of starvation, significant weight loss, and the use of dangerous methods of weight control are well documented.[34] Deliberately restricting food intake over long periods can lead to growth failure, delayed sexual development and puberty, amenorrhea and delayed menarche, osteoporosis, and psychological disturbances such as depression and irritability. Harmful weight-loss practices have been reported among girls as young as 9 years old.[35]

Many young people believe, and accurately so, that smoking is associated with lower weight and that cessation of smoking can lead to weight gain. One study[36] reported that 39% of white female adolescents who were regular smokers admitted to using smoking to control their appetite and weight. Concerns about body image among young people seem to be a strong predictor of which smokers do not have a history of trying to quit and do not intend to quit in the future.

ASSESSMENT OF THE ADOLESCENT FEMALE'S BODY IMAGE

A number of psychological tests are available to assess a young person's body image.[37] However, for the busy clinician, the initial exploration may proceed with a series of questions that are intended to elicit the young girl's own views about her body and the potential impact they may have upon her life (Table 2). Assessment of body image should be a routine part of any medical evaluation of the adolescent patient.

There is no right or wrong way to initiate this investigation and determine how the young girl feels about her body. The clinician may begin by asking, "Is there anything about your body (size, shape, weight) that you wish you could change?" A reply indicative of body dissatisfaction (e.g., "I am really unhappy about it.") or one indicative of an objective misperception of actual size (e.g., "I need to lose weight, even though you say I am at a healthy weight.") warrants further exploration. Specifically, the relative importance that the young girl

TABLE 2. Assessment of Body Image*

- Is there anything about your body that you wish you could change?
- How important is your body size to how you feel about yourself as a person?
- Do you spend a lot of time thinking about your body?
- Are there things you intentionally avoid because of the way you feel about your body?
- Do you try to do something about your weight? Are you trying now?
- What are you doing to control your weight?

* Body image = perception of body size/shape/weight.

places on her size or weight in her overall scheme of self-evaluation should be explored with a question like "How important is your body size to how you feel about yourself as a person?" A reply signifying undue importance (e.g., "Nothing is more important.") should be followed up with questions that will help characterize the girl's body dissatisfaction, along with an exploration of the consequences of the unhealthy body image (e.g., "Do you spend a lot of time thinking about your body?", "Does the way you feel about your body affect your life?", "Are there things that you intentionally avoid because of the way you feel about your body?").

In addition, the clinician must explore other behaviors indicative of body dissatisfaction. Girls who are dissatisfied with their body shape, weight, or size may frequently compare their appearance with that of others; check their appearance in a mirror or, alternatively, avoid mirrors; camouflage their bodies with clothing; seek reassurance about their weight or attempt to convince others of how terrible they look; report excessive exercise or frequent dieting; or avoid social situations because they are discontent with their appearance.

It is vital for the clinician to explore the way the adolescent deals with her body dissatisfaction with questions such as "Do you try to do something about your weight?", "Are you trying now?", or "What are you doing to control your weight?".

Clinicians should be aware that girls involved in competitive sports and dancing are at particular risk for unsafe weight-control practices.[38]

HELPING YOUNG PEOPLE TO MODIFY AN UNHEALTHY BODY IMAGE

Health care providers who work with adolescent girls need to be sensitive to the effect that sociocultural standards and pressures may have upon the body image of adolescent girls. Clinicians need to promote healthy eating, realistic weights, and a healthy body image. There is a great need to educate young girls about realistic body images. Knowledge can help shape the attitudes of young girls and teach them to develop skills that will help them acquire healthy behaviors. Health care professionals can help adolescent girls resist the pressure to conform to unrealistic and unattainable standards of appearance, learn to eat more healthfully, participate in exercises, and develop a sense of self-esteem and self-worth that is not centered on body size and shape.

It is fairly obvious how a negative attitude about the body can produce a negative feeling associated with that attitude, as is the case in Ema's statement, "I really feel fat and it depresses me." Less obvious, however, is how a negative feeling from one source can actually produce a negative judgment about the body: for example, "I am depressed and I really feel fat." A person's emotional state can have a direct impact on the perception of the body. Feelings that arise out of daily experiences in work, study, or relationships can also get translated into feelings specifically about the body.[39]

Called *displacement*, this transfer of feelings is a common reaction of those young people who are particularly self-conscious about their body size.[40] For example, if a person feels bad because she perceives that she is not popular with her peers, as in Ema's case, she may misdirect the understandably negative feelings that may arise out of this experience toward her body: "No boy asked me to be his date for the party because I'm fat. . . . If only I could lose weight, then people would take notice of me." Sadly, some people are actually the victims of such culturally sanctioned prejudices about weight. Many others may falsely make the same attribution to such a negative experience: "This happened to me because I'm fat."

It is natural for young people to want to find answers to the important things they experience in life, whether they are negative or positive. For those people with a poor body image, blame for a negative experience is frequently attributed to body size, and the solution seems immediately clear—lose weight. By displacing feelings about a difficult or distressing situation onto something that now seems manageable—like weight—these young people attempt to solve a problem that may otherwise seem insurmountable. In fact, controlling weight will not solve the original problem if it has nothing whatsoever to do with weight in the first place. Furthermore, it may only compound that problem with all of the negative consequences that weight control holds for the person's physical and emotional well-being.[41]

The physician can help a young person to understand this mechanism of displacement by counseling her to examine her beliefs and feelings about the root problems. For instance, if the emotions that arise from a failed relationship are displaced onto the body and then weight is subsequently lost, the young person may indeed see an improvement in her social life. But the correlation between weight loss and interpersonal happiness may be illusory. By directing her energy to an area other than the true source of her emotional distress, she ultimately sets the stage for ongoing emotional difficulties. If her new relationships falter, she may repeatedly blame her body. It may then be time for her to look at other causes for the difficulties that she experiences. For example, the real difficulties may lie in the expectations that she has about relationships or in the way that she works so hard to please others and overlooks her own needs in the process. Most people would agree that these interpersonal issues have little, if anything, to do with weight. And while these issues may seem to be more difficult to solve than the misperceived weight problem, they nevertheless can be resolved through an examination of the beliefs and feelings about the real problems at hand.

The key to breaking this type of mind–body cycle is to consciously separate body-image issues from the other emotional aspects of the young person's life. Sample exercises that physicians may use with young people who have unhealthy body images are presented in Figures 1 and 2.

Health care professionals are not the only powerful influence on teenage girls. Both the family and peers can greatly affect how a young girl views her body. Families play a central role in the adolescent's developing body image.[42] Cultural standards are transmitted from parent to child. Parents tend to be less positive about their child's appearance and eating and exercise habits as their child grows older. In addition, the parent's own body image can exert a powerful influence on that of the child. Young people who are exposed within the family to a culture of unhealthy body images and eating behaviors are themselves likely to adopt similar attitudes and behaviors. By the same token, parents with healthy body images and eating behaviors provide a very positive

Getting on with My Life

The purpose of this exercise is to help you to separate body image issues from other emotional aspects of your life.

Step 1. Jot down a few things about yourself that you would like to change or do. Restrict your list to realistic issues that have no connection whatsoever with your body image. *Change my hair style* would not count because it is a "body" issue. *Join a club* definitely counts as long as it is something that (1) you really want, and (2) you have been putting off for whatever reason. Construct your own personal list of things that you want to do in getting on with your life.

Goals I want to accomplish . . .

FIGURE 1. Sample exercise that helps adolescents separate body image issues from other emotional aspects of their lives. (From Davis R, Phillips W: Turning Points: A Psychoeducational Video Program for Overcoming an Eating Disorder. Toronto, Multi-Health Systems Inc., 1996, with permission.) *(Continued on following page.)*

learning experience for the adolescent. Importantly, such a positive experience can prepare young people to deal with the harmful societal standards for thinness that they will inevitably be exposed to. Practitioners can help parents in this important modeling task by sharing information about healthy body images, diets, and lifestyles.

School programs also can play an important role in promoting healthy body images and healthy diets because schools reach most adolescents, provide opportunities to practice healthy eating behaviors, and help adolescents resist social pressures.[43] School programs can educate adolescents about the concept of body image using developmentally appropriate and culturally relevant activities.

Clinicians, parents, and teachers should be aware of the impact of the mass media on young girls. Television, films, videos, magazines, newspapers, fashion

Step 2. Choose one goal from your list to work on this week. Use these problem-solving steps:

1. Identify and define the goal. Be specific.

____
____
____

2. List alternative ways to achieve your goal. More is better.

____
____
____

3. Review the implications of each alternative. Select the one that you believe will lead to the achievement of your goal without creating any new problems.

____
____
____

4. Specify a plan to carry out the solution. Outline each step in detail. Rehearse the plan in your mind or even role-play it out with someone else.

____
____
____

5. Act on your plan. Carry it out just the way you rehearsed it. Objectively evaluate the outome of your actions. Compare the outcome to your original goals. What have you learned?

____
____
____

FIGURE 1. Sample exercise *(Continued)*.

designers, and books continue to emphasize the importance of being thin and beautiful. One study[44] examined 50 undergraduates who each rated 54 third-grade text pictures using a thinness scale and found that there was a significant trend toward thinness for girls but not for boys. These unrealistic images and glamorization of thinness imposed on young girls symbolize success, self-control, competence, and strength. The role of the health professional, family, and school in the prevention of these media influences is particularly important.

Health professionals, teachers, and parents must also evaluate their own attitudes about their own body images so that they can have a positive influence on the attitudes of young adolescent girls. After all, we are raised in the same society as these young girls, a society in which more than a modicum of body fat is considered undesirable from a social, psychological, and even medical perspective. Although being overweight or obese has well-documented health risks, the specific form and severity of the risk and the corresponding degree of heaviness is frequently misunderstood, and the data are rather controversial.[41]

A State of Mind

The purpose of this exercise is to illustrate that body image is a state of mind, one that can have a powerful influence on your emotions and your actions if you let it. Start by imagining that you have just entered a party room that is filled with people your age. In the room there is furniture, and a long table at one end filled with the usual festive food and drinks. At the other end of the room people are dancing and mingling. Imagine that you are just entering the room as fat as you can possibly imagine yourself to be. Then imagine that you are entering the room as thin as you would like to be.

Fat me . . . **Thin me . . .**

This is what I am wearing . . .
This is how and where I am standing . . .
This is how I am relating with the other people . . .
This is how I am feeling . . .
This is what I am thinking . . .
Will I dance?
Will I eat or drink?
How long will I stay?
Which one of me is having the better time?

Body image . . . it is only a state of mind; don't let it control you.

FIGURE 2. Sample exercise that helps adolescents to recognize that body image is a state of mind. (From Davis R, Phillips W: Turning Points: A Psychoeducational Video Program for Overcoming an Eating Disorder. Toronto, Multi-Health Systems Inc., 1996, with permission.)

It is especially critical that health care providers remain cognizant of their personal and professional views about body size, since intentionally or inadvertently, their views may have an impact on the formative body images of their adolescent patients. In our institution, we work with young people who suffer from anorexia and bulimia nervosa. Sadly, a number of them have recounted experiences in which a practitioner's opinion or advice about their weight had a profound impact on them, initiating an intensification of their pursuit of thinness. Even the seemingly benign act of weighing the patient can prove to be a much more critical psychological experience for our patients than we may think. In one intriguing study,[45] medical students were weighed and then given false feedback about their weight status according to a fictional height–weight chart. Compared with students who were told that they were of average weight or were underweight, those students who were given false feedback about being overweight subsequently reported feeling more depressed and heavier than they wanted to be. Of greatest concern was the finding that these so-called overweight students reported lower self-esteem after the feedback about their weight.

By being aware of our own attitudes about body image, weight, physical fitness, and health, all of us, as health care providers, are in a position to make a difference in how adolescent girls feel and think about themselves.

SUMMARY

Dissatisfaction about body size and appearance and fears of fatness are alarmingly common among adolescent girls. Such concerns cut across racial, socioeconomic, and developmental lines. An unhealthy body image is linked to the adolescent's overall mental health, self-image, and eating behavior. Assessment of body image should, therefore, be a routine procedure in the overall medical assessment of adolescent girls. Counseling young girls about healthy eating behaviors and body image are vital activities for the practitioner.

REFERENCES

1. Garner DM, Garfinkel PE: Body image in anorexia nervosa: Measurement, theory and clinical implications. Int J Psychiatry Med 11:263–284, 1981.
2. Dwyer JT, Feldman JJ, Mayer J: Adolescent dieters: Who are they? Physical characteristics, attitudes and dieting practices of adolescent girls. Am J Clin Nutr 20:1045–1056, 1967.
3. Hill AJ, Draper E, Stack J: A weight on children's minds: Body shape dissatisfactions at 9-years old. Int J Obes 18:383–389, 1994.
4. O'Dea JA: Body image and nutritional status among adolescents and adults—A review of the literature. Aust J Nutr Dietetics 52:56–67, 1995.
5. Fisher S: Development and Structure of the Body Image. Hillsdale, NJ, Lawrence Erlbaum Associates, 1986.
6. Rodin J: Cultural and psychosocial determinants of weight concerns. Ann Intern Med 119:643–645, 1993.
7. Eisele J, Hertsgaard D, Light HK: Factors related to eating disorders in young adolescent girls. Adolescence 21:283–290, 1986.
8. Koff E, Rierdan J: Perceptions of weight and attitudes toward eating in early adolescent girls. J Adolesc Health 12:307–312, 1991.
9. Feldman W, Feldman E, Goodman JT: Culture versus biology: Children's attitudes toward thinness and fatness. Pediatrics 81:190–194, 1988.
10. Garner DM, Garfinkel PE, Olmsted M: An overview of sociocultural factors in the development of anorexia nervosa. In Darby PL, Garfinkel PE, Garner DM, Coscina DV (eds): Anorexia Nervosa: Recent Developments. New York, Allan R. Liss, 1983, pp 65–82.
11. Garner DM, Garfinkel PE, Schwartz D, Thompson M: Cultural expectations of thinness in women. Psychol Rep 47:483–491, 1980.
12. Rodin J, Silberstein LR, Striegel-Moore RH: Women and weight: A normative discontent. In Sonderegger TB (ed): Nebraska Symposium on Motivation: Psychology and Gender, vol 32. Lincoln, NE, University of Nebraska Press, 1985, pp 267–307.
13. Salmons PH, Lewis VJ, Rogers P, et al: Body shape dissatisfaction in schoolchildren. Br J Psychiatry 2(Suppl):27–31, 1988.
14. Davies E, Furnham A: Body satisfaction in adolescent girls. Br J Med Psychol 59:279–287, 1986.
15. Moore DC: Body image and eating behavior in adolescent girls. Am J Dis Child 142:1114–1118, 1988.
16. Kann LC, Warren CW, Harris WA, et al: Youth risk behavior surveillance. United States, 1995. MMWR CDC Surveillance Summaries 45:1–84, 1996.
17. Killen JDS, Hayward C, Litt I, et al: Is puberty a risk factor for eating disorders? Am J Dis Child 146:323–325, 1992.
18. Folk L, Pedersen J, Cullari S: Body satisfaction and self-concept of third- and sixth-grade students. Percept Mot Skills 76:547–553, 1993.
19. Wilson DB, Sargent R, Dias J: Racial differences in selection of ideal body size by adolescent females. Obes Res 2:38–43, 1994.
20. Desmond SM, Price JH, Hallinan C, Smith D: Black and white adolescents' perceptions of their weight. J Sch Health 59:353–358, 1989.
21. Abrams KK, Allen L, Gray JJ: Disordered eating attitudes and behaviors, psychological adjustment, and ethnic identity: A comparison of black and white female college students. Int J Eat Disord 14:49–57, 1993.

22. Schreiber GB, Robins M, Striegel-Moore R, et al: Weight modification efforts reported by black and white preadolescent girls: National Heart, Lung, and Blood Institute growth and health study. Pediatrics 98:63–70, 1996.
23. Parnell K, Sargent R, Thompson SH, et al: Black and white adolescent females' perceptions of ideal body size. J Sch Health 66:112–118, 1996.
24. Story M, French SA, Resnick MD, Blum RW: Ethnic/racial and socioeconomic differences in dieting behaviors and body image perceptions in adolescents. Int J Eating Dis 18:172–179, 1995.
25. Story M, Fowenwinkel K, Himes JH, et al: Demographic and risk factors associated with chronic dieting in adolescents. Am J Dis Child 145:994–998, 1991.
26. Dornbusch SM, Carlsmith JM, Duncan PD, et al: Sexual maturation, social class, and the desire to be thin among adolescent females. Dev Behav Pediatr 5:308–314, 1984.
27. Leon GR, Fulkerson JA, Perry CL, Cudeck R: Personality and behavioral vulnerabilities associated with risk status for eating disorders in adolescent girls. J Abnorm Psychol 102:438–444, 1993.
28. Button EJ, Sonuga-Barke EJ, Davies J, Thompson M: A prospective study of self-esteem in the prediction of eating problems in adolescent schoolgirls: Questionnaire findings. Br J Clin Psychol 35:193–203, 1996.
29. Killen JD, Taylor CB, Hayward C, et al: Weight concerns influence the development of eating disorders: A 4-year prospective study. J Consult Clin Psychol 64:936–940, 1996.
30. de Castro JM, Goldstein SJ: Eating attitudes and behaviors of pre- and postpubertal females: Clues to the etiology of eating disorders. Physiol Behav 58:15–23, 1995.
31. French SA, Perry CL, Leon GR, Fulkerson JA: Dieting behaviors and weight change history in female adolescents. Health Psychol 14:548–555, 1995.
32. Serdula MK, Collins ME, Williamson DF, et al: Weight control practices of United States adolescents and adults. Ann Intern Med 119:667–671, 1993.
33. Neumark-Sztainer D, Story M, Resnick MD, et al: Body dissatisfaction and unhealthy weight-control practices among adolescents with and without chronic illness: A population-based study. Arch Pediatr Adolesc Med 149:1330–1335, 1995.
34. Fisher M, Golden NH, Katzman DK, et al: Eating disorders in adolescents: A background paper. J Adolesc Health 16:420–437, 1995.
35. Maloney MJ, McGruire J, Daniels SR, Specker B: Dieting behavior and eating attitudes in children. Pediatrics 84:482–489, 1989.
36. Camp DE, Klesges RC, Relyea G: The relationship between body weight concerns and adolescent smoking. Health Psychol 12:24–32, 1993.
37. Thompson JK, Heinberg LL, Altabe M, Tantleff-Dunn S: Exacting Beauty: Theory, Assessment, and Treatment of Body Image Disturbance. Washington, DC, American Psychological Association, 1999.
38. Beals KA, Manore MM: The prevalence and consequences of subclinical eating disorders in female athletes. Int J Sport Nutr 4:175–195, 1994.
39. Davis R, Phillips W: Turning points: A Psychoeducational Video Program for Overcoming an Eating Disorder. Toronto, Multi-Health Systems Inc., 1996.
40. Jasper K: Out from under body-image disparagement. In Brown C, Jasper K (eds): Consuming Passions: Feminist Approaches to Weight Preoccupation and Eating Disorders. Toronto, Second Story Press, 1993, pp 195–218.
41. Ciliska D: Why diets fail? In Brown C, Jasper K (eds): Consuming Passions: Feminist Approaches to Weight Preoccupation and Eating Disorders. Toronto, Second Story Press, 1993, pp 80–90.
42. Striegel-Moore RH, Kearney-Cook A: Exploring parents' attitudes and behaviors about their children's physical appearance. Int J Eat Disord 15:377–385, 1994.
43. Levine MP: How Schools Can Help Combat Student Eating Disorders: Anorexia Nervosa and Bulimia. Washington, DC, National Education Association of the United States, 1987.
44. Davis J, Oswalt R: Societal influences on a thinner body size in children. Percept Mot Skills 74:697–698, 1992.
45. Ogden J, Evans C: The problem with weighing: Effects on mood, self-esteem and body image. Int J Obes Rel Metab Disord 20:272–277, 1996.

CHAPTER 5

Psychosexual Development

Susan L. Rosenthal, Ph.D.
Lisa M. Lewis, Ph.D.
Frank M. Biro, M.D.

Adolescent girls face challenges to their development of sexual health: (1) to their experience of positive feelings about the body and newly developed secondary sexual characteristics; (2) to their management of feelings of sexual arousal and desire; and (3) to their implementation of psychologically and medically healthy decision making when managing sexual behaviors (Table 1). They must make decisions about when to engage in both coital and noncoital behaviors; about with whom to engage in a given behavior; and, for those adolescents having intercourse, about which methods to use as protection against both sexually transmitted infections and undesired pregnancy.[1] These challenges occur during a period of biologic, psychologic, and cognitive change that provides both risk-taking and health-promoting opportunities for the adolescent.

This chapter begins with a discussion of dating and sexual behaviors and reviews various influences on psychosexual development, including onset of puberty, identity development, social and cultural construction, intimate relationships, cognition/decision making, and family influences. It concludes with a discussion of ways to promote sexual health among adolescents.

DATING AND SEXUAL BEHAVIORS

Dating relationships provide opportunities for individuals to express and experience intimacy. Perceived norms of dating age within school or social environments and the timing of puberty are important issues in the initiation of dating practices. Some adolescent girls begin dating as early as 12 years old, and most adolescents have dated at least once by age 16.[2]

Although dating is a common activity among adolescents, there has been limited focus on dating behaviors and their relationships to engagement in sexual activity. Studies examining these relationships would have to consider the various types of dating. Dating can include activities involving a group of teenage boys and girls, an occasional date involving a couple, or a date within the context of a steady relationship.[2] The type of dating may have different effects on sexual behavior. For example, girls may limit their dating to group

TABLE 1. Healthy Adolescent Psychosexual Development

• Positive feelings about body changes
• Appropriate management of sexual arousal and desire
• Responsible decision making about sexual behavior

situations because they are less likely to be alone with a boy and, therefore, are less vulnerable to engaging in unwanted sexual behaviors.

With regard to sexual behaviors, researchers and clinicians have focused primarily on the adolescents who begin having intercourse during the teenage years. Although there has been an increase in the number of adolescents initiating intercourse at earlier ages, the majority (62%) of 15–17-year old-girls are not sexually experienced. It is important to note, however, that being sexually experienced is not necessarily the same as being sexually active. Many adolescents who report having had sexual intercourse do not necessarily report being currently sexually active.[3] Unfortunately, in medical care settings and research, adolescents are often categorized either as having had or not having had sexual intercourse. Such classifications disregard the range and frequency of sexual behaviors. For example, adolescents who have had sexual intercourse only one time may be more similar to those who have never had sexual intercourse than to those who have had regular sexual involvement with either one or multiple partners.[4] Examining both noncoital behaviors and frequency of sexual intercourse allows further understanding of the sexual context and its influence on psychosexual development.

Most adolescents have had their first kiss by age 15 years, and one-third of girls have had their breasts touched by age 14 years. Although masturbation remains a more common activity for boys than for girls, 24% of 13–18-year-old girls have masturbated.[5] It has been suggested that white adolescents are more likely than African-American adolescents to engage in a predictable series of noncoital sexual behaviors before engaging in intercourse.[6] Research exploring these differences, however, is based solely on racial groupings, which contributes to the difficulties in identifying sociocultural differences within racial groups. Clearly, both socioeconomic status and varied cultural aspects (e.g., religion and peer norms) influence behavior and are important to consider in examining noncoital behaviors.

With regard to sexual experience, 22% of adolescent girls have had sexual intercourse by age 15 years, 52% by age 18 years, and 75% by age 20 years. The rates of sexual experience, particularly among younger adolescents, vary according to race, ethnicity, and socioeconomic status. For example, 35% of 15–17-year-old white adolescents are sexually experienced compared with 48% of African-American adolescents and 50% of Hispanic adolescents.[7]

Factors that influence the initiation of sexual intercourse include the onset of puberty, sociocultural expectations, and family environment (Table 2). These factors do not operate in isolation. For example, girls who become pubertal at a young age may initiate intercourse not because of burgeoning hormones, but rather because of societal expectations for sexually mature young women, including pressure from older males. Reasons for having intercourse that demonstrate cultural influences include curiosity, a wish to feel grown,

TABLE 2. Influences on Initiation of Sexual Intercourse

• Timing of onset of puberty
• Sociocultural expectations
• Family environment

and a desire to be accepted by female friends. Furthermore, reasons such as "I was alone with my partner and it just happened" support the relevance of parental supervision. Not all adolescent girls choose to have intercourse. Girls may experience date rape or more subtle forms of coercion, such as the fear of losing a boyfriend.

INFLUENCES ON PSYCHOSEXUAL DEVELOPMENT (Table 3)

Age at Onset of Puberty

The onset of puberty is a biologic, psychologic, and social phenomenon which causes the adolescent girl to look and feel different and prompts society to respond to her in a different way. In the United States, puberty typically begins between the ages of 8 and 13 years, and the expected age of menarche ranges from 11–15 years. Puberty includes hormonal changes, development of secondary sexual characteristics, and increase in body fat. During this time, the pubertal girl is increasingly aware of her body and of sexual feelings. The relative roles of hormonal influences and the development of secondary sexual characteristics on affect and behavior are not entirely clear. For example, one study of white adolescent girls found that body image was positively associated with the rate of change in breast stage development; however, among the same girls, body image was negatively associated with serum follicle-stimulating hormone (FSH) levels.[8]

Although adolescents experience physical changes of puberty roughly in the same sequence, timing and tempo may vary. The timing of puberty relative to one's peers may be more important than the onset of puberty. Girls who develop early are more likely to have a negative body image, engage in sexual activity and problem behaviors earlier, have a more negative affect and depression, and be at greater risk for eating disorders.[1] The impact of the increased body mass associated with the onset of puberty may differ by racial group; white adolescents may experience a greater decrease in self-worth than African-American girls.[9]

Adolescents who initiate sexual intercourse at an early age tend to accumulate more sexual partners, may use less discretion when selecting sexual partners, are less likely to use condoms at first intercourse, and are less effective when using contraception in the first months of sexual experience.[3] When adolescents engage in sexual intercourse at an early age, they are biologically more susceptible to sexually transmitted infections because of the presence of

TABLE 3. Influences on Psychosexual Development

• Age of onset of puberty	• Intimate relationships
• Identity development	• Cognition/decision making
• Social and cultural constructs	• Family influences

columnar epithelial cells on the exterior portion of the cervix (ectropion or eversion of the cervix, a normal developmental stage).[3] In addition, adolescents may not have acquired immunities to pathogens that can be transmitted by either sexual or nonsexual routes, such as herpes simplex virus; thus they are more likely to acquire genital infections.[4]

Identity Development

Developing a sense of identity involves the establishment of a consistent and congruous perception of self, which incorporates past and present experiences and a sense of future orientation. Identity formation has multiple facets, including occupational, sexual, and religious realms. Progress in establishing one's identity is marked by the degree to which one has made personal commitments in each area, although these commitments may not occur simultaneously. For example, a young girl may have a goal-directed plan to be a physician while continuing to struggle with her sexual orientation. For some adolescents, the identity formation process may be especially challenging. Adolescents who are members of disenfranchised groups based on either socioeconomic status or ethnic characteristics may have considerable struggles in establishing an identity.

Sexual identity is an inherent component of how an adolescent girl perceives herself, and it includes gender identification and sexual orientation and behavior. Gender roles are influenced by socialization and societal stereotypes. Early in adolescence, stereotypical gender roles are intensified and manifested in extreme feminine behavior. During late adolescence, however, the intensification of gender-linked behavior diminishes and is replaced by more androgynous behavior.[10]

As with nonsexual aspects of identity, the adolescent may explore different ideas about her sexual orientation during adolescence. Some young people are aware of their homosexual orientation before actually engaging in homosexual behavior. However, self-proclaimed sexual orientation and actual behavior may differ. For example, it is possible for an adolescent girl to have engaged in homosexual behavior in the past, but not consider herself a lesbian. A young adolescent who "comes out" as homosexual often experiences an increase in maladaptive risk behavior (e.g., suicide attempts). These negative risks are believed to be related to the difficult task of openly accepting oneself as a homosexual during a time in which stereotypic gender roles are intensified.[10]

Cultural and Social Constructs

Sexuality is socially and culturally constructed. Adolescents from different environments may have different expectations regarding the timing of transition to adult roles, including engagement in sexual intercourse. For some adolescents, intercourse during the early teen years may represent a syndrome of problem behavior; for others, it may be part of normative behavior and not associated with other problem behaviors. The media may influence the way in which adolescents define physical attractiveness and interpret sexual behaviors. Prime-time commercials using young, attractive women to sell products constitute at least one-third of advertisements. These types of media images depict unrealistic standards of beauty and behavior which lead some women to feel objectified and marginalized. Explicit references to sexuality also are displayed frequently, and despite continual intimations of nonmonogamous, unprotected intercourse, acquisition of sexually transmitted diseases (STDs) is rarely mentioned.[1]

The messages that society provides adolescents about their sexuality may be gender-linked. Both girls and boys have gender-linked sexual scripts that include beliefs about the appropriateness of indicating a desire for intercourse, males' unwillingness to use condoms, males' inability to stop once aroused, and females' need to offer token resistance. These gender-linked scripts can lead to miscommunication and may underlie the concerns of girls about the potential negative repercussions (e.g., aggression) from her male partner should she request condom use. Additionally, heterosexual relationships often are characterized by differences in power, which construct and influence women's sexual decisions. For example, some adolescent girls from inner-city environments have described a need to use sexual behavior to gain power.[6]

Intimate Relationships

Dating relationships may play a significant role in fostering the development of intimacy skills. There are developmental differences in the reasons adolescents date. For younger adolescents, dating may be a means of social interaction. Dating also may be perceived as important to adolescents because it gives them status with their peers and makes them feel "grown up." As adolescents mature, they become more interested in the quality of the relationship, particularly the degree of intimacy.

An intimate relationship should signify emotional attachment and a level of caring that is reciprocal. These qualities and the perception of their meaning may influence the implementation of "safer-sex" behaviors. Intimacy defined as trust and love may be perceived by the adolescent to be inconsistent with engaging in protective behaviors. However, intimacy and mutual sexual exclusivity may not coincide with each other. With regard to exclusivity, many adolescent girls, regardless of their sexual experience or inexperience, state that either they or their "boyfriend" saw someone else during their relationship. Adolescent girls who have had sex within their relationship spend more time with their boyfriends outside of school and describe the relationship as lasting longer into the future than girls who are sexually inexperienced. However, it is not clear whether these differences lead to sexual activity or whether adolescents describe their relationships differently after they initiate sexual intercourse.[11]

Cognition/Decision Making

During adolescence, the capacity for abstract reasoning develops. This newly developed ability (formal operational thinking) is characterized by hypothetical thinking, formal and systematic logic, the use of abstract concepts, and consideration of the future. Thus, younger adolescents and those without formal operational thinking may be limited to perceptions based solely on their own experience, rather than through deliberation and inference. The transition from concrete to formal operational thinking is task-dependent and believed to occur somewhere around 14 years of age.

While advanced developmental skills are useful in all problem solving and decision making, they may not lead to implementation of safer sexual behaviors. For example, a study examining condom negotiation from a developmental perspective evidenced little variance in the developmental level of negotiation skills. Most of the adolescents described strategies that focused on the needs or desires of one person. Both experience and emotions may lead to less advanced decision making in sexual situations, which may explain the inconsistent associations between variables of chronologic age, time since sexual debut, condom use, STD history, and negotiation of condom use in adolescents.[12] Adolescents often are inexperienced in the sexual situations in which they find themselves, and their decision making is influenced by the intensity of emotions in such situations.

More advanced reasoning skills also have implications for social reasoning. The *personal fable,* which is the concept that natural laws do not apply to oneself, has been the aspect of adolescent egocentrism that has received the most focus. The personal fable leads to faulty assumptions such as the belief that the adolescent will not become pregnant—"It won't happen to me." Sexually experienced adolescents who have not acquired an STD, compared with those who have acquired an STD, perceive STDs to be less prevalent among their friends and adolescents in general.[13]

Family Influences

Parents and other family members play a critical role in the adolescent girl's psychosexual development and her ability to develop the skills to make healthy decisions. Adolescents may describe adults and parents as not having the ability to understand their problems; this judgment may reflect their need to feel independent and autonomous, rather than reflecting a true distance between parent and adolescent. Adolescents do argue more with their parents than when they were children, but the degree of closeness to their parents continues. However, there are adolescents whose parents are not able to provide the support and guidance the adolescent needs.

In general, adolescents who are engaging in less sexual risk taking have parents who are available and who supervise them, and with whom there is closeness and communication.[6] The importance of parental relationships also is evident for the management of sexual risk for sexually experienced girls. These girls believe that their parents would help them should they acquire an STD.[14] The parent–adolescent relationship also may play an important role in the location of services that adolescents utilize. Adolescents with less involved parents may benefit from access to school-based or community-based (such as Planned Parenthood) clinics.

PROMOTION OF SEXUAL HEALTH

Knowledge of the various influences on psychosexual development of adolescent females can be integrated into our efforts to support adolescents in the development of psychosexual health. These influences interact with one another, creating risks and opportunities for adolescent girls. In our efforts to prevent adverse outcomes, we need to incorporate culturally and developmentally sensitive issues into our understanding and our interventions.

Adolescents need adults, including health care providers, who are interested in them holistically and who attend to the concerns they raise, no matter how trivial these appear to the adult. The care provider must take the initiative in discussing sensitive information because adolescents may not ask questions, even when interested in discussing these topics. Assessment begins with an understanding of the nature the adolescent girl's relationships and her perceptions about them. Consideration of her support system and the availability of significant adults to provide guidance and supervision is also important. Parents of prepubertal girls may benefit from discussions of how they plan to supervise their adolescents as they mature.

Care providers may ask young teens how much time they spend with significant friends outside of school, and where and how they spend that time. A teenager who has a boyfriend with whom she talks on the phone for hours may need a different type of intervention than a teenager who has no identified boyfriend, but who is alone regularly with male peers. Obtaining this information provides the clinician with an opportunity to assess the adolescent's risk-taking behaviors and decision-making skills. For example, one might explore with the teenager the issues of being alone with a boy to whom she is attracted.

As girls begin to demonstrate romantic interests, it is important to consider the possibility that they may be struggling with same-gender sexual feelings. Simple strategies, such as using gender-neutral language or asking about both same-sex and opposite-sex behavior, can be critical. Early in the adolescent's romantic relationships, clinicians should explore experiences with noncoital behaviors; too often the focus is primarily on sexual intercourse and adverse outcomes. It would be helpful for the care provider to feel comfortable about saying, "We are not sure that, at your age, intercourse is a good choice, but we will help you protect yourself if you do choose to engage in sex." When faced with a 15-year-old, a clinician may be likely to say, "Don't do it," and cut off communication, or may undermine efforts to postpone engagement by jumping immediately to discussing condoms and forgetting the precursors to sexual intercourse. Finding ways to master these conversations is the art of listening and responding nonjudgmentally.

One approach will not work for all adolescent girls. Sexually inexperienced girls, particularly those who mature early, may need help postponing the initiation of sexual intercourse. These efforts may include helping parents to provide appropriate supervision, helping adolescents to identify pressures to become sexually active, supporting their ability to say "no" to unwanted intercourse, and helping them to focus on the future. Fear tactics and lack of information about sex and contraception are not helpful. For girls who are already sexually experienced, providing access to health care and information about STD prevention and contraception is necessary but not sufficient to avoid adverse outcomes. For all girls, sexually experienced or inexperienced, our attention must focus on their feelings about their bodies and romantic relationships. Finally, it is critical that we improve our ability to discuss the whole range of sexual experiences, not just intercourse between consenting heterosexual couples.

Efforts should not be limited to office-based interventions, but must include a broader scope. If adolescents do not perceive opportunities for their future, there is little to gain through delaying immediate gratification. If girls are not protected from sexually exploitative or harassing school and work situations, sexual health will be difficult to obtain. Individual practitioners can contribute to societal and public health efforts by adding their voices in advocating for adolescent girls.

REFERENCES

1. Brooks-Gunn J, Paikoff RL: "Sex is a gamble, kissing is a game": Adolescent sexuality and health promotion. In Millstein SG, Peterson AC, Nightingale EO (eds): Promoting the Health of Adolescents: New Directions for the Twenty-first Century. New York, Oxford University Press, 1993, pp 180–208.
2. Steinberg L: Adolescence, 3rd ed. New York, McGraw-Hill, 1993.
3. Biro FM: Adolescents and Sexually Transmitted Diseases. Maternal and Child Health Technical Information Bulletin. Washington, DC, National Center for Education in Maternal and Child Health in cooperation with the Maternal and Child Health Bureau, Health Resources and Services Administration, Public Health Service, U.S. Department of Health and Human Services, 1992.
4. Miller KS, Clark LF, Wendell DA, et al: Adolescent heterosexual experience: A new typology. J Adolesc Health 20:179–186, 1997.
5. Koch PB: Promoting healthy sexual development during early adolescence. In Lerner RM (ed): Early Adolescence: Perspectives on Research, Policy, and Intervention. Hillside, NJ, Lawrence Erlbaum Associates, 1993, pp 293–307.
6. Rosenthal SL, Petersen AC, Hein K: Adolescent psychological development and STD acquisition. In Hitchcock PJ (ed): Adolescents and Sexually Transmitted Diseases. Oxford University Press [in press].
7. National Center for Health Statistics: Fertility, family planning, and women's health: New data from the 1995 National Survey of Family Growth. Vital and Health Statistics, Series 23, No. 19. Hyattsville, MD, National U.S. Department of Health and Human Services, DHHS Publication No. (PHS) 97-1995, May 1997.
8. Slap GB, Khalid N, Paikoff RL, et al: Evolving self-image, pubertal manifestation, and pubertal hormones: Preliminary findings in young adolescent girls. J Adolesc Health 15:327–335, 1994.
9. Brown KM, McMahon RP, Biro FM, et al; Changes in self-esteem in black and white girls between the ages of 9 and 14: The NHLBI Growth and Health Study (NGHS). J Adolesc Health 23:7–19, 1998.
10. Petersen AC, Leffert N, Graham BL: Adolescent development and the emergence of sexuality. Suicide Life Threat Behav 25:4–17, 1995.
11. Rosenthal SL, Burklow KA, Lewis LM, et al: Heterosexual romantic relationships and sexual behaviors of young adolescent girls. J Adolesc Health 21:238–243, 1997.
12. Rosenthal SL, Cohen SS, Biro FM: Developmental sophistication among adolescents of negotiation strategies for condom use. J Dev Behav Pediatr 17:94–97, 1996.
13. Rosenthal SL, Lewis LM, Succop PA, et al: Adolescent girls' perceived prevalence of sexually transmitted diseases and condom use. J Dev Behav Pediatr 18:158–161, 1997.
14. Rosenthal SL, Cohen SS, Biro FM, DeVellis RF: How do family characteristics relate to interpersonal expectations regarding STD acquisition among adolescent girls? Families, Systems, and Health. J Collab Fam Health Care 14:465–474, 1996.

CHAPTER 6

Negotiating Confidentiality

Elizabeth M. Alderman, M.D.

One cornerstone of providing optimal, accessible health care for adolescents is establishing confidentiality within the practitioner–patient relationship. The most prevalent causes of adolescent morbidity are related to high-risk behaviors. Adolescents may conceal information out of fear of disclosure if confidentiality is not guaranteed. In fact, adolescents are more likely to seek timely medical treatment if confidentiality has previously been established.[1] Most states have statutes guaranteeing adolescents the right of confidential health services for sexuality and drug-related issues. Sometimes, however, ensuring confidentiality in an office setting may be complicated by payment issues and informed consent.

WHY CONFIDENTIALITY IS IMPORTANT

Decision Making and Adolescent Development

To appreciate the importance of confidentiality when gathering medical information from the adolescent and implementing an effective health plan with her, it is important to understand that adolescent development is a continuum of progressing cognitive abilities and decision-making skills. Ages 11 years through 21 years represent a time of rapid changes in abstract thinking, moral development, and cognitive reasoning. Three of the most important tasks of adolescence are establishing autonomy, developing mature decision-making skills, and, ultimately, gaining emancipation from parents.

In descriptions of psychosocial development, adolescence is usually divided into three phases—early adolescence (ages 11–13 years), middle adolescence (ages 14–17) and late adolescence (ages 18–21), corresponding to junior high, high school, and college/employment, respectively. The early adolescent, preoccupied with her changing body, often strives for privacy. She also begins to spend more time with peers than with parents and family. Decisions are often shaped by peer norms and concrete thinking.[2] The middle adolescent has increased intellectual capabilities and begins to conceptualize abstractions, although peer norms are still strong in shaping behaviors. In fact, risk-taking behaviors are extremely common during the middle adolescent years because of a sense of omnipotence, curiosity and a continued attempt to establish independence from parents and authority figures. Conflict with parents is at its height. However, at this stage, the adolescent is still unable to fully appreciate the consequences of risk-taking behaviors.

The development of formal operational thinking with a fuller appreciation of the consequences of actions is the cornerstone of late adolescence. The young adult woman has established personal values, which are usually a hybrid of her own and her family's value system. She has a more developed future-time perspective than her younger peers and can consider alternatives effectively when making health care decisions.

Confidentiality in the practitioner–patient relationship is the basis for the development of trust. Working with adolescents and young adults is a challenge for primary care providers who are accustomed to dealing mostly with parents or caregivers in health-related decisions. However, it is important, once adolescence is reached, that the practitioner begin to address the adolescent, herself, in private, when discussing behaviors that might compromise her health. Girls and young women should be encouraged to discuss these behaviors with their parents. But the amount of detail required to assess health risk is not usually shared with parents, and there are some circumstances in which parental involvement is not possible or advisable.

The Limits of Confidentiality

An adolescent girl may not be able to involve her parents in health care decision making because it is dangerous for the parents to know or the adolescent fears parental alienation if such issues are disclosed.[3] The adolescent may be afraid of parental violence in certain situations. Many adolescents are uncomfortable discussing their sexual behaviors or personal problems with parents or have poor communication with parents. Furthermore, because of physical and mental incapacity, some parents may not be able to be involved in the health care of the adolescent.

CONFIDENTIALITY AND THE LAW

There is a legal basis for allowing adolescents to participate in their own health care decisions (see also chapter 9). In the United States, adolescents aged 18 years and older are considered legally to be adults and are able to give informed consent to medical treatment. However, the emancipated minor doctrine allows female adolescents younger than 18 years who are married, are in the armed forces, live away from parents, and are financially independent, or who have a child, to give consent for medical care. The mature minor principle allows adolescents younger than age 18 who have demonstrated that they have the cognitive abilities and have accepted responsibility for many of their personal matters to give informed consent for medical care.[4]

Most states have enacted laws designed to assure confidential care for adolescents for certain types of medical care, specifically care related to sexuality, contraception, pregnancy (including termination), sexually transmitted diseases (STDs), and HIV testing. These statutes reflect the sensitive and private nature of these issues and appreciation of the developing autonomy of the adolescent. The legal precedent reflected by these statutes is the adolescent's right to privacy.[4] Specific laws regarding access to contraception, prenatal care, HIV testing, treatment for STDs, and termination of pregnancy vary from state to state. If no state statute exists, the mature minor doctrine is evoked.

Contraception

There are no state laws that prohibit the prescription of contraception to a minor; however, in some states, there are lower age limits. An adolescent, regardless of age, is assured confidential access to contraception in all federally funded clinics and Planned Parenthood clinics.[4] However, private physicians are not covered by the federal law that mandates these services. The private practitioner must determine if an adolescent has the cognitive skills and is mature enough to understand the risks and benefits of taking prescribed hormonal medications such as oral contraceptives or medroxyprogesterone acetate. The adolescent should be able to provide a complete medical history, because these contraceptive options may be contraindicated in certain situations. However, the mere fact that an adolescent girl is requesting contraception should be evidence of maturity, for she clearly understands the consequences of sexual activity and is taking responsibility for pregnancy prevention. Parental involvement should be encouraged, particularly for young girls.

Many states have separate laws regarding sterilization. It is the exceptional adolescent who can weigh the pros and cons of sterilization and foresee the future consequences of such a procedure. Parental consent for sterilization of mentally subnormal individuals evokes tremendous ethical controversy, and many states prohibit this practice.

Sexually Transmitted Diseases (STDs)

Confidential diagnosis and treatment of STDs for minors is generally allowed in all states that have either statutes specifying this or no law prohibiting it, reflecting public health concerns. Some states may have lower age limits. A few states allow confidential HIV testing of adolescents, but most states do not have any specific statutes. Practitioners in states with no law cite the specific state laws regarding STD prevention and treatment when providing confidential HIV testing to minors. During pre-test counseling, assessment of the adolescent's competence is extremely important because informed consent must be obtained for HIV testing. Treatment of adolescents for HIV infection or AIDS without the knowledge of a parent or guardian is controversial and should be decided on a case-by-case basis.

Pregnancy

Most states allow adolescent girls under age 18 years to consent for the confidential diagnosis of pregnancy and prenatal care.[1] However, parental involvement is strongly encouraged, and this encouragement should be stressed to adolescents. Parental notification is not required once a pregnancy is diagnosed; but if the adolescent wishes to enter into prenatal care, she should be assisted and encouraged to tell her family, because the pregnancy will become obvious at some point.

Termination of Pregnancy

No issue in confidential health care for adolescents has evoked as much controversy as a minor's consent for termination of pregnancy. Many professional organizations have published position papers supporting a minor's ability to consent for termination of pregnancy if she is judged competent to understand the procedure and appreciate the consequences.[1] Position statements by the AMA Council on Ethical and Judicial Affairs and the American Academy of Pediatrics strongly encourage parental involvement, if possible, but recognize that parents may respond in an abusive fashion and their involvement may mean delay in seeking appropriate medical care.[5,6]

In some states, access to abortion services by minors is not entirely confidential.[1] As of 1994, parental notification of termination of pregnancy is required in 8 states and parental consent is required in 10 states[1] (Table 1). Each state has variations in its laws regarding absent parents, so it is mandatory that the practitioner be familiar with his or her individual state law. The states that require parental consent or parental notification do have a judicial bypass system to maintain confidentiality. Notification and judicial bypass may be waived in certain states if a second physician determines that a minor is mature enough to give consent or that parental notification would not be in her best interest. In states where no law exists, girls younger than 18 years may consent to termination of pregnancy via the mature minor doctrine. Under no circumstances may parents force an adolescent to terminate a pregnancy without her consent.[3]

Sexual Abuse

Sexual abuse is one circumstance in which confidentiality is not assured, because states require health professionals to report sexual abuse and incest of minors under 18 years of age to state authorities.[4] Statutory rape is a criminal offense in most states, involving a minor girl (usually 16 years old and under)

TABLE 1. States that Require Parental Consent or Notification for Termination of Pregnancy

Parental Consent	Parental Notification
Alabama	Arkansas
Indiana	Georgia
Louisiana	Idaho
Massachusetts	Minnesota
Michigan	Nebraska
Missouri	Ohio
North Dakota	Utah
Rhode Island	West Virginia
South Carolina	
Wyoming	

From Gans JE (ed): Policy Compendium on Confidential Health Services for Adolescents. Chicago, American Medical Association, 1994, with permission.

and a male partner (usually 10 years older or more), and does not consider whether the sexual contact was consensual or not. However, there is no mandatory reporting for this crime.

Substance Abuse

Surreptitious laboratory testing of a competent minor for illicit substances is strongly discouraged by the American Academy of Pediatrics.[7] In most states, minor adolescents are allowed to consent for diagnosis and treatment of drug abuse. However, effective treatment may not be possible without parental involvement, primarily for health insurance reasons. Some states exclude alcohol abuse treatment from this statute, and others allow only treatment of alcohol abuse. Other restrictions may include lower age limit for the adolescent and a provision for outpatient treatment only.

Mental Health

Many states allow adolescents to receive outpatient mental health services confidentially, but most states require parental consent for minors to receive inpatient psychiatric care and allow parents to admit their child involuntarily to a psychiatric facility.[1] A competent minor may refuse inpatient psychiatric treatment.[3]

School-Based Health Centers

One caveat in the setting of school-based clinics is that each school board sets its own rules regarding confidential services. In fact, schools in New York City have a section of the parental consent form where parents can "opt out" of allowing health care professionals to discuss and/or treat STDs, contraception, pregnancy, mental health problems, and substance abuse. Many school-based clinics do not allow the administration of medroxyprogesterone acetate or the dispensing or prescription of oral contraceptive pills. Practitioners in these settings should be knowledgeable about institutional policies and about alternative strategies to assure appropriate medical care to girls and young women.

AN APPROACH TO NEGOTIATING CONFIDENTIALITY (Table 2)

The best time to set standards for confidentiality in the practitioner–adolescent–parent relationship is well before the need for confidentiality arises. Often, such standards are set at the first encounter or in the preadolescent visit so that everyone understands the rules when the need for confidentiality arises. The ideal way to set standards for confidentiality is to establish a verbal or written agreement during this first visit.[8] The agreement should state the services the practitioner is willing or unwilling to provide and under which circumstances confidentiality will be maintained (i.e., contraception, STDs, pregnancy, substance abuse). The agreement must include the caveat that if a condition threatens the life of the adolescent or anyone else, then confidentiality must

TABLE 2. Tips on Negotiating Confidentiality

1. Lay the groundwork with the parent and patient at the first visit.
2. Establish a verbal or written agreement.
3. Note exceptions to confidentiality, such as suspected abuse.
4. Encourage parental participation.
5. Reiterate your willingness to discuss health-related issues with both patient and parent.

be breached and the adolescent will be informed of this necessity. This condition reflects legal and ethical requirements.[9] If, for example, an adolescent girl is diagnosed with a contagious disease such as hepatitis B or C, it is mandatory that household contacts, including parents, be informed. At this time, it is important to reiterate that parental participation in the health care of their daughter is extremely important and that the practitioner is available to help both parents and adolescent discuss health-related issues.

Challenges to the Confidentiality Agreement

If after discussing confidentiality at the initial visit the adolescent adamantly does not want the parent to know about a condition such as pregnancy or contraception use, the practitioner is obligated to explore the consequences of such a request for confidentiality. This exploration can take the form of posing hypothetical questions to the young woman, e.g., "What will you do if your Mom finds the birth control pills?" When a pregnancy is diagnosed, during the course of options counseling, it is important to emphasize that involvement of a parent or adult relative is important because he or she may provide support both emotionally and financially, regardless of whether the decision is to continue or to terminate the pregnancy.

If the practitioner believes that confidentiality must be breached, he or she is obligated to discuss this with the adolescent before informing the parent. There have been no court decisions in which an adolescent sued a practitioner for revealing confidential information to parents, but gaining the patient's consent is an ethical obligation of the practitioner–patient relationship.

Of note, practitioners are not legally obligated to report criminal activity of a patient to police unless it threatens the life of the patient or another.[9] However, injuries that are a result of violence, such as gunshot wounds or stab wounds, are mandatory reports in most jurisdictions.

Financial Considerations (Table 3)

Although maintaining a confidential relationship with the adolescent may be the gateway for better access to health care for contraception and other sexually related health care needs, the practitioner should always consider the practicality of not informing the parent of a patient visit in terms of billing. Parents are not obligated to pay for services if an adolescent sought confidential care.[9] When setting the stage for the confidential relationship with the adolescent, the practitioner should discuss how the visit will be billed and that letting parents know about the visit may be in the adolescent's best interests in terms of finances.

TABLE 3. Overcoming Financial Obstacles to Providing Confidential Health Care

1. Discuss the realities of payment for services with the adolescent.
2. Schedule small, regular payments by the adolescent.
3. Negotiate lower fees with the laboratory for confidential patients.
4. Obtain an alternative address at which the adolescent can receive bills in confidence.
5. Establish referrals to facilities with free or low-cost reproductive health care and contraceptive services if money is an obstacle to care.

If the adolescent lets her parent know she is being seen by the practitioner, the parents' insurance carrier may be billed without revealing the confidential nature of the encounter.[8] The bigger problem is usually the laboratory bills for STD tests, pregnancy tests, or Pap smears. The practitioner can try to negotiate lower billing rates with the laboratory for such confidential visits and have the bill sent to an alternative address such as that of a friend or relative. The adolescent can then pay the bill herself. If the adolescent absolutely cannot afford the laboratory tests necessary, the practitioner should be aware of clinics such as Planned Parenthood, college health services, and public health services that have lower charges or bill on a sliding scale. Most adolescents, however, are willing and able to pay something for confidential health services, and it is an appropriate developmental milestone to accept this responsibility.[9] If the practitioner does not wish to provide confidential services for adolescents and insists on parental consent or notification for all care, then knowledge of and referral to alternative, confidential health care providers is crucial.

CONFIDENTIALITY OF MEDICAL RECORDS

When a practitioner is requested to release medical information to insurance companies, managed care organizations, or other physicians, he or she should review the adolescent's chart to ascertain whether sensitive information is being disclosed. Many times, a parent will consent to medical record release, unaware of the confidential information contained in the adolescent's record. Results of HIV tests may not be disclosed without the specific consent of the adolescent. To obviate this quandary, some practitioners maintain separate charts, one with nonsensitive information and another that contains information related to confidential issues. A notation in the regular medical record can indicate that confidential information is stored in a separate chart. For example, one may note that "family issues were discussed" without detailing the exact nature of the conversation in the regular chart but note that the data exist in the confidential record. Some practitioners use codes in their notes (e.g., if anticipatory guidance was given regarding contraception, substance abuse, and STDs, one can note that SDRR was covered—sex, drugs, rock and roll).

CONFIDENTIALITY AND THE OFFICE STAFF

Nurses, receptionists, and other personnel are integral participants in creating an environment that provides confidentiality for adolescent patients. Office personnel should receive in-service training on the legal rights of adolescents with regard to reproductive health care. It is also necessary that the practitioners set up specific guidelines for office personnel to follow in terms of confidential billing and contacting a patient without involving a parent if the patient requests confidentiality. The procedure for notifying adolescents of laboratory results in a confidential manner should also be outlined for other health professionals. The general tone of the office is extremely important, and staff should be instructed not to discuss patients' private issues in the general office area.

DISCLOSURE OF INFORMATION TO OTHER HEALTH CARE PROFESSIONALS

Adolescents are often served by a multidisciplinary team when receiving health care. Thus, disclosure of confidential information to other health care providers may be vital and is permissible by ethical and legal standards.[10] However, before sharing confidential medical information with providers outside an institution, the practitioner should obtain written consent from the adolescent and, if applicable, the parent. This process shows the adolescent that she can trust the practitioner to maintain confidentiality and allows the adolescent to participate further in the health care process.

CONCLUSIONS

Independent decision making and personal autonomy are the ultimate accomplishments of adolescence. However, before achieving these milestones, many adolescents participate in behaviors that may lead to substantial morbidity. It is important for the practitioner caring for adolescent girls to provide confidential health care to address these morbidities. The practitioner may attempt to facilitate discussion of sensitive health-related issues between girls and their parents; however, in some cases, this approach is not possible or advisable.

In most circumstances, when addressing high-risk behaviors, the practitioner is empowered to care for the adolescent in confidence. The practitioner should be familiar with local statutes regarding confidential care and explicitly advise the adolescent and parent of the permissible scope of such care.

REFERENCES

1. Gans JE (ed): Policy Compendium on Confidential Health Services for Adolescents. Chicago, American Medical Association, 1994.
2. Battle CU, Kreisberg RV, O'Mahoney K, et al: Ethical and developmental considerations in caring for hospitalized adolescents. J Adolesc Health 10:479, 1989.
3. Greydanus DE, Patel DR: Consent and confidentiality in adolescent health care. Pediatr Ann 20:80–84, 1991.
4. Holder AR: Legal issues in adolescent sexual health. Adolesc Med 3:257– 267, 1992.
5. American Academy of Pediatrics, Committee on Adolescence: The adolescent's right to confidential care when considering abortion. Pediatrics 97:746–751, 1996.
6. Council on Ethical and Judicial Affairs, American Medical Association: Mandatory parental consent to abortion. JAMA 269:82–86, 1993.
7. American Academy of Pediatrics: Policy statement: Drug abuse in adolescents. Pediatrics 84:396, 1989.

8. Alderman EM, Fleischman AR: Should adolescents make their own health-care choices? Contemp Pediatr 10:65–82, 1993.
9. Fisher M, Marks A, Treieller K, Brody R: Are adolescents able and willing to pay the fee for confidential health care? J Pediatr 107:480–483, 1985.
10. English A: Treating adolescents: Legal and ethical concerns. Med Clin North Am 74:1097–1112, 1990.

CHAPTER 7

The Mother–Daughter–Female Clinician Triad

Estherann Grace, M.D.

The old adage "three girls do not play well together" may be confirmed in the mother–daughter–female clinician triad. The success of the triad depends on clear communication of individual needs. In the triad, the female clinician's role is to identify the health-related issues of concern, to prioritize them, and to negotiate an acceptable plan for resolving them with both mother and daughter. Fathers are rarely involved in their adolescent daughters' health care. When they are, it is usually the consequence of the mother's unavailability. Career choices, divorce rates, and shared child care may reverse this trend in the future.

Providing health care to adolescent girls and young women requires an understanding of their physiologic and psychologic stages of development. Because of the dramatic differences within stages, adolescents are grouped according to age: early adolescence (11 to 14 years), middle adolescence (15 to 17 years), and late adolescence (18 to 22 years). A daughter's relationship with her mother evolves as she proceeds through these recognized stages, and the clinician must adapt to these changing relationships (Table 1).

EARLY ADOLESCENCE

The early adolescent often vacillates between total dependence on her mother and the need to be independent. This wavering is demonstrated by the 12-year-old girl who is willing to have a physical examination while her mother sits in the waiting room, but insists that her mother hold her hand when she receives an immunization. At this developmental stage, helping the mother to cope with the adolescent's mood swings, which are typical of perimenarchal hormonal instability, assumes priority in office encounters. Mothers are often confused and, at times, angered by their daughters' erratic behavior. The easy communication of childhood is replaced by the verbal confrontations of early adolescence. One responsibility of the clinician is to prepare mothers for these normal fluctuations in their daughters' moods. Helping mothers to foster their daughters' independent strivings while continuing in a supervisory and supportive role

TABLE 1. Prominent Issues in the Mother–Daughter Relationship

Early Adolescence	Middle Adolescence	Late Adolescence
Dependence vs. independence	Increasing sexual awareness	Maturation of patient–clinician relationship
Pubertal development and hormonal storms	Coital debut	Benefits of parental involvement in young adult's life
Mother's confusion over daughter's erratic behavior	Decision on drugs, alcohol, tobacco, sexual activity	Patient's willingness to allow parent to be involved in medical issues
Withdrawal of teen from family—turning to friends for emotional support	Increasing need for independence	Independent living arrangements
	Diminishing parental control	Commited sexual relationships
		Sexual orientation identified

starts in early adolescence, but does not end there. Healthy mother–daughter relationships are a continual challenge for all members of the mother–daughter–female clinician triad, regardless of the stage.

MIDDLE ADOLESCENCE

Middle adolescence brings an added dimension to the triad. Girls in this age group have an increasing awareness of their own sexuality and sexual identity. Many young women experience their coital debut during this stage. The availability of alcohol and illicit drugs, coupled with the adolescent's need for increasing independence, further contributes to the mother–daughter conflicts so common during the years from 15 to 18. Since many choices made at this stage involve potential life-threatening, risk-taking behaviors, mothers are understandably concerned for their daughters' safety. At the same time, however, a mother's sense of control diminishes as her daughter's independent decision making increases. Such fears usually translate into a tightening of restrictions. The adolescent resents the imposed limits, often with a negative response of further acting-out and risk-taking behavior that strains the mother–daughter relationship.

It is into this strained relationship that the female clinician enters. In this context her role as educator and advocate assumes added prominence. Although grateful that the female clinician is available to address their daughters' needs, mothers frequently resent the easy, confidential relationship between clinician and teen. Viewing themselves at a disadvantage, mothers may see the female clinician as a threat. To avoid maternal ambivalence and maintain mother as an alley, a clear restatement of roles within the triad is critical. "You are the mother, I am the doctor" may actually need to be said to some mothers to ensure the triad's function. In addition, reassuring the other that you are both working toward a similar goal of maintaining her daughter's health can be helpful.

Change characterizes middle adolescence: pubertal development is completed; sexual orientation is established and, for some, acted upon; decisions regarding drug and alcohol use are made; and realistic educational goals are identified. Acting-out behavior in middle adolescence is not limited to psychosocial issues. For those with chronic disease, the assertion of independence can be medically risky. Denial is a normal coping mechanism, but for a young woman with diabetes, cystic fibrosis, or an eating disorder it can be fatal. Trial and error characterize the clinician's attempts to find the balance between adolescent autonomy and reduced parental involvement in disease management. The clinician is asking a parent, the primary caregiver, to relinquish her role and support her daughter's efforts to manage her own disease. For some mothers this new approach is not only difficult, it is impossible. Consequently, a mother may devise strategies to maintain control. She can literally step between the clinician and her daughter in her attempt to jeopardize the relationship. She may call to arrange appointments and refill prescriptions rather than her daughter. This strategy reduces the adolescent's involvement in her own care. A mother may further sabotage the doctor–patient relationship by accompanying her daughter to the visit and insisting on being present for the entire visit. In order to ensure the privacy the adolescent deserves, the clinician must intervene, potentially creating a hostile environment in an already difficult situation. The struggle then ensues involving the over-controlling mother, noncompliant teenager, and harassed clinician: not an optimal dynamic for delivery of good patient care. Resolution is possible by negotiating individually with the mother and daughter, and then as a group with clinician as mediator. A time-consuming process, these sessions are best scheduled at regular intervals in 30-minute blocks with structured guidelines; i.e., each member of the triad speaks for 10 minutes. This tactic avoids individual domination, allowing all voices to be heard. The frequency of the visits prevents the build-up of accumulated grievances. Should the adolescent revert to haphazard compliance, her behavior can be addressed promptly with concerned interest rather than dictatorial control by mother or clinician. It also permits distancing from the over-involved mother.

LATE ADOLESCENCE

During late adolescence (18–22 years of age), the patient–clinician relationship matures and the tone of the triad changes. An 18-year-old is legally an adult. Consequently, parents are informed of medical issues only with their daughter's knowledge and consent. Despite the legal designation, young adults continue to need and benefit from parental involvement in their lives. With the maturing of the clinician–patient relationship, mothers' roles become even more marginalized. Young women in this age group usually come to their appointments alone or with a friend, further distancing their mothers from direct knowledge of their health status. Efforts on the clinician's part to keep mothers appropriately informed depend on the patients' willingness to share the information. Routine health care poses little problem. The dilemma arises when disorders are more severe. Consider the 20-year-old who admits to restricting her food intake and purging several times a week but does not want her parents to know that she has an eating disorder. Adhering to the guideline "patient safety first," the clinician can proceed by negotiating a program with the patient to reduce her unhealthy eating behaviors, with a contingency of the treatment plan being parental notification should her health deteriorate to the point of hospitalization. In order to avoid a negative consequence (hospitalization), the patient often will modify her behavior (eating). This technique appropriately reinstates a sense of control to the young adult patient. When the young woman is too sick to act in her own best interest, legal steps can be taken to guarantee her safety. Understandably, legal steps should be taken with great reluctance.

Many young women move out of the family home during late adolescence, signaling the completion of adolescent dependency. When departure is imminent, the mother–daughter relationship often enters a stage of mutual truce. The vocal conflicts of the early teen years and the acting-out behaviors that occurred during high school cease. Each is tolerant of the other's ideas without necessarily agreeing with them. At this stage, daughters examine their mothers' life choices as women. Critically questioning their mothers' lifestyles, they vow not to repeat their mistakes. Open communication by the mother with her young adult daughter can close the potential gap in the maturing relationship. A daughter's awareness of her mother's own late adolescent experiences may give her a better understanding of the woman her mother has become. The female clinician's role at this phase is support and encouragement as these two women move on to the next stage of their relationship.

CASES DEMONSTRATING THE CLINICIAN'S ROLE

Case presentations demonstrate techniques of mother–daughter–female clinician communication. The case material that follows was gathered from a diverse patient population seen in both private practice and urban clinic settings.

Case 1 (Early Adolescence)

Tasha was 12 years old. She started junior high school four months ago. Her attendance in the lower grades was consistent; she was rarely sick or absent. In mid-September she had a viral upper respiratory infection and missed three consecutive days of school. Over the subsequent weeks she continued to miss school on a regular basis. She complained to her mother that she did not feel well and requested to stay home. Her teachers contacted the mother about Tasha's frequent absences and requested a medical explanation. Mrs. Washington called for the appointment and expressed her concern to the secretary, who relayed it to the clinician. A 30-minute appointment was made for Tasha and her mother.

While Tasha was with the nurse having her height, weight, and vital signs recorded, her mother related her perspective on the problems to the doctor. She described Tasha as a very healthy child who was of normal weight until age 11. At that age her appetite markedly increased; her physical activity decreased; and she gained 30 pounds in 8 months. Her mother reported that Tasha had experienced menarche four months earlier and since then her appetite and inactivity had remained constant while her weight increased another 15 pounds. Mrs. Washington stated that she, herself, was 80 pounds overweight and she was very upset that Tasha was following her pattern. She also realized that she was angry at Tasha for gaining excess weight and replicating her own adolescent behaviors. Tasha's repetitive complaints of "always being tired," "just not feeling well," having a "sore throat," and feeling "achy" greatly concerned her mother. She was worried that Tasha had a serious disease. She wanted her daughter to be well, to go to school, to be happy.

Tasha entered the office and sat next to her mother, handing her the completed encounter form that the nurse had told Tasha to give to the doctor. When addressed directly by the doctor, Tasha looked to her mother to answer the questions. The doctor gently prodded Tasha to explain how she felt. She was asked to describe her symptoms in her own words. Gradually, Tasha warmed to her task and gave a detailed description of her symptoms. At this point, Mrs. Washington was asked to return to the waiting area so that Tasha could change into a gown for the physical examination in privacy. Mother's departure gave the doctor the opportunity to ask the confidential questions necessary to complete her history. The physical examination was done with mother in the waiting room.

No significant pathology other than obesity was found on examination. When Tasha and Mrs. Washington were given the negative findings, both were more disappointed than relieved. The mother demanded to know why, if Tasha was so healthy, she was sick all the time. Tasha wondered why she always felt so tired. When told she needed a blood test to confirm the negative exam, Tasha burst into tears and clutched her mother. After reassurances that butterfly "baby" needles would be used and mother would be with her, she agreed to having the blood drawn. The laboratory results were normal.

The doctor now had to deal with a 12-year-old, obese girl with multiple physical complaints, frequent school absences, no evidence of organic disease, and a mother convinced that something was wrong with her daughter. For a triad to function, each member's agenda must be prioritized and treatment plans discussed. In this case, after elimination of a treatable organic disease, a behavioral approach to Tasha's complaints proved helpful, starting with the issue of obesity. Body size and weight are sensitive areas for most women, including female clinicians. This is particularly true when the clinician herself is struggling to maintain her own weight in a healthy range. By acknowledging both the mother's and daughter's concerns, the clinician validates them. So begins the essential component of the relationship, trust. Mother and daughter have not been abandoned because no organic disease was found; instead, they are encouraged to actively participate in planning coping strategies.

With guidance, Tasha and her mother negotiated the guidelines that would allow Tasha to miss school (i.e., a temperature of 100° or higher). The concept of psychotherapy was introduced to help Tasha and her family deal with recurrent chronic illness. The complexity of Tasha's problems precluded a simple solution. Patience was required on everyone's part as Tasha made her way through early adolescence, hampered by psychosomatic illness and its ramifications.

Case 2 (Middle Adolescence)

Mrs. Reynolds called requesting an appointment to speak privately with the doctor. She refused to give the secretary a specific reason, simply stating it was personal. It was obvious to the doctor that Mrs. Reynolds was agitated when she entered the office. Not waiting for the doctor to speak, she blurted, "This is all your fault. I found this (a condom) in Becky's room when I was cleaning under the bed. You're the one who told her about condoms. You're the one responsible for this (pointing to the condom) and her, if she gets pregnant or a disease. She listens to you. I'm just her mother, and she tells me nothing."

At this point in the encounter Mrs. Reynolds paused to take a breath, and the doctor invited her to sit down. Body language was important at this juncture. The clinician sat back in her chair, put down her pen and gave her full attention to the irate mother. The doctor's first priority was to redefine confidentiality as the backbone of the relationship she shared with Becky. This included issues involving Becky's sexuality: "Yes, Mrs. Reynolds, condoms as well as other safe sex practices, including abstinence, have been discussed. I advocate delay in sexual expression, but for any patient who chooses not to wait, I give her the information to make responsible decisions to protect her health. The individual is responsible for her actions, not the educator."

Mrs. Reynolds was slightly placated, but still agitated. She said, "How can I stop her from having sex? I don't want her to think I condone this type of behavior if I permit her to see you and start on birth control pills. If she asks you for them, I do not want you to prescribe them." The interview with Mrs. Reynolds was stressful for both her and the doctor. The anger, frustration, and lack of control that Mrs. Reynolds felt was directed toward the female clinician: "How dare she diminish may place in my daughter's life?" The doctor needed to clarify the basis of her professional relationship with Becky. She responded, "I am responsible for providing your daughter's health care. In no way does this change your position in Becky's life. I am the doctor; you are the mother." As gently as possible, the doctor reminded Mrs. Reynolds that Becky could receive a prescription for birth control pills confidentially.

Mrs. Reynold's and the clinician were unaware that Becky had called earlier in the week to schedule an appointment. The reason given to the scheduling secretary was "personal." Becky arrived for the appointment with her 17-year-old boyfriend. She declined to give the secretary her insurance card because she did not want her parents to know she had come to the office. She clearly stated her concerns to the doctor. She had become sexually active since her last school physical examination. Her boyfriend used condoms most of the time, but her period was late and she was worried about pregnancy. She was also stressed about school work (junior year), PSATs, the soccer team's performance (captain of the team), and the deteriorating relationship with her mother: "I cannot cope with everything and worry about being pregnant. I want the pill. You always told me you would give me birth control if I needed it; well I do. I don't want my mother to know. She would kill me." Becky had blurted out her agenda. She was uncomfortable discussing her sexual needs, avoided eye contact, and played with a magazine. Again, the clinician leaned back in her chair and discussed Becky's contraception options, including abstinence. She then asked Becky what she wanted to do. Becky was clear: "I want the pill." A pelvic examination with appropriate cultures and Pap smear, as well as a pregnancy test, was done, and the method of payment and the office visit charge was negotiated. Becky agreed to pay $20 per month. She understood that if she defaulted in her payment plan, she would forfeit her confidentiality, and the bills would be sent home. Although respecting Becky's right to confidential care, the doctor encouraged her to share with her mother her decision to take birth control pills. It is difficult for a 16-year-old to maintain this type of secret from her mother. Studies have shown improved compliance when adolescents tell their mothers they are taking the pill.

Three months later Becky returned for her follow-up visit. Her mother accompanied her and requested to speak to the doctor. Becky was seen first for weight, vital signs, and a review of pill use. She told the doctor that her mother knows she is taking birth control pills. Mrs. Reynolds found the pills in Becky's room. She confronted Becky, and flew into a rage, disgusted with her behavior.

Mrs. Reynolds joined Becky and the doctor. Despite the doctor's efforts, the atmosphere remained strained. The doctor commented on the strength of the mother–daughter relationship: although there was discord between them, they were still able to relate and care for one another. Mrs. Reynolds began to cry, and Becky stared at the floor. At this juncture, to help them resolve their differences, the concept of a family therapist was introduced: "Becky, it is clear to me that you and your mother love each other very much. Still, you are both having difficulty getting along. My work with young women has taught me that having someone to talk to helps one to sort out differences. I am giving you the name of a counselor today that I have worked with who is very skilled in working with families." By stressing that the family needed help, the doctor avoided casting individual blame. With reluctance they agreed to the referral.

The confrontational parent can wreck havoc in the clinical setting. Coping with an angry screaming parent distracts the doctor and her team from the delivery of patient care. It also creates an avoidance behavior pattern. The obnoxious mother may find herself unable to effectively communicate with an unresponsive office, further fueling her anger. The clinician needs to intervene on her staff's behalf and defuse this situation, preserving a professional decorum. Since women typically feel on equal footing with one another, mothers are more likely to confront a female clinician than a male. Although this is nerve-racking for the doctor, it does allow for a more open and honest discussion of mutual concerns.

Case 3 (Late Adolescence)

Marlene was 20 years old. She had just finished her sophomore year in college. She had been living in an apartment near the campus with two roommates. When she returned home in May, her parents were shocked by her appearance. She had lost 25 pounds since Christmas. They insisted on an immediate medical evaluation. They were terrified that she had a malignancy. She denied any change in her behavior to explain the weight loss. She was emphatic that she had not restricted her food intake, exercised excessively, vomited, or used laxatives. She could not understand their reaction and thought they were being overly dramatic and treating her like a child.

With resentment she came to the appointment her parents had scheduled. She returned the doctor's initial greeting with a surly, "I don't know why I am here. It wasn't my idea. There is nothing wrong with me; my parents are overreacting." When confronted with the now 30-pound weight loss from her previous visit in December, she admitted she had stopped eating fat and was going to the gym twice a day. Her menstrual period had stopped in February, and she denied any risk of pregnancy. Her physical examination was negative except for bradycardia, hypotension, hypothermia, and marked cachexia. A caloric intake of 1000 calories or less per day coupled with 2 hours of exercise at the gym explained the weight loss and her present metabolic state. Marlene met the criteria for a diagnosis of anorexia nervosa. When told, she immediately denied the diagnosis. Yet when asked how she saw herself at 67 inches and 105 pounds, her answer was, "I could stand to lose another 10 pounds."

Marlene's treatment plan was complicated by her adult status and her parents' anxious involvement. Prioritizing medical stability while organizing a treatment team was the focus of weekly office visits. Mr. and Mrs. Greene accompanied Marlene, asking to be present during the doctor's evaluation. When they were refused, they reluctantly waited in the hall while Marlene was examined. Vacillating between childlike dependence and angry independence, Marlene gave her parents a mixed message, compounding the family's dysfunction. The doctor soon became the focus of the family's frustrations. She did not meet the expectations of curing their daughter. She failed Marlene because she would not leave her alone, insisting on monitoring her weight and vital signs weekly. Marlene resisted all outpatient treatment efforts, continued to lose weight, became medically unstable, and was hospitalized.

It was only with the crisis of the hospitalization that Marlene was finally able to accept her diagnosis of anorexia nervosa. Despite Mr. and Mrs. Greene's efforts, they could not coerce Marlene into stopping her anorexic behavior. It had become part of her identity, and she was not willing to relinquish it. Helping Mr. and Mrs. Greene to accept Marlene's adult status became a treatment goal, which the clinician accomplished by gradually reducing their involvement in the treatment process. Marlene was encouraged to come to her appointments on her own. If her parents insisted on bringing her, they were asked to wait in the car. Medical issues (with Marlene's permission) were discussed with them by phone. It was Marlene's responsibility to follow the meal plan, not her parents'. She was asked to prepare her own meals, rather than having her mother control her portions on the plate. Mrs. Greene had great difficulty allowing Marlene this degree of autonomy, and she blamed the clinician for every pound not gained or, worse, lost. "Responsibility for my behavior" was a recurring theme in Marlene and her parents' therapy sessions.

Mr. and Mrs. Greene were requested not to discuss food or the eating disorder with Marlene. They had constantly quizzed her on what she had eaten and why she refused to eat more. Breaking this pattern of behavior was difficult. If they felt compelled to say something, they were to walk away, leave the room, and, if necessary, leave the house. If they were unable to do this, Marlene was advised to absent herself.

The clinician is treading a fine line as she attempts to extinguish the overcontrolling parental behavior. Frequent communications with all treatment team members is essential to present a unified front. Parents and patients are capable of splitting teams. The team's defeat may unfortunately be the patient's as well. In anorexia nervosa, consistency is the cornerstone of treatment. In Marlene's case, the concept of responsible adult behavior was emphasized as well. Her recovery depends on everyone acting on it.

CONCLUSION

Adolescent girls frequently request a female health care provider. The reasons given range from personal embarrassment to a belief in the clinician's implicit understanding of what a menstrual cramp is. Regardless of the initial reason for the gender preference, patients remain with clinicians because they trust and respect their judgment.

Developing this patient–clinician relationship requires time, commitment, and a firm grasp of the physiologic and psychosexual development of adolescents. Supporting mothers through the stages of their daughters' adolescence remains an integral part of patient care. Maintaining alliances with the mother while providing confidential health care to her daughter truly tests the clinician's skills.

SUGGESTED READING

1. Grace E: Incorporation of adolescent gynecology into general practice. Adolesc Med 2:397–404, 1991.
2. Tolmas HC, Long VA Jr, Grace E: Solutions: Role for the private practitioner. Adolesc Med 1:145–160, 1990.
3. Ross-Lee B: The physician–patient relationship. In Women and Their Health Care Providers: A Matter of Communication. Public Health Rep 101(Suppl):142–144, 1986.
4. Suchman AL, Markakis K, Beckman HB, Frankel R: A model of empathic communication in the medical interview. JAMA 277:678–682, 1997.
5. Schlicht SM, Dunt DR: Women's perceptions of female general practitioners. Community Health Stud 11:176–182, 1987.
6. Bernzweig J, Takayama JI, Phibbs C, et al: Gender differences in physician–patient communication: Evidence from pediatric visits. Arch Pediatr Adolesc Med 151:586–591, 1997.

CHAPTER 8

Issues for the Male Clinician

Robert T. Brown, M.D.

As we enter the 21st century, American women have become increasingly comfortable with self-assertion and self-determination and are increasingly intolerant of male chauvinism. Women have expressed these feelings in many ways, including asserting their right to equal opportunity in participation and funding in college sports, entering the traditionally male medical establishment as physicians, and increasing their penetration of the corporate "glass ceiling." Women as medical patients have also asserted their rights to treatment equivalent to men in research and in clinical venues. This phenomenon is not limited to the pediatric and adolescent population. Women of all ages want their health care to be provided by clinicians who first are competent, but who are also sensitive, compassionate, and interested in them as people, not just as interesting diagnostic or therapeutic puzzles. They want clinicians who are sensitive to the lot of women in modern American society, and they want help in making their lives easier to bear (Table 1). Recently, more and more female patients, both adult and adolescent, have sought this kind of care from female clinicians with the intimation, if not the literal assertion, that only another woman can give this kind of caring attention to issues of health and well-being.

A recent discussion at the internet site of the Society of Adolescent Medicine has pointed out a corollary to this situation. The issue was that so many female adolescents are requesting female clinicians, especially for pelvic examinations and for discussion of intimate topics, that male medical students and residents are not getting enough experience in these most necessary interactions with female patients in this age group.

What, then, is the male clinician to do to make himself sympathetic and benign enough to female patients that they will feel comfortable seeing him for their comprehensive health care? A corollary question is whether the male clinician should abdicate the field of women's health care to female clinicians and just avoid getting involved.

This chapter explores factors that make physicians appealing to patients of either gender and then assesses whether there is hope for male clinicians with female patients. Additionally, it looks at the factors that make female adolescents seek female providers to see if they can be developed by clinicians of the opposite and, more often, weaker sex.

TABLE 1. Qualities that Women Seek in Clinicians

Good listening abilities	Thoroughness
Empathy	Competence
Sensitivity	

ISSUES COMMON TO ALL CLINICIAN–ADOLESCENT PATIENT ENCOUNTERS

Respect

The medical encounter has always implied a contract between the person seeking service and the provider of that service. Implicit in that contractual relationship is the provision of respect given by each participant to the other. The clinician is expected to accord to the patient respect based on the patient's essential worth as a human being and as a person who has need of the clinician's professional expertise. The patient, in turn, is expected to respect the clinician as a human being and as someone with special expertise in maintaining health, alleviating suffering, and curing disease. So it is with the clinician–adolescent patient encounter. No matter whether the patient is male or female, is dressed or decorated appropriately according to the clinician, or has a history of behaving in ways personally sanctioned by that clinician, the clinician must accord the patient respect. Similarly, irrespective of the clinician's ethnic derivation, mode of dress, or style of speaking, the patient must accord respect if the interaction is to be beneficial at all.

The clinician's behavior is the key factor in establishing this mutual feeling of respect. If the clinician does not demonstrate interest in the patient as a person rather than as another "case"; if the clinician makes inappropriate comments regarding the patient's dress, decorations, behaviors, or personal characteristics; if the clinician makes the patient feel more uncomfortable than is necessitated by the needs of the health encounter; and if the clinician does not prevent the adolescent patient from feeling assaulted, then respect between the dyad is not possible. The clinician must explicitly demonstrate attention to cleanliness, sterile technique, and professional competence.

Empathy and Sensitivity

The patient does not expect the clinician to be a buddy or a peer. He or she expects the physician or other provider to display behavior and dress commensurate with his or her age and profession. The patient is reassured that the clinician really is interested in her as a person if the clinician inquires about and engages in conversation about aspects of the patient's life other than the immediate issue which led to the encounter. Even the shortest medical visit for a very focused reason such as an ear infection can provide an opportunity for inquiry about the patient's school situation, interests in television, music, or activities. A system such as the "5 Boxes," through which the clinician explores the patient's life in the medical, home, school/work, peer, and romance "boxes," provides a ready mechanism upon which to base these questions (Fig. 1).

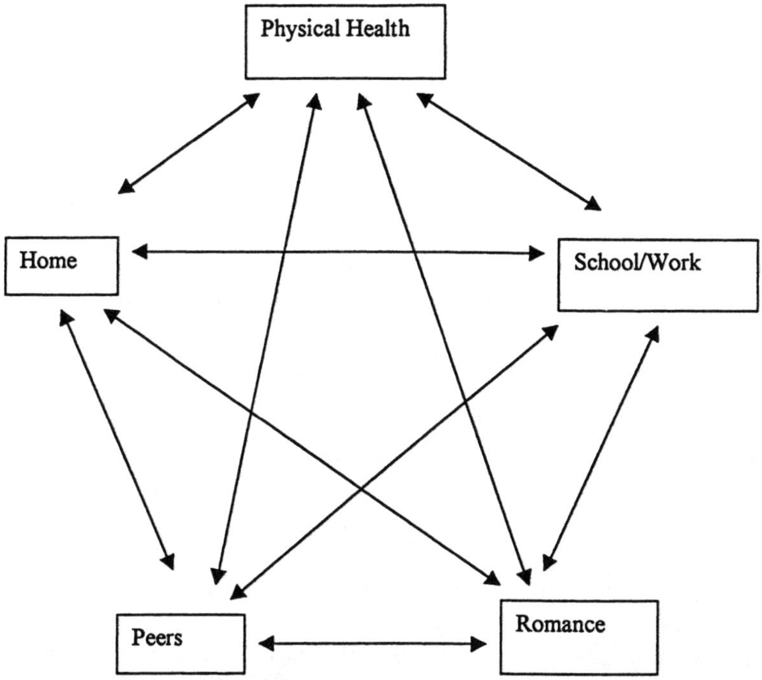

FIGURE 1. The schema illustrates five important areas in an adolescent's life and their interconnections. The medical interview should explore each of these areas because they all can be related to physical health. Inquiring about aspects of the adolescent's life other than physical health helps the clinician to communicate interest in the adolescent as a person.

If the patient's dress or decorations are a health concern, then the physician or other provider should take care to make those comments either complimentary or neutral. Asking an adolescent girl whether having her tongue pierced interferes with any activity such as eating is probably harmless, and the comment can lead to a discussion of the need for sterility in any procedure that compromises the body's defenses. A comment that the patient's shirt or other piece of clothing is attractive or that the written statement on the patient's T-shirt is interesting may be helpful in establishing at least a superficial rapport. The male clinician especially should be cautioned not to make comments that may have double meanings or that may be construed as crossing the boundaries of intimacy. This is particularly true in relation to comments about items such as underwear that may be perceived by adolescent patients as sexually provocative.

Clinicians need to pay particular attention to the patient's unspoken communications, better known as "body language" (Table 2). Does the adolescent convey confidence or does she seem nervous? Is the nervousness out of proportion to the situation, or is it appropriate for a situation in which she will shortly have to disrobe for an examination by a relative stranger? Do seemingly simple and emotionally uncharged questions, such as "With whom do you live?" or "How do you like your new school?," engender excessive withdrawal or tears

TABLE 2. Unspoken Communication Cues

• Eye contact	• Body posture
• Facial expression	• Style of clothing
• Hand gestures	• Use of make-up

or anger? The clinician must be sensitive, i.e., communicate empathy, to those nonverbal cues. These cues can include, among others, facial expression, body posture, hand gestures, clothing style, and make-up.

Commenting on body language or nonverbal cues frequently is very helpful in drawing out any previously unspoken anxiety or issue. Just stating that it is normal to be nervous and anxious about going to the doctor for a physical examination and about discussing sensitive and intimate topics lets the patient know that she does not have to expend energy trying to act as if she is not nervous. Asking why a seemingly neutral comment has evoked an apparent emotion may be all the patient needs to vent about a stressful situation. On the other hand, the physician or other provider needs to be sensitive to the fact that the patient may not want to talk about an issue. There is no harm done in acknowledging that an area of inquiry seems to be stressful, but that it can be talked about at a later time when the adolescent is ready.

The clinician needs to approach sensitive issues such as sexuality-related topics with great care and tact. Usually it is best to preface questions in these areas by stating that topics that may make the patient uncomfortable need to be discussed for the patient's benefit. It is also useful to refer to teenagers in general and to "lots of kids." One can use use these terms in phrases such as "Lots of kids these days are sexually active." And then one can segue into specific questions about the patient herself.

Participating in a conversation, no matter how time-limited, with the adolescent patient rather than cutting off her comments and lecturing, signals to the patient that the clinician respects her and is a willing listener now and whenever the need may arise. The clinician conveys interest in the patient and eases discomfort with the health care experience by being an interested and participatory listener who genuinely seems to care about the adolescent as a person.

THE PHYSICAL EXAMINATION

Male or female, any patient can, and usually does, feel some anxiety and discomfort when having to disrobe for a physical examination. This anxiety is accentuated when the examiner must view and/or touch intimate body parts such as the breasts or genitalia. The keys to easing the female adolescent's anxiety in this situation are first to acknowledge that such anxiety exists and, indeed, is perfectly normal and to be expected, and then to take as much care as possible to make the patient feel covered and to limit touches to those areas that are absolutely necessary to the task at hand. These touches should be neutral, gentle, and efficient. In each instance, care should be taken to engage the patient in an educational dialogue concerning the area being touched. This process helps the adolescent shift into her "student" mode and helps to diffuse anxiety. Educating the patient about what the clinician is doing can also decrease the patient's fear of the unknown. Covering the young woman means that the clinician should take full advantage of gowns and sheets to screen any area not being examined at that moment.

Mention needs to be made of chaperones. The basic rule for any examination of an adolescent is to offer a female chaperone and to have one present whenever the adolescent wishes it. Equally as important, the clinician, male or female, should have a chaperone present in any situation in which he or she feels uncomfortable being alone with the patient. Even when the clinician is interviewing the patient, if the need for a chaperone is felt, then one should be present. In order to have a productive interview, the chaperone should be a neutral party. For the younger adolescent, her mother is an excellent choice as a chaperone during the physical examination, although this choice is less appropriate for the middle and late adolescent. There are rare occurrences, however, when the clinician may feel that a neutral chaperone is necessary in addition to the patient's relative. Should the male physician have a chaperone present for all examinations in which the patient disrobes or in which the patient's breasts or body will be touched? A sensitive, caring, and mature clinician usually does not need such assistance, but in our litigious society, this may be a necessary option. The author, however, has found that a chaperone is not necessary unless a genital examination, i.e., inspection of the external genitalia, rectal examination, or pelvic examination, is to be performed. Again, the option for a chaperone always should be offered to the patient and should always be an option for the clinician who feels uncomfortable for any reason when alone with a particular patient.

Elsewhere in this volume, considerable mention is made of female adolescent growth and development. The cognitive and psychosocial developmental level of the patient always must be considered by the clinician. Younger adolescents may be highly sensitive about their recent and ongoing bodily changes, and they may be much more sensitive than older adolescents about allowing anyone, let alone an adult male who is a veritable stranger, to see and/or touch their unclothed bodies. These girls also are struggling with their burgeoning sexuality, and issues having to do with fantasies about older men and about ideal partners may interfere with their ability to distance themselves enough from the interview and examination to allow it to proceed. In addition, for girls who are struggling with issues of sexual orientation, any intimate assessment by a practitioner may be unwelcome. Cognizance by the clinician of these and other developmental issues is mandatory.

FACTORS WHICH LEAD ADOLESCENT GIRLS AND YOUNGER WOMEN TO BE MORE COMFORTABLE WITH FEMALE CLINICIANS

As women have felt and become more empowered in American society, assumptions about propriety of interactions between the genders in various venues have come under scrutiny. Issues as weighty as sexual harassment in the work place and in the military have demanded national attention. Other issues recently discussed in the media include date rape, spousal abuse, and even female sports reporters in the locker rooms of male teams.

Women also have come to ask whether they need unquestioningly to accept health care from male physicians. As adult women have explored their feelings and opinions on this issue, so have adolescent girls. Several factors have come together to produce this situation in the United States. As stated above, women have become more empowered to determine their preferences in many venues over the past 20–30 years. In conjunction with this evolution, women have felt freer to select medicine as a career, and medicine, in fits and starts, has come to solicit more women as members of the profession. In addition, women in nursing have increasingly chosen to become practitioners, and a whole new profession—physician assistants—has provided an even greater pool of female clinicians.

What can female clinicians provide to female adolescents that is lacking from male clinicians? Just by being female, the clinician may have a ready-made rapport with a female adolescent patient. The male clinician may have to work hard to get to this same point, and he may never do so. Girls feel that women clinicians are better listeners, are more empathic, and are less judgmental about intimate issues than are their male counterparts. Male physicians, in previous reports, tend to be more science-oriented than their female counterparts, and they tend to be more directed in their diagnostic investigatory style. They may be more inclined to discount the patient's desire to feel more at ease and instead head right for the problem to be solved. Their unspoken communication style may be more abrupt and less accepting. Women and female adolescents may expect easier communication with a female clinician because most of their "easy" communications have always been with women. Traditionally, men have had power over women in almost every aspect of women's lives. Women, therefore, may find that it is very difficult to enter an interaction with any man as an equal. With women clinicians, feelings of powerlessness are not such an important issue.

ISSUES SPECIFIC FOR MALE CLINICIAN–FEMALE ADOLESCENT PATIENT INTERACTIONS

So how can the male clinician overcome these handicaps, so many of which may not be of his own making? Should every female patient be assigned to a female clinician whenever possible, thereby making the issue moot? For the purposes of this volume, the author assumes that many girls need to have their care provided by male clinicians. Therefore, the male clinician needs to do all within his power to make such encounters as positive as possible (Table 3).

The male clinician needs to pay special attention to the issues discussed above. The male physician or other provider must realize that, until a female adolescent patient has gotten to know him and has become comfortable with him, he is working at a disadvantage. He has to be very assiduous in conveying an accepting, nonthreatening persona. He has to be keenly aware of the developmental level of his female adolescent patient and the issues that are paramount at each stage of her physical, cognitive, and psychosocial development. He must be very conscious of the image he conveys and of the nonverbal communications demonstrated by his facial expression, body posture, and hand movements. The male physician should never make comments that can be

TABLE 3. Essential Behavior of the Male Clinician

• Be respectful	• Be nonthreatening
• Be sensitive and empathetic	• Be a teacher

construed as being suggestive sexually, and he should be careful about using sarcasm with a patient who may be functioning at a very concrete cognitive level. Every encounter should begin with a discussion of nonthreatening issues, even during visits for illness. In those circumstances, such nondirected discussion may be held to a minimum, but it still helps to ask such usually benign questions as "How is school going?" or "What's your favorite subject or activity?"

The issues pertaining to the physical examination are important for any clinician, but they are even more important for the male clinician. To repeat some of the essential ones: always use a chaperone when examining the genitalia or anal areas; if you or the patient seems uncomfortable with other parts of the examination, always use a chaperone; always drape the girl in a gown and sheet to keep as much of her covered as possible; and always educate while examining. Teaching about self-examination of the breast makes a breast examination much easier.

The male clinician never can be a female clinician. But even given that handicap, he can take many steps to assure that his patient has as thorough and as comfortable and productive a visit as is possible. The goal of each encounter should be to have the girl leave feeling better in all ways than when she walked in—if not about the diagnosis or treatment, then at least about herself and about her relation with the clinician.

SUGGESTED READING

1. Gabbard GO, Nadelson C: Professional boundaries in the physician-patient relationship. JAMA 273:1445–1449, 1995.
2. Ginsburg KR, Slap GB, Cnaan A, et al: Adolescent's perceptions of factors affecting their decisions to seek health care. JAMA 273:1913–1918, 1995.
3. Kelly JM: Sex preference in patient selection of a family physician. J Fam Pract 11:427–430, 1980.
4. Korsch BM, Freemon B, Negrete VF: Practical implications of doctor–patient interaction analysis for pediatric practice. Am J Dis Child 121:110–114, 1971.
5. Lurie M, Slater J, McGovern P, et al: Preventive care for women: Does the sex of the physician matter? N Engl J Med 329:478–482, 1993.
6. Magee J: The pelvic examination: A view from the other end of the table. Ann Intern Med 83:563–564, 1975.
7. O'Connor SJ, Shewchuk RM, Carney LW: The great gap: Physician's awareness of patient service quality expectations fall short of reality. J Health Care Marketing 14:32–39, 1994.
8. Orzano AJ, Cody RP: Gender concordance between family practice residents and diagnoses in an ambulatory setting. Fam Med 27:440–443, 1995.
9. Ross-Lee B: The physician–patient relationship. In Women and Their Health Care Providers: A Matter of Communication. Public Health Reports 101(Suppl):142–144, 1986.
10. Society for Adolescent Medicine: Access to health care for adolescents: A position paper of the Society for Adolescent Medicine. J Adolesc Health 13:162–170, 1992.
11. Suchman AL, Markakis K, Beckman HB, Frankel R: A model of empathic communication in the medical interview. JAMA 277:678–682, 1997.
12. Wilson MD, Joffe A: Step-by-step through the pelvic exam. Contemp Pediatr 5:92–104, 1988.
13. Weisman CS: Research findings and unanswered questions. In Women and Their Health Care Providers: A Matter of Communication. Public Health Reports 101(Suppl):147–151, 1986.

CHAPTER 9

Ethical and Legal Issues

M. Max Quinn, J.D.
Nancy Neveloff Dubler, L.L.B.

In western cultures, including the United States, adolescence is a time of emotional and behavioral turmoil. From a developmental perspective, adolescents are in the final stage of becoming adults and functioning independently of their parents. This is a major developmental step for at least two reasons. First, although the adolescent has been taking small steps towards independence almost since birth, full independence is contrary to the major assumptions and habits of the adolescent's life so far. Second, childhood has become, through experience and concrete evidence, a familiar place, whereas adulthood has been glimpsed only vicariously and is still uncharted territory.

Adolescence precipitates a developmental transition for the parent as well, and foists upon the parent a new and unfamiliar role. Parents have a lifelong habit of care, responsibility, and surrogate decision making for the child. It is a habit that is difficult to break, especially since the adolescent is likely to make errors of judgment or to base decisions on values and preferences that may be very different from those of his or her parents. Parental reaction to this transition is likely to be a mixture of excitement at seeing the child blossom into an adult and fear of the consequences that might ensue from the adolescent's potential or actual errors of judgment. The fear may at times give rise to an uncontrollable urge to step in and usurp the adolescent's decision making, especially when parents feel that the adolescent is choosing a misdirected route. There are times when this urge should be followed and times when it should be suppressed, challenging the parent to choose correctly when to intervene.

Added to this mix of complex and troubling emotions, needs, and impulses on the part of both the adolescent and the parents is the adolescent's burgeoning sexuality. Adolescence is a time of sexual awakening. The internal forces driving this awakening, whether encouraged or discouraged by culture and family, are unquestionably powerful, perhaps even overpowering. Although American culture has increasingly acknowledged adolescent sexuality, it is at the same time somewhat uncomfortable with it. We also are a culture, like most other cultures, with a double standard—we do not view or treat the sexuality of the adolescent girl the same as that of the adolescent boy. Thus, when the adolescent girl seeks medical care, especially care for matters connected with sexual activity, the provider is injected into the middle of a potentially volatile situation. Even seemingly innocuous circumstances can present ethical difficulties, fear of alienating the adolescent patient or her parents, and concerns about legal reprisals.

This chapter, using hypothetical cases and principled discussion, examines the ethical and legal issues that arise when parents (most often mothers) attempt to influence health care providers and make decisions that either violate ethical protections due their adolescent daughters or are in conflict with the wishes of the adolescent. These circumstances can be delicate and difficult for the provider because they create a tension among several areas of concern. One concern is with the provider's views about the appropriate course of action, e.g., whether the provider thinks that the adolescent or the parent (or neither) is advocating the correct treatment choice. This concern overlaps with the provider's ethical obligations to his or her patient—the adolescent girl. Another concern is the provider's sense of obligation toward the parent, which has a complex provenance involving (1) ethical concerns, (2) the assumption that parents ought to and do speak for and in the best interests of their children, and (3) the interpersonal dynamics of the patient–parent–provider relationship. When parents feel strongly about their adolescent daughter's treatments, they are likely to defend vigorously their "right" to make decisions for those daughters. Resisting a parent under these circumstances can be both difficult and uncomfortable for the provider. The final concern is over the uncertainty in the law regarding the parents' legal rights over the adolescent. When the parent threatens to sue, how much should the provider be concerned?

The following discussion addresses each of these areas and concludes, not surprisingly, that (1) the provider's primary ethical responsibility is to the patient; (2) a great deal of patience and skill is required to serve the patient's best interests in the face of an opposing parent; and (3) providers in this country operate in a legal environment that is disposed to encourage providers to serve the best interests of their adolescent patients, rather than the interests of the parents, when there is a conflict. Not every circumstance that a provider will encounter is covered by the clear letter of a statute or by favorable cases. Even so, the general climate is friendly, and the absence of suits against providers in this area is an indication that the fear of legal reprisals need not interfere with good and ethical care of adolescent girls.

THE ETHICAL PERSPECTIVE

The Principles

Four basic ethical principles—respect for autonomy, beneficence, nonmaleficence, and justice—govern the health care provider's treatment of adult patients (Table 1). These same principles generally apply to the treatment of adolescents,

TABLE 1. Basic Ethical Principles

• Respect for autonomy	• Nonmaleficence
• Beneficence	• Justice

TABLE 2. Ethical Principles Specific to Adolescents

• Respect for uniqueness	• Privacy
• Support for autonomy	• Freedom from abandonment or aloneness

but require expansion and modification to take into account the special developmental circumstances of adolescence (Table 2). A recent study that focused on the adolescent alone identified additional principles of respect for the adolescent's need for support and guidance and freedom from abandonment or aloneness.[1] In the context of a disagreement about treatment between the wishes of the adolescent and those of the parent, the most relevant principles are respect for autonomy and respect for the adolescent's need for support and guidance.

Respect for Uniqueness and Support for Autonomy

The health care provider has a moral obligation to respect the adolescent as a unique person and to support the adolescent's developing autonomy. Although analogous to the general principle applicable to the care of adults, during adolescence the principle must be adapted to take into account the developmental differences between adolescents and younger children, on the one hand, and adolescents and adults on the other. All children are engaged in the process of developing their own unique identities and becoming autonomous persons, but adolescents have reached the stage at which they need, want, and should be encouraged to test their decision-making skills in making the increasingly important decisions in their lives. They have also reached the stage at which their basic cognitive skills are likely to be substantially similar to those of an adult, even though they lack the experience of adults in living and in decision making. Moreover, they have a well-developed system of preferences and values. These values may to some extent reflect the special pressures of adolescence, especially the need for peer approval, and may evolve as the adolescent matures; nevertheless, they are the contemporaneous system by which the adolescent defines himself or herself and the foundation from which the more refined set of adult preferences, values, and behaviors will grow. If we accept that as adults we have general moral obligations to the younger generations, we must acknowledge that one of these moral obligations is to help them grow into the best adults they can be. We discharge this obligation with a combination of respect for their individuality and autonomy, just as we do for an adult, and support in the face of their relative lack of experience and the evolving nature of their values and preferences.

Privacy

One corollary of respect for autonomy is respect for privacy. The adolescent's fight for autonomy and need for decreased emotional dependency on parents often translates into a strong need to withhold information, especially from parents. Violation of this privacy by a health care provider sends the message to the adolescent that his or her involvement alone is inadequate, i.e., that the adolescent is not autonomous but is dependent upon and needy of parental involvement. It is a statement that the health care provider does not fully trust the adolescent. Legitimate disclosures, such as the adolescent's suicidality, are in fact based in part on such reasoning. This message of mistrust certainly damages the relationship between the adolescent and the health care provider; but, equally important, it may work to the detriment of the adolescent's developing autonomy. Disclosures to parents may also bring a parent into the adolescent's decision-making process in a way that is detrimental to the adolescent's growing independence. Parental involvement should be judiciously encouraged, but the adolescent's need and right to become an autonomous adult should not be sacrificed.

One author has illustrated the connection between privacy and respect for personhood and autonomy using the image of the individual at the center of a series of concentric circles that represent, from smallest to largest, the most intimate to the least intimate of the individual's relationships.[2] The individual at the center controls the access to each circle by being the primary, sometimes the sole, determiner of who has access to personal information. Those in the innermost circle are privy to the private secrets and thoughts of the individual; those in the outermost circle are told only what they need to know to accomplish whatever the individual wants them to accomplish. This control over disclosure "constitutes a large part of what it means for us to have control over our lives and our identities."[3] It follows from this premise, however, that when a health care provider discloses private information—information that the individual would disclose only to those in the innermost circle—the provider has robbed the individual of an important aspect of control and of a part of his or her identity or personhood.

The violation is especially profound because, in most cases, people are admitted to the inner circle of intimate information because the individual in the center has or desires an intimate relationship with them. Lovers, family, and close friends are people to whom we want to grant access to our more private thoughts and feelings. Our desire to grant such access is based on our feelings of warmth and trust toward the persons admitted. Health care providers, however, gain access to this intimate information by virtue of their *role*, rather than their *relationship* with the patient. Moreover, health care providers often learn things about the patient that even those closest to the patient do not know. To the patient, the health care provider is a person in the outer circle who is entitled to only that information required to perform the task the patient wishes him or her to perform. Unfortunately, at least part of the information necessary for fulfillment of the desired task is intimate information that the patient would otherwise guard from many of his or her acquaintances. In many cases when this information is disclosed, the patient and the health care provider are meeting for the first time, and the bonds of trust that can only develop over time as a result of observing a person's behavior and character have not been formed. The trust that the patient places in the health care provider is based on the patient's understanding of the health care provider's role and amounts to a much greater leap of faith than trust based on relationships.

Adolescents in the health care setting are taking new and unfamiliar steps into the adult world and are uncertain of the consequences that are likely to follow from any given action. The game is new and the rules are to a great extent unknown, or at least not experienced. Adolescents have also just begun to realize that some information is personal and to feel entitled to withhold it from their parents. For the first time, the adolescent's relationship with the health care provider excludes the parents. In past medical interactions, the mother usually described the child's symptoms to the provider, who then performed an examination, made a diagnosis, and prescribed a treatment. A few questions might have been directed to the child—"point to where it hurts," "did you fall down?"—but most of the conversation was adult to adult, with the child as the object under investigation. Under the new rules, the adolescent begins to take over the role played by the mother. This gives the adolescent a greater sense of ownership and control over the information being provided: "If mom is telling my story, it must, in part, be her story too; if I am telling my story, I can tell it to whom I like and even exclude mom or anyone else altogether." This control is one of the ways in which the adolescent develops a concept of self and exercises developing autonomy. The developing nature of these traits makes them unstable and fragile and thus entitled to additional care and respect.

Cases

The cases of Ann, Barbara, and Christine all raise issues of respect for autonomy and support for the adolescent.

Ann

Ann is a 16-year-old girl who has not yet begun to menstruate, although other secondary signs of sexual maturity have developed. Upon examination it was discovered that Ann's chromosomal structure is XY rather than XX, meaning that genetically she is male. She has not developed male genitalia, however, because the relevant portion of the Y chromosome is inactive. She has a uterus and a vagina, but in place of ovaries are undeveloped gonads. Ann's providers explained to her that she has a chromosomal problem that has resulted in improper maturation of her reproductive system and that she will never be able to have children. They did not, at this point, tell her that her chromosomal structure is male rather than female. In addition, it was necessary to remove the gonads because of the significant risk of their becoming cancerous. Ann understood the problem as it was explained to her, including that she would be unable to bear children.

A few months after the operation, Ann's physician received a request from Ann's mother asking that Ann's medical record be forwarded to the mother's gynecologist, because the mother was having some problems that the gynecologist believed might be genetically caused and the mother thought that the daughter's records might be useful.

Ann is entitled to have the private facts of her medical record remain confidential. Her mother should not automatically have access to Ann's records, especially when the purpose of the access is not a question of making decisions with respect to Ann's health care. Parents' access to their children's medical records is in large part derived from their need to make medical decisions for their children. In this case, even though Ann is not aware of the exact nature of the chromosomal abnormality, the health care provider should take the position that Ann would not want this information disclosed, until such time as Ann can make the decision for herself. As will be discussed later, the health care provider in this circumstance is generally protected by the legal environment in withholding the information from the parent.

The health care provider should keep in mind that Ann should be told the nature of her condition as soon as she is developmentally able to understand it. In addition, support should be available to help her with questions and feelings she may have when she is told. It is important for her to know as soon as possible because she is developing sexually and her condition is likely to be relevant to her sexuality.

Barbara

Barbara is a 15-year-old who is sexually active. She had previously discussed the fact of her sexual activity with her family physician, but had sought care from a women's health clinic rather than through the family physician. The family physician had not discussed her sexual activity with her parents. Barbara's mother brought Barbara to see the family physician because she had been complaining of abdominal pain and had a slight fever. The doctor performed an external examination and then began making preparation for a pelvic examination. At this point, Barbara's mother stopped him and said she would not consent to the pelvic examination. In a case such as Barbara's, what is the physician's responsibility?

The health care provider has a duty to see that Barbara's abdominal pain is properly diagnosed as well as a duty not to reveal confidential information about Barbara's sexual activity to her mother. In addition, Barbara is both ethically and legally entitled to give her own consent for treatment for sexually transmitted diseases. How to fulfill the ethical duties in the face of an adamant parent presents the true challenge for the health care provider in this situation. One possibility is to tell Barbara and her mother that legally the decision is for Barbara to make, without being specific about the basis of the legal right. It may become necessary to talk to Barbara alone and suggest either that she return without her mother or that she get treated at the clinic she has been using.

Christine

Christine is a 17-year-old who is pregnant. Her mother has five other children, all of whom are younger than Christine. Christine and her siblings have three different fathers, none of whom lives with them or takes substantial financial or other responsibility for them. Christine, as the oldest, has always had a lot of responsibility for her younger siblings and has taken very good care of them. They are always clean and very well-behaved, mostly as a result of the discipline imposed by Christine. She has often expressed the feelings of satisfaction that she gains from caring for them and from seeing them do well in school. She believes that her contribution to their well-being is valuable and gives meaning to her life. She says that she would like to help them grow up, get a good education, and have good jobs.

Christine has been involved with John, the father of her child, for over two years. They regularly used protection when having sex, but she became pregnant in spite of this precaution. Christine and John do not live together. He is

19 years old and has graduated from high school. He is about to finish some computer training and has been offered an entry-level position upon completion. He has expressed his desire to be a father to his child and would like to marry Christine if she is willing.

Christine does not want to leave her mother to care for the other children by herself. Christine not only derives a lot of satisfaction from her role as caregiver, but also does not want to abandon her mother. She feels that at some point she will be happy to marry John, but it does not have to be right away, and she does not want to marry him if it will mean leaving her current home. Christine had considered what she would do if she were to become pregnant, although she had not discussed it in depth with John because she believed the possibility to be remote. She briefly considered and rejected, in turn, the options of abortion and adoption. She clearly knows that she loves children and wants children of her own. Even though she understands that this child will arrive before she has planned it, she is happy and excited about the prospect of being a mother and raising her own child.

Christine's mother, on the other hand, does not want her daughter to bear this child. She has been trying to convince Christine to have an abortion and has tried to enlist the help in achieving that goal of the doctor who has begun to care for Christine during her pregnancy. She has gone so far as to suggest that the abortion be performed over Christine's objections.

Christine's position is slightly more complicated ethically, but still does not present a true dilemma, i.e., a situation in which two "goods" are pitted against each other. The health care provider in this case should assure himself or herself that Christine is making a truly considered choice based on her values. The fear, of course, is that having a baby at such a young age will foreclose many options for a career and a life in the future. Christine seems to be quite aware of the pleasures and disadvantages of raising children from her experiences with her siblings. The health care provider, in the interest of providing support for her decision to have the child, should try to ferret out hidden resentments and dissatisfactions that Christine might be harboring. There should be no question, however, of honoring the mother's wishes to perform an abortion over Christine's objections. The legal status of such a decision on the part of the health care provider is also of great concern and is discussed below.

Freedom from Abandonment or Aloneness

Unlike the other principles, the principle of freedom from abandonment or aloneness does not have an easy adult analogue among well-established bioethical principles, even though the principle is equally applicable to the socially isolated adult. According to this principle, it is ethically unacceptable to require an adolescent to make decisions on his or her own, without the possibility of consultation with a trusted adult. Because adolescents are almost, but not fully, adults, it is important that they have access to adult guidance and support. Even the most street-wise and grown-up teenager may need the wisdom and succor of a trusted adult. Sometimes the mere presence is sufficient, and the adolescent is able to make decisions on his or her own bolstered simply by the knowledge that the net is there if needed. In other cases, adolescents need adult consultation and advice. This need is not surprising; very few adults hope to make weighty decisions without consulting their spouses, a trusted friend, or some other significant person in their lives. If a health care provider is aware that his or her adolescent patient is without such support, the provider should work to help the patient find a person who can be a wise guide and companion. In some cases heightened provider involvement with the child may be the only possibility.

THE LEGAL CLIMATE

There are four potential decision-makers involved in making decisions regarding the medical treatment of minors: the health care provider, the parent, the child, and, at times, the state. The health care provider evaluates the child's condition and reaches a professional opinion regarding the course of treatment that is most advisable. The parent either agrees and consents or disagrees and refuses. If the parent disagrees and the failure to provide the child with the recommended treatment meets the legal definition of medical neglect, the state can intervene, usurp the parent's authority, and offer judicial consent to the treatment. Very young children have little or no involvement in decision making, but as children get older and more capable of making their own decisions, getting assent to treatment is appropriate; gradually the balance of power in the decision-making group shifts (or should shift) to grant them more and more real power. The laws of this country acknowledge this developmental stage in adolescents' lives by granting them certain legal rights to make health care decisions before the age of majority, which, in most states, is 18 years.

Minors' Rights to Treatment

Emancipated and Mature Minors

The laws of all states support the notion of minors' right to some extent through *emancipated minor* statutes and the *mature minor* doctrine. Emancipated minor statutes provide that persons under the age of majority who are no longer under parental control may give consent for medical treatments. What constitutes no longer being under parental control varies among the states but generally includes being married or being financially self-supporting and living away from the parents.[4]

The mature minor doctrine emerges from numerous cases in which parents have tried to sue when a health care provider treated their child without obtaining their consent. In general, parents have fared poorly in these suits. Courts have routinely held in favor of health care providers when the child treated was over 15 years old and the treatment was for the child's benefit. Courts have been unsympathetic to parents of younger children, especially when the circumstances involved the withholding of life-sustaining treatment.[5]

Sexually Transmitted Diseases, Contraceptives, and Abortion

All states make some provision for children under the age of majority to give their own consent for medical diagnosis and treatment of sexually transmitted diseases and, in some cases, for any disease considered dangerous to public health, such as tuberculosis. In most states, minors can consent for HIV testing without involving their parents. A few states allow minors to consent to treatment for HIV infection without notification of, or consent from, the parents. Although some states provide that minors of any age may give consent, others restrict the right to minors over a certain age, sometimes as young as 12 years old. In Massachusetts, a health care provider who believes a minor's condition endangers her life is required to inform parents of infection with a sexually transmitted disease, but not to obtain their consent for treatment.

Minors also have the right in all states to obtain contraceptives without the consent or notification of their parents* and the right in many states to consent to abortion, although notification of parents is sometimes required. The Supreme Court has decided numerous cases in which states have attempted to pass laws placing constraints on a minor's right to have an abortion. Most of these statutes involve a requirement that a minor's parent or parents consent to the procedure. Such statutes are deemed unconstitutional only if they impose an "undue burden on a woman's ability to make [a] decision" regarding abortion.[6] Statutes that impose a parental veto on a minor's abortion have been held unconstitutional.[7] Statutes requiring the consent of one parent with adequate provisions for bypass of such consent through judicial procedures, however, have withstood constitutional scrutiny.[8]

Sterilization

The cases and laws governing sterilization are directed toward protecting women from being sterilized against their wishes. Many of the laws deal with protections for institutionalized women. Current regulations of the Department of Health and Human Services absolutely prohibit the use of federal funds for the sterilization of any person under 21 years of age.[9] The age limitation holds notwithstanding a lower age of majority in a particular state or the maturity, desire for sterilization, or family circumstances of the person involved. The constitutionality of the regulation has been unsuccessfully challenged several times.[10]

Protection of Minor's Confidentiality

There is more to treating an adolescent, however, than obtaining consent. As the cases above demonstrate, often parents do not recognize their adolescent children's right to privacy. This right is, however, supported by the laws of many states. In New York, for example, the public health law governing access to patient information, defined as "any information concerning or relating to the examination, health assessment . . . or treatment" of a person, limits parents' rights to obtain the patient information of their children in several ways. First, parents are entitled to such information only with respect to care and treatment for which they gave consent or emergency care resulting from an

---

* On September 10, 1997, a bill presented in the House of Representatives failed to pass by a vote of 220 to 201. The bill would have required all federally funded health clinics to give parents written notice five business days before providing contraceptives to a minor. On February 12, 1998, a substantially similar bill (H.R. 3230) was introduced in the House. To date this bill is still pending.

accident or the unexpected onset of a serious illness. Thus parents are not entitled in New York to obtain information relating to treatment that was not emergency treatment for which the child alone gave consent, neither are parents entitled to their children's medical information if the health care provider determines that "access to the information . . . would have a detrimental effect on the provider's professional relationship with the [child], or on the care and treatment of the [child], or on the [child's] relationship with his or her parents or guardian." A health care provider in New York is also entitled to inform any child 12 years old or older of a request by her parents for patient information; if the child objects, the health care provider is entitled to deny the parents' request. There are also general provisions that limit access to patient information that apply both to adults and minors. A health care provider can deny access to information if he or she determines that revealing it would "reasonably be expected to cause substantial and identifiable harm" to the patient or others or if the "material requested is personal notes and observations."[11]

No cases have been reported in which a minor has sought protection or redress under this statute. The only case mentioning a parent's right to access involved a father who sued for emotional damages in connection with the disclosure to his ex-wife that he had undergone a paternity test to determine if he was the father of her two children.[12] The court was unsympathetic to the father's view and stated that the mother was entitled to "full and complete disclosure of any records concerning tests and procedures involving [her] children."[13] The case does not disclose the ages of the children, and the facts of the case as presented do not involve the exceptions contained in the law for the protection of the minor's confidentiality.

Not all states provide the same kind of protection to minors, and health care providers should consult the relevant laws in their own state.

Legal Applications

Where do these legal provisions leave the health care provider in terms of legal support when faced with situations like the cases presented earlier? In New York or any state with similar laws, Ann is afforded protection by statute. Legally, the clearest option is to discuss the situation with Ann and ask her whether she wants her records disclosed or not. In order to fully protect Ann's rights, however, the health care provider must disclose to Ann the exact nature of her chromosomal abnormality. The health care provider has to make a judgment about Ann's maturity and ability to cope with the information balanced against disclosure to her mother. If the health care provider is reluctant to inform Ann fully, he or she may resort to the other statutory exceptions for withholding patient information. These are less clearly applicable; for example, disclosure to Ann's mother may or may not have a detrimental effect on the health care provider's relationship, on treatment, or on Ann's relationship with her mother.

Legally, the health care provider is also empowered in the case of Barbara. Barbara has the legal right in every state to consent for diagnosis and treatment of sexually transmitted diseases. What the health care provider does with this power is not so easy to determine. As presented above, it will not be easy for the health care provider to let Barbara know about her legal rights in front of her mother without disclosing a confidence. At least the health care provider can be assured that those legal rights exist and can be assured of support in the law for treating Barbara appropriately.

Christine presents a different situation. In general, a minor's right to refuse treatment is not as clearly delineated as the minor's right to consent, although at least one author has suggested that if a minor can give consent in a particular case, he or she also should be able to refuse under the same circumstances.[14] Others believe that the minor's right to refuse probably depends on the nature of the treatment—its invasiveness, necessity, permanence, and long-term effects.[15]

Although existing Supreme Court cases deal with factual circumstances involving the right to have an abortion rather than to avoid one, they generally discuss the right in terms of reproductive freedom or the right to choose whether or not to bear a child. Beginning with the decision in *Roe v. Wade*, the cornerstone abortion case, the Court stated that the right of privacy protected and guaranteed by the United States Constitution extended to "a woman's decision *whether or not* to terminate her pregnancy" (emphasis added). In *Missouri v. Danforth*, the Court concluded that "the State may not restrict the *decision* of the patient and her physician regarding abortion during the first stage of pregnancy" (emphasis added).[16]

Several lower courts have used the language of the Supreme Court cases to hold that a pregnant minor has the right to choose to bear a child. In 1972, a Maryland Juvenile Court determined that a 16-year-old pregnant female was a "child in need of supervision" and ordered her to "obey her Mother in submitting to the medical procedures . . . to terminate her pregnancy."[17] The Maryland Court of Appeals agreed that the teenager was a child in need of supervision, but reversed the order to terminate the pregnancy. The court's reasoning in this case is important. It held that it was not within the legislative intent of the abortion statute to grant a parent of a child 16 years old or older the right to "compel that child over the child's opposition to submit herself to procedures which may lead to an abortion."[18] The court stated that the relevant law led to the conclusion that a "female minor over 16 years of age is emancipated . . . with respect to matters concerning pregnancy," has "the same capacity to consent as an adult," and "may not be forced, more than an adult, to accept treatment or advice concerning pregnancy."[19]

This case was decided before the Supreme Court's decision in *Roe v. Wade*, which changed abortion laws all over the country, including Maryland's. Two cases since *Roe v. Wade* have agreed with the Maryland decision. In 1981, the Family Court of New York addressed a mother's petition to have her pregnant, 15-year-old daughter, Mary, declared a "person in need of supervision" (PINS), in part because Mary was refusing an abortion. Citing *Roe v. Wade*, the Family Court stated that "the Fourteenth Amendment envisions a freedom of personal choice" that "extends to a woman's decision *whether or not* to have an abortion."[20] The Family Court also stated that it was "quite obvious" that the right to give birth necessarily followed from the right to abort. The Family Court did not stop there, however. In addition to rejecting a minor's refusal to have an abortion as grounds for a PINS adjudication, the Family Court issued an order of protection against the mother which specifically stated that the mother was not to "interfere with Mary's determination to deliver her child nor attempt to force Mary to have an abortion."[21]

Finally, the Federal Court of Appeals for the Eleventh Circuit determined that "coercing a minor to abort a child violates the minor's constitutionally protected freedom to choose whether to abort or bear her child."[22] In that case, a parent brought suit alleging that a guidance counselor had coerced her daughter into having an abortion. In its opinion, the court cited several Supreme Court cases involving abortion and contraception as having established that "it is freedom in the *decision-making process* which receives constitutional protection" (emphasis added).[23] The court stated that even though most cases dealt with the right to choose abortion, there was no need to create a new constitutional right to protect the freedom to bear a child because "the attention given the decision to abort" does not diminish "the protection which should be given the decision to carry the child to term," but merely refocuses the emphasis of the freedom of choice.[24] The court clearly found its conclusion to be essentially self-evident, stating: "There simply can be no question that the individual must be free to decide to carry a child to term."[25]

Each time the question of a minor's right to choose to bear a child has arisen, the court in question has had little difficulty determining that such a right exists. Should the question arise in the same context in other jurisdictions, we are confident that the same conclusion would follow.

THE REAL WORLD

Ethical and legal considerations, however, do not tell a complete story. Further complicating the picture are interpersonal dynamics. It is very simple to write about an adolescent's legal and ethical rights in a paper or a chapter of a book. It is quite different to confront an adamant parent like Barbara's mother, who, with righteous indignation and the belief that God, justice, right, and the law are on her side, *forbids* a pelvic examination on her 17-year-old daughter, who is complaining of abdominal pain.

The difficult position that the health care provider finds himself or herself in is that of, on the one hand, having ethical obligations toward the patient and, on the other hand, having to deal with a parent who believes that he or she has certain rights and entitlements by virtue of being the parent. Parents who attempt to usurp their children's right to privacy and autonomous decision making are not necessarily bad parents or worthy of censure. They are going through a difficult developmental stage as well, and one in which their definition of themselves as parents must change. This transition can be as difficult as the transition from child to adult that takes place in the adolescent years. It may be relatively easy to say that a physician's primary obligation is to his or her adolescent patient and that the best interests of the patient should prevail over parental wishes. It is an entirely different matter to put this succinctly stated moral principle into action in the face of angry parents who are threatening administrative or legal action if their wishes are not honored.

On the side of personal relations, a physician who believes that a parent is requesting or demanding action that is not in the best interests of the adolescent patient is in much the same position as a physician who is morally opposed to abortion but has a patient demanding that he or she perform an abortion. One option for the health care provider is first to confidently disabuse the parent of the belief that the legal threat has bite. Then, with understanding and compassion for the parent, whose position is not enviable and who may truly believe that his or her wishes will lead to a better result for the child, explain that what the parent is requesting is not something the physician can, in good conscience, perform.

Health care providers should also understand that treatment of the sexually active adolescent female is a dynamic process that requires balancing the interests of the patient, parent, health care provider, and the state. When those interests clash, it will almost always be the case that there are some common interests to be found. It is incumbent on the health care provider to identify both what the patient and parent believe to be their interests and alternative views of what may actually be in their interests. Sometimes a reluctant teenager is better off if the health care provider encourages and supports more open communication with parents. Sometimes parents can come to understand that their baby is growing up and her best interests are in fact served by the parents having respect for her privacy. This is in no way an invitation to neglect the ethical duties the health care provider has towards his or her patient. It may help to let the parent know early in the treatment process, without alienating him or her, that the adolescent girl is the patient and the health care provider's primary ethical responsibility is towards her.

CONCLUSION

A health care provider treating a sexually active adolescent girl faces many challenges, often the least of which is the patient's medical condition. The ethical responsibilities toward the patient must remain primary, but it is important as well to maintain understanding for the parents' position and respect for what they believe to be their rights. This approach is not only for the parents' sake; the adolescent needs independence, but also needs the protection and nurturing of a harmonious home. In the eyes of the law, the adolescent has rights to consent for treatment in some circumstances, and, in some states, the adolescent has significant protections of privacy. These legal rights and protections should be of some comfort to the health care provider when faced with conflicts from parents.

REFERENCES

1. Blustein J, Dubler NN, Levine C (eds): The Adolescent "Alone": Decision Making in Health Care [in press].
2. Veatch RM (ed): Medical Ethics, 2nd ed. Sudbury, MA, Jones and Bartlett Publishers, 1997.
3. Brody H: Confidentiality. In Veatch RM (ed): Medical Ethics, 2nd ed. Sudbury, MA, Jones and Bartlett Publishers, 1997, p 90.
4. English A, Dubler NN, Quin MM, Rebensdorf A: Legal and Ethical Issues: Delivery of Adolescent STD Services and Conduct of Research. Adolescent STD Monograph, National Institute of Allergy and Infectious Diseases, in press.
5. Belcher v. Charleston Area Medical Center, 422 S.E. 2d 827 (W. Va. 1992).
6. Planned Parenthood v. Casey, 305 U.S. 833; 112S. Ct. 2791 (1992) @ 2819.
7. Missouri v. Danforth, 428 U.S. 52; 96 S. Ct. 2831 (1976).

8. Planned Parenthood v. Casey, Planned Parenthood v. Ashcroft.
9. 42 CFR 50.203.
10. Peck v. Califano, 454 F. Supp. 484, (Utah 1977); Voe v. Califano, 434 F. Supp. 1058, (DC Conn 1977), California Medical Association v. Lackner, 177 Cal. Rptr. 188, Cal 1981.
11. New York Consolidated Laws, Public Health Law, Article 1, Title II, § 18.
12. Rosen v. Arden Hill Hospital, 163 Misc. 2d 70; 622 N.Y.S. 2d 662 (Sup. Ct. 1993).
13. Rosen v. Arden Hill Hospital, 163 Misc 2d 70, 622 N.Y.S. 2d 663 (Sup. 1993).
14. Holder AR: Legal Issues in Pediatric and Adolescent Medicine, 2nd ed. Yale University Press, 1985.
15. Macdonald MG, Meyer KC, Essig B: Health Care Law: A Practical Guide. New York, Matthew Bender & Company, 1997.
16. 428 U.S. 52 @ 66 (1976).
17. Matter of Cindy Lou Smith, 16 Md. App. 209; 295 A. 2d (Sp. App. 1972).
18. Id. @ 19.
19. Id. @ 19.
20. Matter of Mary P, 111 Misc. 2d 532; 444 N.Y.S. 2d 545 (Family Court, Queens 1981) @ 532-3.
21. Id. @ 536.
22. Arnold v. Board of Education of Escambia County, 880 F. 2d 305 (11th Cir. 1989).
23. Id. @ 311.
24. Id. @ 311.
25. Id. @ 311.

CHAPTER 10

The Health Maintenance Visit

Wendy Neal, M.D.

The majority of health problems encountered by young women stem from preventable high-risk behaviors such as unplanned pregnancies, substance abuse, eating disorders, and STDs, including HIV. This fact has led to a change in our health care philosophy from diagnosis and treatment to a focus on preventive care policies for this population.[1–3] The goals of routine health care–maintenance visits are to detect problem areas early in an effort to prevent morbidity and mortality as well as to promote healthy behaviors. Key elements of the health maintenance visit are health guidance, preventive screening history, physical assessment, routine screening tests, and immunizations (Fig. 1).

Health care providers serving the adolescent population must evaluate their current practice environment to ensure that it is accessible and adolescent-friendly.[4] In order to increase the teens' utilization of and compliance with health care visits, providers must address several issues about access. Teenagers may need after-school appointments; clinical settings should be accessible by public transportation; and issues of reimbursement/confidentiality must be clearly resolved. If these issues are not resolved, patients may not come for routine health visits. They will seek services, if required to, for school immunizations, employer-working papers, sports clearances demanded by coaches, or resolving a problem that has developed (e.g., pregnancy or STD symptoms).

Clinical settings serving teenagers should employ adolescent-sensitive staff and, if possible, have a separate waiting room or separate clinical session for the teens. Adolescence is a period of rapid developmental and physical change; staff working with teens must be able to communicate in a clear, respectful, developmentally appropriate manner. It is also important to have a telephone triage system available to address questions or concerns that may arise (e.g., "I forgot my oral contraceptive pill; what do I do?"). A study of 6821 ninth-graders in the Philadelphia area revealed that their selection of health care centers were most influenced by provider characteristics of cleanliness (e.g., washing hands, wearing gloves) and interpersonal communication (e.g., speaking in nontechnical terms and directly to the teens, as well as maintaining confidentiality).[5] Providers can use mirrors, anatomical models, and diagrams to help facilitate concepts that appear to be difficult for the patient.

Age of adolescent

<table>
<tr><th rowspan="2">Procedure</th><th colspan="4">Early</th><th colspan="3">Middle</th><th colspan="4">Late</th></tr>
<tr><th>11</th><th>12</th><th>13</th><th>14</th><th>15</th><th>16</th><th>17</th><th>18</th><th>19</th><th>20</th><th>21</th></tr>
<tr><td>Health guidance</td><td colspan="4"></td><td colspan="3"></td><td colspan="4"></td></tr>
<tr><td>Parenting*</td><td colspan="4">■</td><td colspan="3">■</td><td colspan="4"></td></tr>
<tr><td>Development</td><td>■</td><td>■</td><td>■</td><td>■</td><td>■</td><td>■</td><td>■</td><td>■</td><td>■</td><td>■</td><td>■</td></tr>
<tr><td>Diet & physical activity</td><td>■</td><td>■</td><td>■</td><td>■</td><td>■</td><td>■</td><td>■</td><td>■</td><td>■</td><td>■</td><td>■</td></tr>
<tr><td>Healthy lifestyles**</td><td>■</td><td>■</td><td>■</td><td>■</td><td>■</td><td>■</td><td>■</td><td>■</td><td>■</td><td>■</td><td>■</td></tr>
<tr><td>Injury prevention</td><td>■</td><td>■</td><td>■</td><td>■</td><td>■</td><td>■</td><td>■</td><td>■</td><td>■</td><td>■</td><td>■</td></tr>
<tr><td>Screening history</td><td colspan="4"></td><td colspan="3"></td><td colspan="4"></td></tr>
<tr><td>Eating disorders</td><td>■</td><td>■</td><td>■</td><td>■</td><td>■</td><td>■</td><td>■</td><td>■</td><td>■</td><td>■</td><td>■</td></tr>
<tr><td>Sexual activity***</td><td>■</td><td>■</td><td>■</td><td>■</td><td>■</td><td>■</td><td>■</td><td>■</td><td>■</td><td>■</td><td>■</td></tr>
<tr><td>Alcohol & other drug use</td><td>■</td><td>■</td><td>■</td><td>■</td><td>■</td><td>■</td><td>■</td><td>■</td><td>■</td><td>■</td><td>■</td></tr>
<tr><td>Tobacco use</td><td>■</td><td>■</td><td>■</td><td>■</td><td>■</td><td>■</td><td>■</td><td>■</td><td>■</td><td>■</td><td>■</td></tr>
<tr><td>Abuse</td><td>■</td><td>■</td><td>■</td><td>■</td><td>■</td><td>■</td><td>■</td><td>■</td><td>■</td><td>■</td><td>■</td></tr>
<tr><td>School performance</td><td>■</td><td>■</td><td>■</td><td>■</td><td>■</td><td>■</td><td>■</td><td>■</td><td>■</td><td>■</td><td>■</td></tr>
<tr><td>Depression</td><td>■</td><td>■</td><td>■</td><td>■</td><td>■</td><td>■</td><td>■</td><td>■</td><td>■</td><td>■</td><td>■</td></tr>
<tr><td>Risk for suicide</td><td>■</td><td>■</td><td>■</td><td>■</td><td>■</td><td>■</td><td>■</td><td>■</td><td>■</td><td>■</td><td>■</td></tr>
<tr><td>Physical assessment</td><td colspan="4"></td><td colspan="3"></td><td colspan="4"></td></tr>
<tr><td>Blood pressure</td><td>■</td><td>■</td><td>■</td><td>■</td><td>■</td><td>■</td><td>■</td><td>■</td><td>■</td><td>■</td><td>■</td></tr>
<tr><td>BMI</td><td>■</td><td>■</td><td>■</td><td>■</td><td>■</td><td>■</td><td>■</td><td>■</td><td>■</td><td>■</td><td>■</td></tr>
<tr><td>Comprehensive exam</td><td colspan="4">■</td><td colspan="3">■</td><td colspan="4">■</td></tr>
<tr><td>Tests</td><td colspan="4"></td><td colspan="3"></td><td colspan="4"></td></tr>
<tr><td>Cholesterol</td><td colspan="4">1</td><td colspan="3">1</td><td colspan="4">1</td></tr>
<tr><td>TB</td><td colspan="4">2</td><td colspan="3">2</td><td colspan="4">2</td></tr>
<tr><td>GC, Chlamydia, Syphilis & HPV</td><td colspan="4">3</td><td colspan="3">3</td><td colspan="4">3</td></tr>
<tr><td>HIV</td><td colspan="4">4</td><td colspan="3">4</td><td colspan="4">4</td></tr>
<tr><td>Pap smear</td><td colspan="4">5</td><td colspan="3">5</td><td colspan="4">5</td></tr>
<tr><td>Immunizations</td><td colspan="4"></td><td colspan="3"></td><td colspan="4"></td></tr>
<tr><td>MMR</td><td colspan="2">■</td><td></td><td></td><td colspan="3"></td><td colspan="4"></td></tr>
<tr><td>Td</td><td colspan="2">■</td><td></td><td></td><td colspan="3"></td><td colspan="4"></td></tr>
<tr><td>Hep B</td><td colspan="2">■</td><td></td><td></td><td colspan="3">6</td><td colspan="4">6</td></tr>
<tr><td>Hep A</td><td colspan="4">7</td><td colspan="3">7</td><td colspan="4">7</td></tr>
<tr><td>Varicella</td><td colspan="4">8</td><td colspan="3">8</td><td colspan="4">8</td></tr>
</table>

1. *Screening test performed once if family history is positive for early cardiovascular disease or hyperlipidemia.*
2. *Screen if positive for exposure to active TB or lives/works in high-risk situation, eg, homeless shelter, health care facility.*
3. *Screen at least annually if sexually active.*
4. *Screen if high-risk for infection.*
5. *Screen annually if sexually active or if 18 years or older.*
6. *Vaccinate if high risk for hepatitis B infection.*
7. *Vaccinate if at risk for hepatitis A infection.*
8. *Vaccinate if no reliable history of chicken pox.*

* *A parent health guidance visit is recommended during early and middle adolescence.*

** *Includes counseling regarding sexual behavior and avoidance of tobacco, alcohol, and other drug use.*

*** *Includes history of unintended pregnancy and STD.*

FIGURE 1. Guidelines for Adolescent Preventive Services (GAPS). (From American Medical Association: GAPS Recommendations Monograph, 2nd ed. Chicago, American Medical Association, 1995, with permission.)

ADOLESCENT HEALTH MAINTENANCE

Health Guidance and Preventive Screening History

A complete, accurate history from the patient and parents is one of the most important elements of the health care–maintenance visit. A complete history includes current medical problems, past medical problems, family history, review of systems, and a thorough psychosocial history. Complete screening histories should be done annually, and the psychosocial history should be updated at each patient encounter, because this area of the teenager's life is fluid. As discussed in chapter 6, it is very important to maintain the adolescent's confidentiality and to assure her that she is your patient, while not alienating her parents. The adolescent may not know key elements of the history, such as family history and childhood illnesses; thus this part of the history can be obtained with all parties in the room. The psychosocial history should almost always be asked when the adolescent is alone because of the sensitive nature of some questions.

In the sexually active adolescent female close attention and care in gathering information from the psychosocial history are imperative. The *Guidelines for Adolescent Preventive Services* (GAPS) shown in Figure 1 gives an overview of the components of the screening history, and chapters one, two, and three address taking a history from these young women. One important aspect of the psychosocial history that is not included in the GAPS recommendation is exposure to violence. Young women are exposed to various forms of violence, and health care providers must inquire about exposure to acquaintance/date rape, domestic violence, witnessing violent acts, and gang associations. Most often adolescent girls do not reveal a history of victimization or involvement in gangs unless they are asked in a nonjudgmental way and feel safe and comfortable with the health care provider.

Additional areas of preventive health care guidance not addressed by the GAPS are breast self-examination and skin protection. Because of the low incidence of breast cancer in the adolescent population (< 1%), experts argue the pros and cons of teaching adolescents self-breast exam (Table 1). The effectiveness of sunscreen in the prevention of skin cancer is debatable. Fair-skinned teenagers should be advised to avoid intense ultraviolet rays by wearing protective clothing and staying indoors during the early daytime hours. If the protective measures are not possible, then use of a sunscreen of at least an SPF of 30 is advisable.

Physical Assessment

As shown in Figure 1, GAPS recommends a comprehensive physical examination once during each stage of adolescent development, with annual blood pressure (BP), height, and weight measurements for the healthy adolescent. Healthy adolescents usually require annual comprehensive physical examinations if they are still in high school, participating in any organized sports activity, beginning college, or entering the work force. Teenagers with chronic illnesses usually require more frequent monitoring, depending on their disease and current state of health (see chapter 12).

TABLE 1. Breast Self-Examination

Pros	Cons
Familiarizes adolescent with her breast contour	Unnecessary because rate of breast cancer in adolescents is very low
Initiates healthy pattern of behavior early	May frighten the adolescent unnecessarily
Empowers the young woman	Most will not do breast self-examinations

Anticipatory guidance addressing weight, exercise, and healthy eating habits is crucial to the adolescent female, especially in American culture, which promotes the thin body image as ideal, while bombarding the media with high-fat, high-sodium foods. American adolescents consume way too much fat and sodium in their meals; thus it is important to routinely monitor BP, height, and weight.

Elevated BP should be rechecked on three separate occasions within one month using the proper-size BP cuff (the bladder of the cuff should cover 75% of the arm between the shoulder and the olecranon). If systolic or diastolic BP is ≥ 95% for age, gender, and height, the patient is hypertensive. The new guidelines for defining hypertension from the Task Force on High Blood Pressure in Children and Adolescents consider height as well as gender and age (Fig. 2).[6] Hypertensive adolescents should initially be evaluated with a urine analysis and creatinine; if abnormal, a referral is indicated. For the asymptomatic obese adolescent with borderline essential hypertension who has normal laboratory values, a weight reduction program should be initiated if the adolescent is ready to lose weight (see chapter 14).

Routine Screening Tests

The tests in Table 2 should be performed on all asymptomatic, sexually active adolescent girls. Other tests such as hormonal testing, liver function studies, and serum chemistries are done in special cases at the discretion of the health care provider, based on the history and physical exam.

HEMOGLOBIN/HEMATOCRIT

The adolescent female is susceptible to iron deficiency anemia due to poor nutritional habits, menstrual blood loss, and rapid bone growth during puberty. Most guidelines recommend a hemoglobin test at the initial visit and another at

TABLE 2. Routine Screening Tests

Test	Recommendation
Hemoglobin	At the initial visit Annually in girls with malnutrition, heavy menses, impoverished background
Urinalysis	Annually in sexually active girls
Pap smear	Annually in all sexually active girls; if abnormal, more frequently
Cervical gonorrhea and chlamydia test	Annually in sexually active, asymptomatic girls; if prevalence rates are high, may do every 6 months
Syphilis	Annually
HIV testing	Should be offered to all sexually active girls; frequency of test determined by risk factors
Cholesterol	Controversial (see text) 1. Parent or grandparent (< 55 yrs old) has heart disease 2. Family history unknown 3. Patient has risk factor (obesity, smoking) 4. Parent has cholesterol ≥ 240
Sickle cell	Once in Hispanic and African-American youth

the end of puberty. Health care providers working with high-risk impoverished youth do hemoglobin levels yearly. Adolescents who are severely malnourished or afflicted with heavy menstrual blood loss need closer monitoring.

Urinalysis

There are no formal recommendations for urinalysis. Some sexually active teens are prone to recurrent urinary tract infections (UTIs). Many health care providers perform urine dipstick as a screen for UTIs (leukocyte esterase) and diabetes (glucose).

Pap Smears

Pap smears should be performed annually in the sexually active adolescent because of high rates of human papillomavirus infection. If a Pap smear is abnormal, more frequent monitoring is indicated (see chapter 22).

Cervical Gonorrhea and Chlamydia Test

Cervical testing should be done at least annually in the asymptomatic, sexually active girl. Some adolescent health facilities that serve high-risk youth and/or have high rates of chlamydia infection do testing every 6 months. Symptomatic patients should be tested at each visit.

Syphilis

Syphilis screening should be done annually.

HIV Testing

The official recommendation is to test high-risk adolescents. Many experts in the adolescent HIV arena feel HIV testing should be offered to all sexually active adolescents. With advances in drug therapy, early detection of the virus, and treatment, patients can live symptom-free, productive lives.

Cholesterol Screening

The decision about whom to screen for elevated cholesterol and what type of screening test to use is controversial. The current recommendation is to screen adolescents based on high-risk family history. However, family history may not be reliable, as was shown in a Boston study that found family history to be a poor predictor of elevated cholesterol levels in the adolescent.[7] Thus, some health care facilities screen all adolescents every 5 years.

Sickle Cell Screening

At the initial visit, sickle cell screening should be done on all Hispanic and African-American youth who are not known to have sickle cell disease or trait.

Tuberculin Testing

The Mantoux test, a protein-purified derivative (PPD), should be administered at the initial visit to all adolescents with no past history of a positive PPD. Frequency of PPD monitoring is governed by the environment in which the adolescent lives. The local health department sets guidelines for its areas. CDC recommendations for interpretations of PPD reaction are illustrated in Table 3.

TABLE 3. CDC Recommendations for 5TU PPD Intradermal (Mantoux test) Interpretation

Induration < 5 mm	Negative
Induration ≥ 5 mm	Positive in the following people: • HIV-infected patients • Patients who are recent close contacts of person with active TB • Patients who have fibrotic changes on chest radiograph
Induration ≥ 10 mm	Positive in the following people: • HIV-negative patients who are injecting drugs • Immunocompromised patients (e.g., severe anorexia, malignancies, diabetes, etc.) • Patients born in areas with high rates of TB (e.g., Africa, Asia, Caribbean) • Patients from impoverished, medically underserved areas • Patients in long-term care facilities (e.g., correctional facilities, group homes, mental institutions) • Patients from high-risk communities as determined by the local health department
Induration ≥ 15 mm	Positive in low-risk patients

Adapted from Centers for Disease Control and Prevention: Core Curriculum on Tuberculosis: What the Clinician Should Know. Atlanta, Centers for Disease Control and Prevention, 1994.

For treatment guidelines, contact the local health department, because there are different resistance patterns.

Immunizations

Ensuring completion of vaccinations in the adolescent population significantly decreases the prevalence of childhood diseases. Adolescents accounted for 51% of the measles cases, 30% of the mumps, and 21% of the rubella cases in 1994. Recent serologic surveys reveal that approximately 20% of 11–12-year-old adolescents are susceptible to varicella, while children aged 9–13 years lack protective levels of tetanus antitoxin. Since the introduction of the hepatitis B vaccine, the incidence of hepatitis B infection has decreased.

All currently recommended vaccines are presented in Table 4. Table 5 covers timing of vaccinations in the unvaccinated adolescent or one who does not

TABLE 4. Previously Immunized Adolescent: Vaccines to Be Given at 11–12 Years*

Immunizations	Dosage/Frequency
Measles, mumps, rubella† (2nd shot if not given previously)	0.5 cc subcutaneously
Tetanus and diphtheria booster	0.5 cc intramuscularly, every 10 years
Hepatitis B (patients from countries with high prevalence of hepatitis or known contact with an infected person should be screened before vaccination)	Must use appropriate microgram dosage for the particular preparation Dose given at time 0, 1 month, 6 months‡
Varicella† (individuals who are susceptible)	0.5 cc subcutaneously in one dose (2 doses separated by 1–2 months for adolescents > 13 years)

* Vaccines should be targeted for this age group, but can be given at any time.
† Should not be given to a pregnant adolescent because of small theoretical risk to the fetus.
‡ The interval between doses does not have to be exact; no need to repeat doses or restart series.

TABLE 5. Required Vaccines for Previously Unimmunized Adolescent

Immunization	Interval
Measles-mumps-rubella vaccine: 2 doses must be given	At least 1 month from first dose
Tetanus-diphtheria toxoid: 3-dose series must be given	At time 0, 2nd dose 2 months later, 3rd dose 6–12 months later
Oral polio vaccine:* 3-dose series that can be given with tetanus-diphtheria toxoid	Same as that for tetanus-diphtheria toxoid

* Inactivated polio vaccine should be given if > 19 years or living in household with an immunocompromised person.

have documentation of her immunization record. If the adolescent is attending school, the school should have documentation of the childhood vaccines: measles-mumps-rubella vaccine (MMR) × 2, diphtheria-pertussis-tetanus vaccine (DPT) × 4 and oral polio vaccine (OPV) × 4. The teenager should make an effort to get documentation of previous immunizations from her parents, schools, and previous health care providers to avoid duplication of vaccines. However, there are no known deleterious effects of receiving duplicate vaccines.

During the health maintenance visit, adolescents with chronic illness should be offered the influenza vaccine. Pneumococcal vaccine should be administered to those with sickle cell disease, functional or anatomic asplenia, or who are immunosuppressed, and hepatitis A vaccine to those living in high-risk areas in the United States or those who travel routinely to countries where hepatitis A infection is prevalent. Routine serologic testing for antibodies to MMR, hepatitis B, and varicella is not recommended, but serologic testing should be considered in adolescents immigrating from countries where hepatitis B infection is endemic or youth in very high-risk environments, such as the homeless teenager.

CONCLUSION

Health care maintenance serves many functions in the care of the sexually active female. It is an important time to gather information about the life and experiences of the youth, while providing health care guidance and education to the young women. Appropriate time should be allowed for the initial visit so that the patient does not feel you are rushing to get her out of the office. During these visits, it is important to convey to the adolescent that you care and to empower her to be a partner in the management of her health care.

REFERENCES

1. Elster A, Kuznets N: AMA Guidelines for Adolescent Preventive Services (GAPS): Recommendations and Rationale. Baltimore, Williams & Wilkins, 1994.
2. American Academy of Pediatrics: Committee on Psychosocial Aspects of Child and Family Health. Guidelines for Health Supervision III. Elk Grove Village, IL, American Academy of Pediatrics, 1996.
3. Green M (ed): Bright Futures: Guidelines for Health Supervision of Infants, Children, and Adolescents. Arlington, VA, National Center for Education in Maternal and Child Health, 1994.
4. Goldfarb A: Symposium: Making your office adolescent-friendly. Contemp Adolesc Gynecol 3:4–10, 1998.

5. Ginsburg KR, Slap GB, Cnaan A, et al: Adolescents' perceptions of factors affecting their decisions to seek health care. JAMA 273:1913–1918, 1995.
6. National High Blood Pressure Education Working Group on Hypertension Control in Children and Adolescents: Update on the 1987 Task Force on High Blood Pressure in Children and Adolescents: A Working Group Report from the National High Blood Pressure Education Program. Pediatrics 98:649–658, 1996.
7. Gagliano NJ, Emans J, Woods ER: Cholesterol screening in the adolescent. J Adolesc Health 14:104–108, 1993.
8. Centers for Disease Control and Prevention: Core Curriculum on Tuberculosis: What the Clinician Should Know. Atlanta, Centers for Disease Control and Prevention, 1994.
9. Neinstein LS, Schubiner HH: Health screening and evaluation. In Neinstein LS (ed): Adolescent Health Care: A Practical Guide, 3rd ed. Baltimore, Williams & Wilkins, 1996.
10. Division of Viral and Rickettsial Diseases, Hepatitis Branch, National Center for Infectious Diseases and National Immunization Program: Immunization of Adolescents with Hepatitis B Vaccine: An Educational Resource. Atlanta, Centers for Disease Control and Prevention, 1997.
11. Centers for Disease Control and Prevention: Vaccine-Preventable Diseases: Improving Vaccination Coverage in Children, Adolescents and Adults. MMWR 48(RR-8):1, 1999.
12. Burstein GB, Gaydos CA, Diener-West M, et al: Incident *Chlamydia trachomatis* infections among inner-city adolescent females. JAMA 280:521–526, 1998.

CHAPTER 11

The Preparticipation Sports Physical

Eric Small, M.D.

Each year millions of adolescent athletes take to the playing fields, and this number continues to grow. The 1990s has seen an explosion of young women participating in sports. All of these athletes must undergo a preparticipation physical evaluation (PPE). The PPE is a three-step process requiring a medical questionnaire, completed and signed by the athlete and parent, a physical examination, and a determination of clearance (Fig. 1).[1] These evaluations usually are not performed in a uniform fashion and may last from several minutes up to half an hour. Most often, the physicians conducting PPEs are not sports medicine specialists and thus have limited formal training in performing this specialized examination. In addition, most are males, have little professional experience dealing with adolescent females, and may not be sensitive to or comfortable with the particular medical needs of female athletes. Clinicians performing preparticipation evaluations of adolescent girls and young women must take into account the unique musculoskeletal injuries of females, e.g., patellofemoral pain syndrome, shin-splints, chronic ankle sprain, and how these relate to sports participation. Medical concerns such as the female athlete triad also must be highlighted. This chapter discusses a systematic approach to the PPE as well as specific injuries and medical concerns unique to the female athlete.

GOALS OF THE PREPARTICIPATION PHYSICAL EVALUATION

The first and most important goal of PPE is to screen for the possibility of sudden death (Table 1). Males are far more likely than females to die suddenly during athletic events. The most common causes of sudden death are hypertrophic cardiomyopathy, idiopathic hypertrophic subaortic stenosis (IHSS), myocarditis, and arrhythmia.[2] In addition, the athlete often has persistent injuries that are untreated, unrecognized, and not addressed (e.g., chronic ankle sprain, knee pain, or shoulder pain). The PPE is the ideal time to identify the weakness or problem and prescribe a set of rehabilitation exercises. Ideally, the

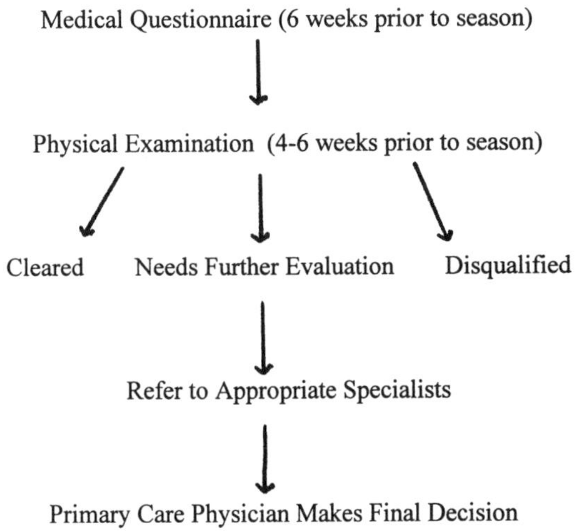

FIGURE 1. Outline of preparticipation physical evaluation.

evaluation should be done 4–6 weeks before a season begins so that any chronic injuries can be addressed and rehabilitated. Certain conditions, such as exercise-induced asthma, may be exacerbated by athletic participation, and such conditions should be identified and treated. Other conditions, if present, may disqualify the adolescent from playing a particular sport. For example, athletes with a single kidney or one eye may be prohibited from playing contact sports. These athletes may be steered toward playing a noncontact sport. In the PPE, fewer than 2% of athletes are disqualified, and only 3–14% require further consultation.

An additional goal of PPE is to provide the athlete with information to improve performance. For example, athletes participating in endurance events can be counseled to increase their carbohydrate intake for several days before the event. Also, the importance of sufficient hydration should be discussed. Many adolescents do not receive routine periodic health care, so the PPE provides an opportunity for the adolescent girl to discuss any ongoing health concerns and for the clinician to promote regular exercise and good nutritional habits. The experience is a good opportunity to reintegrate the athlete into the health care system while using sports as the major focus. Lastly, a goal of the PPE is to satisfy insurance requirements. States have different requirements for clearance for sports participation. Some states require a yearly PPE; others require an evaluation twice during high school; and the most liberal requirement is one evaluation only during the high school years. It is this author's opinion that PPE should be done yearly because of the many health- and sports-related issues that can change over this period in the rapidly developing adolescent.

TABLE 1. Goals of Preparticipation Physical Evaluation

• To prevent sudden death	• To improve performance
• To prevent injury	• To promote health
• To screen for medical conditions	• To satisfy insurance requirements

TABLE 2. Individual Versus Station-by-Station Preparticipation Physical Examination

	Advantages	Disadvantages
Individual	Individual attention Privacy Counseling	Costly Time-consuming Poor communication with athletic staff
Station-by-station	Cost-effective Athletic staff present Immediate feedback to athlete and coach	No privacy No personal attention Insufficient time to address risk-taking behavior

The individual PPE usually takes place in the private office setting. This examination often takes about 30–40 minutes but allows time for various personal health issues to be addressed (Table 2). There is limited contact or follow-up with the coaching staff, however. In contrast, a time-efficient method of completing PPEs on large numbers of adolescents simultaneously is to use a station-type examination procedure. The station examination may have anywhere from 6–8 stations, and many can be staffed by non-physicians, e.g., athletic trainers, exercise physiologists, physical therapists, or nurses. Mandatory stations, including vital signs, cardiorespiratory, extremity, and abdominal examinations, are indicated in Figure 2. Optional stations may include body-fat testing, nutrition, and an assessment of aerobic fitness. The stations may be set up in a school gym or in a clinic with separate examination rooms.

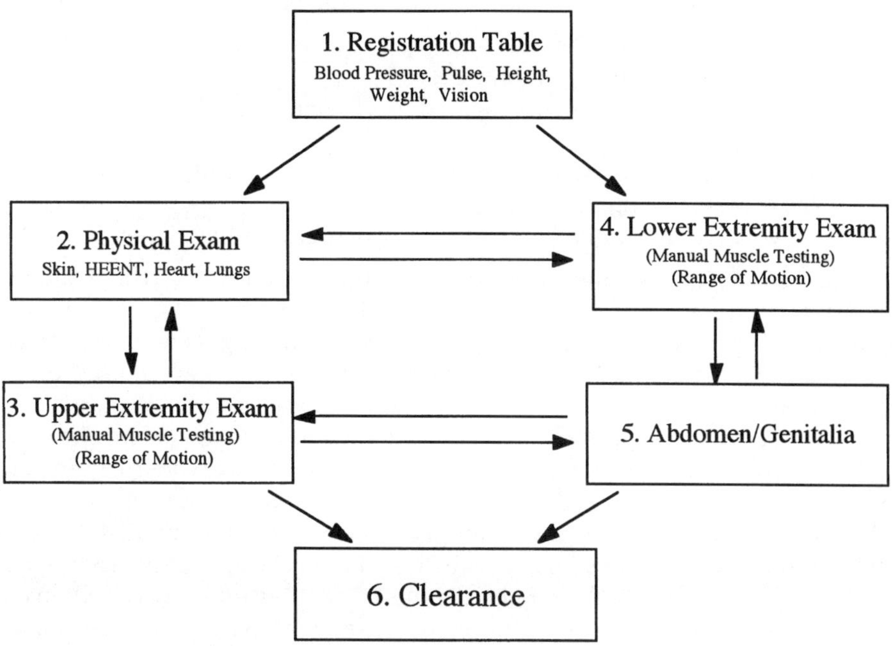

FIGURE 2. Station-by-station preparticipation physical examination.

COMPONENTS OF THE PREPARTICIPATION PHYSICAL EVALUATION

History

Before arrival at the examination site, a medical questionnaire should be completed by the parent of the athlete in conjunction with the adolescent. The best questionnaire is the one endorsed by the American Academies of Pediatrics and Family Physicians as well as several sports medicine organizations (Fig. 3). Ideally the physician receives the completed questionnaire about one week before the scheduled evaluation. If the athlete notes anything significant in her history, the physician has a better idea of how to focus the line of questioning. The majority of the abnormalities are picked up by the medical history (Table 3).

General questions inquiring about recent or chronic injury or illness, hospitalization or surgery, medication use, and allergies should be asked to identify those athletes with a chronic condition or a medical problem that may require further evaluation. Immunization status should be checked.

Questions about chronic skin rashes are important, especially for athletes who are involved in contact and collision sports. Common skin conditions that may be present in adolescent athletes include herpes simplex, scabies, pubic lice, furunculosis, and impetigo. Herpes simplex is a reason for temporary disqualification from wrestling or martial arts until the lesions have healed. Spread of infection via a fomite (mat, towel, or helmet) can occur, and skin infections should be treated before entry into contact sports.

It is crucial to evaluate the cardiovascular system. Important questions to ask either in person or on the questionnaire include the following:

- Have you ever passed out during or after exercise?
- Do you feel dizzy during or after exercise?
- Has a family member died at age 50 or younger from heart problems or sudden death?
- Has a physician ever denied or restricted you from athletic participation because of heart problems?
- Have you ever been told you had high cholesterol or high blood pressure?

The first three of these questions are mandatory to screen for risk of sudden death. It is important to remember, when taking a history of cardiovascular complaints, that chest pain in children and adolescents is generally not cardiac in origin. The majority of cases are related to asthma or costochondritis, or are psychogenic in nature.

Assessment of the pulmonary system is also important during the PPE. Athletes who have asthma, one of the most common chronic conditions in adolescence, can participate in all sports so long as the condition is well-controlled. The young athlete with exercise-induced asthma should be reminded that premedication 10–15 minutes prior to exercise with a beta-agonist or cromolyn is helpful. If the athlete has not been diagnosed with asthma yet complains of cough or shortness of breath with exercise, she may have exercise-induced asthma and should be further evaluated. The appropriate testing includes baseline pulmonary function tests, followed by an 8-minute bout of exercise

Preparticipation Physical Evaluation

HISTORY

DATE OF EXAM ______________

Name ______________ **Sex** ____ **Age** ____ **Date of birth** ______________

Grade ___ **School** ______________ **Sport(s)** ______________

Address ______________ **Phone** ______________

Personal physician ______________

In case of emergency, contact

Name ______________ **Relationship** ________ **Phone (H)** ____________ **(W)** ____________

Explain "Yes" answers below.
Circle questions you don't know the answers to.

	Yes	No
1. Have you had a medical illness or injury since your last check up or sports physical?	☐	☐
Do you have an ongoing or chronic illness?	☐	☐
2. Have you ever been hospitalized overnight?	☐	☐
Have you ever had surgery?	☐	☐
3. Are you currently taking any prescription or nonprescription (over-the-counter) medications or pills or using an inhaler?	☐	☐
Have you ever taken any supplements or vitamins to help you gain or lose weight or improve your performance?	☐	☐
4. Do you have any allergies (for example, to pollen, medicine, food, or stinging insects)?	☐	☐
Have you ever had a rash or hives develop during or after exercise?	☐	☐
5. Have you ever passed out during or after exercise?	☐	☐
Have you ever been dizzy during or after exercise?	☐	☐
Have you ever had chest pain during or after exercise?	☐	☐
Do you get tired more quickly than your friends do during exercise?	☐	☐
Have you ever had racing of your heart or skipped heartbeats?	☐	☐
Have you had high blood pressure or high cholesterol?	☐	☐
Have you ever been told you have a heart murmur?	☐	☐
Has any family member or relative died of heart problems or of sudden death before age 50?	☐	☐
Have you had a severe viral infection (for example, myocarditis or mononucleosis) within the last month?	☐	☐
Has a physician ever denied or restricted your participation in sports for any heart problems?	☐	☐
6. Do you have any current skin problems (for example, itching, rashes, acne, warts, fungus, or blisters)?	☐	☐
7. Have you ever had a head injury or concussion?	☐	☐
Have you ever been knocked out, become unconscious, or lost your memory?	☐	☐
Have you ever had a seizure?	☐	☐
Do you have frequent or severe headaches?	☐	☐
Have you ever had numbness or tingling in your arms, hands, legs, or feet?	☐	☐
Have you ever had a stinger, burner, or pinched nerve?	☐	☐
8. Have you ever become ill from exercising in the heat?	☐	☐
9. Do you cough, wheeze, or have trouble breathing during or after activity?	☐	☐
Do you have asthma?	☐	☐
Do you have seasonal allergies that require medical treatment?	☐	☐
10. Do you use any special protective or corrective equipment or devices that aren't usually used for your sport or position (for example, knee brace, special neck roll, foot orthotics, retainer on your teeth, hearing aid)?	☐	☐
11. Have you had any problems with your eyes or vision?	☐	☐
Do you wear glasses, contacts, or protective eyewear?	☐	☐
12. Have you ever had a sprain, strain, or swelling after injury?	☐	☐
Have you broken or fractured any bones or dislocated any joints?	☐	☐
Have you had any other problems with pain or swelling in muscles, tendons, bones, or joints?	☐	☐

If yes, check appropriate box and explain below.

☐ Head	☐ Elbow	☐ Hip
☐ Neck	☐ Forearm	☐ Thigh
☐ Back	☐ Wrist	☐ Knee
☐ Chest	☐ Hand	☐ Shin/calf
☐ Shoulder	☐ Finger	☐ Ankle
☐ Upper arm		☐ Foot

	Yes	No
13. Do you want to weigh more or less than you do now?	☐	☐
Do you lose weight regularly to meet weight requirements for your sport?	☐	☐
14. Do you feel stressed out?	☐	☐

15. Record the dates of your most recent immunizations (shots) for:

Tetanus ____________ Measles ____________

Hepatitis B ____________ Chickenpox ____________

FEMALES ONLY

16. When was your first menstrual period? ____________

When was your most recent menstrual period? ____________

How much time do you usually have from the start of one period to the start of another? ____________

How many periods have you had in the last year? ____________

What was the longest time between periods in the last year? ____

Explain "Yes" answers here: ______________

I hereby state that, to the best of my knowledge, my answers to the above questions are complete and correct.

Signature of athlete ______________ Signature of parent/guardian ______________ Date ________

FIGURE 3. Preparticipation physical evaluation. (From American Academy of Family Physicians, American Academy of Pediatrics, American Medical Society for Sports Medicine, American Orthopaedic Society for Sports Medicine, and American Osteopathic Academy of Sports Medicine: Preparticipation Physical Evaluation (PPE), 2nd ed. New York, McGraw-Hill, 1997, with permission.)

TABLE 3. The Preparticipation Physical Evaluation Medical History

The athlete	
• Skin rashes	• Sports injuries
• Fainting or dizziness after exercise	• Disordered eating
• Symptoms of exercise-induced asthma	• Menstrual dysfunction
• Head injury or concussion	• Bone pain/stress fractures
• Heat stroke	• Emotional stress

The family
- Sudden death
- Cardiovascular death at age 50 years or younger
- Congenital disorders (e.g., Marfan's, sickle cell)

(treadmill or bicycle ergometer) at heart rate of 150–160 beats per minute. A drop of 15% in FEV_1 signifies exercise-induced asthma. Active tuberculosis is rare in adolescents but, if found, is a contraindication to all participation in competitive sports because of risk of transmission to other participants.[3]

A careful screening for neurologic symptoms is essential. The following questions are important:

- Have you ever had a head injury or concussion?
- Have you ever become unconscious or lost your memory?
- Have you ever had numbness or tingling in your arms, hands, legs, or feet?

The examining clinician should be particularly concerned about any residual neurologic symptoms after a head injury (e.g., headache, dizziness, weakness) because of the risk of second-impact syndrome. If a second head trauma occurs in an athlete who has already suffered a concussion from which the symptoms have not totally cleared, there is a risk of death due to loss of vascular autoregulation, resulting in vascular engorgement, swelling, and herniation. The following guidelines for management of head trauma in young athletes should be used. If there is no loss of consciousness, the athlete may return to competition within 20 minutes provided there are no residual symptoms. If there is brief loss of consciousness and the athlete is free of symptoms, the minimum time before return to play is 1 week. Other common neurologic symptoms experienced by athletes are those of brachial plexus injury (stinger, burner, or pinched nerve), which are especially common in contact sports.

Heat-related illness is another area that should be explored in the history. Problems while exercising in the heat may range from mild nausea and cramps to death. As with musculoskeletal injury, there is a predisposition to heat injury once a heat-associated problem has occurred. An athlete who has had problems with the heat should drink extra fluids before practice or competition and allow heat acclimatization over 10–14 days by gradually increasing training time and level of exertion. Often adolescents do not take in enough fluids before, during, and after competition or practice. A guideline is to drink one extra glass of fluid just beyond thirst level before competition. Contrary to many anecdotal reports, there are no studies indicating that fluid intake will induce muscle cramps. Quite the contrary, a relatively dehydrated individual is more likely to suffer from cramps. Athletes generally do not need sports drinks unless the sporting event lasts more than one continuous hour.

The musculoskeletal system is the part of the history in which the athlete is most likely to have had a problem. Detailed inquiry should be made about any past or recent injury (strain, sprain, subluxation, or fracture). Probably the most important fact to ascertain is what the course of treatment was and whether the injury was fully rehabilitated, resulting in return of full strength, range of motion, and proprioception.

Eating disorders are very common in female athletes. Disordered eating may occur in up to 60% of adolescent female athletes. Girls engaging in certain sports, particularly gymnastics, dance, and figure skating, have a high prevalence of eating disorders. The majority of these athletes do not fulfill DSM-IV criteria for eating disorders. However, they may binge and purge, skip meals, or not take in adequate calories. One interesting observation is that athletes may believe they are consuming enough calories if they eat about 2000 kilocalories per day, the norm for nonathlete adolescent girls. They do not realize that physical training for 4–5 hours per day, 5–6 days per week, in a sport such as gymnastics or ballet may require 3000 or more kilocalories per day. All female adolescents should be screened for eating disorders. Important questions to ask include the following:

- Are you happy with your weight?
- What was your lowest and highest weight in the past year?
- Are you on any kind of special diet?

Obsession with exercise may be part of the eating disorder, so it is useful to ask about the number of hours spent per week exercising; this includes training for the current sport as well as exercise not related to the sport.

The female athlete triad is a term that was introduced by the American College of Sports Medicine in 1992. It consists of disordered eating, amenorrhea, and osteopenia. Up to 60% of female athletes have menstrual disturbances ranging from primary and secondary amenorrhea to irregular infrequent periods (oligomenorrhea). The combination of excessive training, low body fat, stress (physical and emotional), and inadequate caloric intake appear to be the most important factors contributing to athletic amenorrhea. The menstrual dysfunction is a result of hypothalamic suppression and is associated with reduced secretion of estrogen from the ovaries. Athletes with primary or secondary amenorrhea should be investigated further to determine the cause, because athletic amenorrhea is a diagnosis of exclusion. It is important to remember that the most common cause of secondary amenorrhea in the young athlete is pregnancy and that other congenital and acquired disorders of the genital and endocrine systems may occur. Sexually active female athletes should be encouraged to seek gynecologic care.

Athletes who admit to chronic shin pain or have more than one stress fracture in a year may be suffering from osteopenia related to low estrogen levels and low calcium in the diet. In extreme cases an athlete in her teenage years or in her twenties may experience hip and vertebral fractures. Many girls who are dieting consume only 1000 to 1500 kilocalories per day, which makes it nearly impossible to take in enough calcium to meet requirements. Adequate calcium intake for an adolescent is 1200 mg. For the amenorrheic athlete the recommended intake is 1500 mg. The best sources of calcium are yogurt or milk. The equivalent of 3–4 portions per day is required to achieve optimal bone density. Calcium supplements may be indicated for those girls who cannot tolerate dairy products.

Many female athletes, particularly endurance athletes, are susceptible to iron deficiency anemia. Iron deficiency may hamper performance in endurance sporting events. Vegetarian and fad diets are popular among adolescent girls, and most do not provide adequate iron. Good sources of iron include lean meats, beans, and legumes. Testing for iron deficiency with a serum ferritin level may be indicated if the history indicates a low iron intake.

The history should include a brief screen for emotional problems. Questions about self-esteem, happiness, and perceived stress level are important screening tools. Girls with low self-esteem and high stress levels may participate in health-risk behaviors. Specific areas of risk include alcohol and drug use, sexual activity, and use of ergogenic aids. Certain athletes train excessively and place undue pressure upon themselves. Parents and coaches may place unnecessary demands on the young athlete. In these circumstances the youngster may suffer from overtraining syndrome or burn-out. Characteristics of this syndrome are excessive fatigue, loss of interest in the sport or other activities, frequent infections, and high injury rates. The syndrome is more common in certain sports in which technical proficiency is required, such as dance, figure skating, and gymnastics.

Physical Examination

As with any medical encounter, the physical examination must be performed using a systematic approach. The most important part is the musculoskeletal examination, which is the part most likely to generate a positive finding. The 2-minute orthopedic exam is frequently done (Table 4). It is recommended that the exam be further focused depending on the sport played. For example, with runners the focus should be on the lower extremities, whereas for tennis and baseball players examination of the upper extremity should receive more focus. There are standard parts to the PPE, and it is important to know the salient features of each system.

The general appearance and behavior of the athlete should be noted. Does she appear well-nourished, hydrated, and calm, or is she particularly thin or nervous? Both height and weight should be accurately measured. If the young woman is significantly under- or overweight, appropriate referral to a physician, nutritionist, and/or mental health professional should be entertained.

The skin should be examined carefully to identify any rashes or lesions that may be infectious in origin. Visual acuity should be tested using a Snellen near chart to screen for visual impairment, which is defined as corrected vision poorer than 20/40. In addition, those athletes who wear glasses should be advised to obtain the correct eye guards or protective lenses. For athletes participating in a water sport, examination of the ears to rule out a perforated tympanic membrane is necessary to determine the need for protective ear plugs. Examination of the mouth may provide clues to abnormal eating behaviors and purging (oral ulcers, gingival atrophy, and decreased tooth enamel).

The lungs and cardiovascular system should be carefully examined. Wheezes, rubs, rales, or other abnormal breath sounds may need further evaluation.

TABLE 4. The Two-Minute Orthopedic Examination

Instructions	Points of Observation
Stand facing examiner	Acromioclavicular joints, general habitus
Look at ceiling, floor, over both shoulders; touch ears to shoulders	Cervical spine motion
Shrug shoulders (examiner resists)	Trapezius strength
Abduct shoulders 90° (examiner resists at 90°)	Deltoid strength
Full external rotation of arms	Shoulder motion
Flex and extend elbows	Elbow motion
Arms at sides, elbows 90° flexed; pronate and supinate wrists	Elbow and wrist motion
Spread fingers; make fist	Hand or finger motion and deformities
Tighten (contract) quadriceps; relax quadriceps	Symmetry and knee effusion; ankle effusion
"Duck walk" 4 steps (away from examiner with buttocks on heels)	Hip, knee, and ankle motion
Back to examiner	Shoulder symmetry, scoliosis
Knees straight, touch toes	Scoliosis, hip motion, hamstring tightness
Raise up on toes; raise heels	Calf symmetry, leg strength

Adapted from Dyment PG (ed): Sports Medicine: Health Care for Young Athletes, 2nd ed. Elk Grove Village, IL, American Academy of Pediatrics, 1991, p 54.

Blood pressure should be taken with the appropriately sized cuff. An athlete with a high blood pressure reading should have the measurement repeated at least 10 minutes later. If the blood pressure is also elevated on the second reading, the athlete should be questioned about the use of stimulants such as caffeine, nicotine, or ephedrine, and the examiner should consider referral for further investigation. Innocent heart murmurs are common in adolescents. However, it is important to identify the murmur of hypertrophic cardiomyopathy (HCM) and that of aortic stenosis because both of these conditions disqualify an athlete from some sports. The murmur of HCM increases with the Valsalva maneuver and decreases with squatting; the opposite holds true for the murmur of aortic stenosis. An arrhythmia detected on physical examination requires an electrocardiogam (EKG). An arrhythmia that disappears with exercise is generally benign; an arrhythmia that becomes more prominent with exercise requires a consultation with a cardiologist. An athlete with known structural heart disease or one with suspected heart disease based on PPE should have the following tests: 12-lead EKG, echocardiogram, and exercise treadmill or ergometer test. Further evaluation should be performed by a cardiologist. In the peripheral vascular examination both radial and femoral pulses should be palpated. Absence of femoral pulses suggests coarctation of the aorta.

The abdominal examination should be done with the athlete in the supine position. Primarily, the clinician is screening for abdominal masses, tenderness, or enlargement of the liver or spleen. Screening for a pregnant uterus should be accomplished by palpating from the xiphoid process to the symphysis pubis. For females, a genital examination is not a required part of PPE.

The examination of the musculoskeletal system should be thorough. Asymmetry of muscle bulk, loss of range of motion, or pain upon provocative maneuvers may signify recent or chronic injury. When an injury has been identified by history, the clinician performing the musculoskeletal examination should spend more time looking for residual swelling, problems with strength, and limited range of motion. A systematic approach to examining the musculoskeletal system is important. A good approach to take is the 2-minute orthopedic examination (see Table 4). This is the minimum that should be done. In certain sports in which a particular body part is more likely used and therefore injured, that part should be examined more thoroughly. For example, swimmers may experience a great deal of shoulder pain while athletes involved in track may experience problems in their lower extremity (knee, shin, and foot/ankle). Particular attention should be paid to examining the spine for scoliosis, because this deformity is common in adolescent girls.

Routine laboratory tests such as complete blood count and urinalysis are not a standard of PPE. If the PPE is used in place of a yearly preventive check up, screening laboratory tests are recommended (see chapter 10).

Disposition

Once the evaluation is completed, the athlete must be assigned to one of three categories: namely, cleared to participate, needs further evaluation, or unable to participate (see Fig. 1). It is a good idea to have a network of physicians to whom referrals can be made. For example, the cardiologist is an invaluable resource to determine medical clearance for suspected cardiac conditions. Other health care professionals who should be available for the athlete's care include psychiatrists, psychologists, and nutritionists.

Clearance

According to the American Academy of Pediatrics, sports may be classified as contact and noncontact. Contact sports are then subdivided into contact/collision and limited contact/impact (Table 5). In addition, sports may be classified by strenuousness into three categories: strenuous, moderately strenuous, and nonstrenuous. Common reasons for disqualification from contact sports include cardiac conditions, one eye, one kidney, enlarged liver, enlarged spleen, and poorly controlled seizure disorder. In the majority of medical conditions encountered, the decision for clearance must be individualized by weighing the potential risks to the athlete.

SPECIFIC MEDICAL CONDITIONS OF IMPORTANCE IN THE ATHLETE

Sudden Death

The biggest fear of any parent and coach is sudden death. Causes of sudden death in the young athlete include both cardiovascular and noncardiovascular conditions. Cardiovascular conditions include hypertrophic cardiomyopathy, dilated cardiomyopathy, myocarditis, coronary artery abnormalities (anomalous origin of left coronary artery), valvular disorders (congenital aortic stenosis), aortic disorders (aortic dissection and/or rupture secondary to

TABLE 5. Classification of Sports by Contact

Contact/Collision	Limited Contact	Noncontact
Basketball	Baseball	Archery
Boxing	Bicycling	Badminton
Diving	Cheerleading	Body building
Field hockey	Canoeing/kayaking (white water)	Canoeing/kayaking (flat water)
Football (flag, tackle)	Fencing	Crew/rowing
Ice hockey	Field (high jump, pole vault)	Curling
Lacrosse	Floor hockey	Dancing
Martial arts	Gymnastics	Field (discuss, javelin, shot put)
Rodeo	Handball	Golf
Rugby	Horseback riding	Orienteering
Ski jumping	Racquetball	Power lifting
Soccer	Skating (ice, in-line, roller)	Race walking
Team handball	Skiing (cross country, downhill, water)	Riflery
Water polo	Softball	Rope jumping
Wrestling	Squash	Running
	Ultimate frisbee	Sailing
	Volleyball	Scuba diving
	Windsurfing/surfing	Strength training
		Swimming
		Table tennis
		Tennis
		Track
		Weightlifting

Adapted from American Academy of Pediatrics: Medical Conditions Affecting Sports Participation. Elk Grove Village, IL, American Academy of Pediatrics, 1994.

Marfan's syndrome), and cardiac arrhythmias (Wolff-Parkinson-White syndrome, idiopathic Q-T syndrome). Noncardiovascular conditions associated with sudden death include exertional hyperthermia, exertional rhabdomyolysis and sickle cell trait, status asthmaticus, and exercise-induced anaphylaxis. Fortunately, sudden death in young athletes is an extremely rare event, occurring in 1- to 2-dozen high school and college athletes per year in organized sports. For unknown reasons the majority are male.

Marfan's Syndrome

The characteristics of this congenital disorder involve at least three organ systems: cardiac (enlargement of aortic root), musculoskeletal (hyperflexible/hypermobile joints), and ocular (dislocated lenses). Not all people with the syndrome necessarily fulfill all criteria. With regards to the PPE, if the athlete is known to have Marfan's syndrome, she should have a yearly echocardiogram. If the diagnosis of Marfan's syndrome is entertained, a consultation with a geneticist should be sought. An athlete with Marfan's syndrome and a dilated aortic root is generally not permitted to participate in strenuous activity.

Mitral Valve Prolapse

Athletes with uncomplicated mitral valve prolapse (MVP) may participate in any physical activity. Complications would include a history of syncope due to arrhythmia, a family history of sudden death due to MVP, arrhythmia worsened by exercise, or moderate-to-marked mitral regurgitation. If any of these are present, high-intensity sports are not recommended. Participation in low-intensity sports (e.g., bowling, golf) may be possible if evaluated on an individual basis.

Infectious Mononucleosis

Infectious mononucleosis occurs relatively frequently in adolescents and young adults. In moderate-to-severe cases the spleen will become enlarged. The physician performing the PPE must decide whether and when the athlete may participate in her sport. Most experts agree that the spleen must return to normal size before participation in any contact sport is permitted. This usually occurs 4–6 weeks after onset of symptoms. However, for noncontact sports the athlete may participate even with an enlarged spleen if she has normal energy.

Human Immunodeficiency Virus

With increased attention to the acquired immunodeficiency syndrome (AIDS) in the general public and scientific community, many coaches, parents, and adolescents fear that athletes may become infected with human immunodeficiency virus (HIV) through contact with small amounts of blood or saliva. To date, there has not been a documented case of HIV transmission during sports participation. Coaches and athletes should be educated that HIV is not transmitted through sports participation. However, an athlete with HIV who is immunocompromised with symptoms of AIDS must be precluded from participating in strenuous activity.

Asthma

Asthma, a common chronic disease affecting 6% of the population, is not a contraindication to sports participation. Conversely, regular aerobic activity may decrease the rate of school absenteeism and lessen frequency of attacks. The physician performing the PPE should counsel the athlete to premedicate with a beta agonist or cromolyn 10–15 minutes before exercise. Athletes frequently neglect to do this.

Hyperflexibility/Hypermobility Syndrome

Many young athletes suffer from pain in the elbows, wrists, knees, or ankles during and after sports competition. Most often, they do not suffer from a systemic disease such as juvenile rheumatoid arthritis, systemic lupus erythematosis, or any other collagen vascular disease. Instead, they have hyperflexible/hypermobile joints. More girls than boys appear to suffer from this condition, which has been described in up to 10% of adolescents who complain of joint pain.[4] To make the diagnosis, three out of four of the following physical findings must be present: thumb opposition, genu recurvatum, elbow hyperextension, and/or wrist hyperextension. There is no reason for disqualification, but the athlete should be counseled about appropriate strengthening exercises and conditioning.

Osgood-Schlatter Disease

A common condition found in adolescent athletes is a painful tibial tubercle (Osgood-Schlatter disease). This disease may be detected by medical history or on physical examination. There are many physicians who do not allow sports participation and treat the condition with rest. However, others recommend activity modification or limited competition, as does this author. The adolescent should be instructed to try to avoid squatting and jarring activities. If the limb is immobilized or activity severely restricted, muscle atrophy ensues and aerobic fitness diminishes. Management includes a reduction of 30–50% of training load, quadriceps/hamstring flexibility and strengthening exercises, a protective knee brace, and icing of the painful tibial tubercle 3–4 times per day.

Patellofemoral Pain Syndrome

Patellofemoral pain syndrome (runner's knee, chondromalacia patellae) is one of the most common musculoskeletal conditions affecting females aged 15–25 years. It is characterized by nonspecific anterior knee pain. Precipitating factors appear to be increasing running mileage or intensity too quickly, an anatomic malalignment (hyperpronation of feet when running, pes cavus, or genus varum or valgum). Other factors include worn running shoes and running on hard surfaces (concrete vs. grass or a paved track). In some cases, there appears to be a lack of development of the vastus medialis oblique muscle (VMO). The condition is bilateral in > 50% of cases and occurs most commonly with impact sports such as running, basketball, gymnastics, or ballet. Physical examination findings may range from a completely normal knee to parapatellar swelling, positive patella compression test, and unwillingness to hop on one foot or bend over and do a duck walk secondary to pain.

Management includes strengthening of VMO, altered training regimen, and occasionally knee bracing. If this condition is discovered during the PPE, appropriate exercises can be instituted before the season begins. As with many conditions, reassurance is especially important. Many athletes believe they have arthritis or chronic disability in their knee. Because of the frequency of patellofemoral pain syndrome, it is extremely important to make the diagnosis and provide appropriate rehabilitation and guidance.

"Shin-Splints"

Chronic shin pain is another common entity encountered in young athletes. Athletes and their coaches often refer to these pains as "shin-splints." This is really a layman's term and refers to several diagnoses, including medial tibial stress syndrome, tibial stress fracture, and exercise-induced compartment syndrome.

Medial tibial stress syndrome is generally what is referred to as "shin-splints." The typical history is chronic shin pain that begins at the start of the season but usually improves as the season progresses. On physical examination there is diffuse tenderness over the posteromedial aspect of the tibia. This is the location of the posterior tibialis muscle insertion and the microscopic fibers become inflamed and tender. Treatment includes decreasing training by 30–50%, improving plantar flexion and dorsiflexion strength. If these methods fail, a trial of orthotics may be indicated.

A tibial stress fracture is diagnosed by the presence of exquisite tenderness over one particular area of the tibia. The athlete usually has had pain and diffuse mild tibial tenderness for at least 1 month. Fewer than 25% of stress fractures are diagnosed radiographically. A bone scan is the recommended imaging modality for diagnosis. There is a focal area of increased uptake corresponding to the area of pain. Treatment consists of 2–4 weeks of nonimpact activities, i.e., no running or jumping. Stationary biking and swimming are encouraged to maintain aerobic fitness. If a diagnosis of tibial stress fracture has been made and the athlete has other chronic bone pains or is underweight and amenorrheic, there may be a problem with low bone density, and a DEXA scan should be obtained.

In exercise-induced compartment syndrome the history is significant for exquisite shin pain only while exercising, usually during running or a high-impact activity. There is no pain before or after exercise. Usually there are no positive findings on physical examination unless the athlete is examined immediately after intense exercise. To make the diagnosis, it is necessary to measure compartment pressure before and after exercise. A positive test is one in which there is elevated pressure after exercise. Treatment includes avoidance of the inciting activity or four-compartment fasciotomy.

Anterior Cruciate Ligament Injuries

A 1992 National College Athletic Association (NCAA) study revealed an epidemic of anterior cruciate ligament (ACL) injuries in female athletes.[5] For Division I college athletes playing varsity basketball and soccer, women suffered 3–5 times more ACL injuries than men. The proposed causative factors are inadequate hamstring strength, prior injury, narrow femoral groove, impaired proprioception, and joint/ligament laxity. Physicians performing the PPE should advise girls with a significant prior knee injury or significant knee laxity of the potential risk of ACL injury.

Pregnancy

Pregnancy is not a contraindication to sports participation. However, it is not advisable to begin a new exercise program or participate in a sport that was not previously tried. Sports with a high risk of abdominal trauma such as skiing or soccer are not recommended. Pregnant women should be cautioned to ensure adequate hydration when participating in sports. In addition, they should be advised to stop any activity if they experience dizziness or fatigue.

CONCLUSION

The preparticipation physical evaluation can be an informative and enjoyable experience for both the athlete and physician alike. The entire process should be taken seriously, and each athlete should be evaluated individually. Generally, few conditions present an absolute contraindication to sports participation. If an athlete is ineligible to play a contact sport, a noncontact sport can be recommended. Clinicians conducting the evaluation should ensure the communication of findings to coaches, athletic trainers, and parents as well as to the young athlete herself.

REFERENCES

1. American Academy of Family Physicians, American Academy of Pediatrics, American Medical Society for Sports Medicine, American Orthopaedic Society for Sports Medicine, and American Osteopathic Academy of Sports Medicine: Preparticipation Physical Evaluation (PPE), 2nd ed. New York, McGraw-Hill, 1997.
2. Van Camp SP, Bloor C, Mueller FO, et al: Nontraumatic sports death in high school and college athletes. Med Sci Sports Exerc 27:641–647, 1995.
3. Tucker JB, Marron JT: The qualification/disqualification process in athletics. Am Fam Physician 29:149–154, 1984.
4. Gedalia A, Person DA, Brewer EJ Jr, Giannini EH: Hypermobility of the joints in juvenile episodic arthritis/arthralgia. J Pediatr 107:873–876, 1985.
5. Arendt E, Dick R: Knee injury patterns among men and women in collegiate basketball and soccer: NCAA data and review of literature. Am J Sports Med 23:694–701, 1995.
6. American Academy of Pediatrics, Committee on Sports Medicine: Sports Medicine: Health Care for Young Athletes. Elk Grove Village, IL, American Academy of Pediatrics, 1991.
7. Moeller JL: Contraindication to athletic participation—cardiac, respiratory, and central nervous system conditions. Physician Sports Med 24:47–58, 1996.
8. Moeller JL: Contraindications to athletic participation—spinal, systemic, dermatologic, paired-organ, and other issues. Physician Sports Med 24:57–75, 1996.
9. 26th Annual Bethesda Conference: Recommendations for determining eligibility for competition in athletes with cardiovascular abnormalities. Med Sci Sports Exerc 26(Suppl 10): S223–S283, 1994.

CHAPTER 12

Reproductive Health for Girls with Chronic Illness

Elizabeth M. Alderman, M.D.

In the United States, it is estimated that approximately 6% of all adolescents have a chronic health condition that results in limitation of daily activities or disability.[1] The most common conditions found in this age group are asthma, mental retardation, diabetes mellitus, cystic fibrosis, sickle cell anemia, malignancies, epilepsy, and human immunodeficiency virus (HIV) infection.

As medical treatments for common chronic illnesses of childhood improve, more children are surviving to adolescence and adulthood. However, the optimal treatment of an adolescent with a chronic medical illness is not limited to biomedical treatment alone. The practitioner caring for an adolescent girl with a chronic medical illness must consider the complex behavioral, psychosocial, and developmental changes of adolescence when working with her.

One of the hallmarks of adolescence is participation in risk-taking behaviors. Initiation of sexual activity is an important contributor to morbidity in the adolescent age group, putting girls at risk of sexually transmitted infections (STIs) and unintended pregnancy. For the adolescent girl with a chronic illness, the health risks of sexual activity may be exacerbated by the illness itself, or by medications used to treat it. Certain forms of contraception may be inappropriate for girls with certain chronic illnesses. STIs may be more virulent or difficult to treat in girls who are immunosuppressed because of illness or medication.

Many practitioners fail to address sexually related issues and focus solely on the medical illness. However, studies show that many adolescents with chronic illness are sexually active and most have concerns about their sexuality. This chapter reviews such studies and discusses specific considerations in reproductive health for adolescent girls with chronic health conditions.

IMPACT OF CHRONIC ILLNESS ON GROWTH AND DEVELOPMENT

The physiologic changes that occur during puberty may be startling or confusing to any young adolescent who is constantly comparing herself to her peers. The onset of puberty and the prospect of childbearing may be more poignant for the adolescent with a chronic medical illness that, either by virtue of the illness or the treatment, delays puberty and affects fertility.

Delayed Puberty

When evaluating a chief complaint of primary amenorrhea or delayed puberty, the practitioner must always consider nonendocrine chronic illness in addition to derangements of reproductive hormone secretion. What is more common, however, is delayed puberty in the adolescent with a known chronic illness. Delayed growth, pubertal development, and menarche are frequent in girls with cystic fibrosis. The delay may be related to a lag in attainment of pubertal levels of sex steroids and gonadotropins, in part due to malnutrition and hypoxia related to severity of disease. A study of girls with cystic fibrosis found that amenorrheic patients were shorter and had less body fat than those who had reached menarche; also they were younger when first diagnosed with the disease.[2] The majority of the girls with menses had irregular periods.

In a study of girls who had undergone bone marrow transplantation for acute lymphocytic leukemia during childhood, half spontaneously entered puberty at an average age of 13 years.[3] Girls with ovarian failure received radiation and chemotherapy treatments at an older age than girls who showed spontaneous pubertal development. The ovaries are quiescent in children prior to puberty and thus less vulnerable to damage by ionizing radiation or chemotherapeutic agents than ovaries in older peri- and postpubertal girls, whose cells are dividing more rapidly.

Impaired Fertility

A large study of survivors of childhood/adolescent cancer demonstrated that radiation therapy below the diaphragm had the greatest effect on fertility in women, compared with sibling controls. There was little effect of alkylating agents.[4] Chemotherapeutic treatment of Hodgkin's disease, the most common malignancy in adolescence, has been associated with impaired gonadal function in girls and a risk of future infertility.[5] Newer techniques for protecting ovaries from damage by surgically pinning them back out of the radiation field or using oral contraceptive pills to reduce cell division during chemotherapy may help to lower the incidence of fertility problems in the future. Illnesses that are known to cause impaired fertility are shown in Table 1.

SEXUAL BEHAVIOR

According to the 1995 Youth Risk Behavior Survey conducted by the Centers for Disease Control and Prevention (CDC) on a representative sample

TABLE 1. Medical Conditions that May Impair Fertility in Girls

Chronic renal failure	Cancer (radiation below the diaphragm)
Thyroid dysfunction	Uncontrolled diabetes mellitus

TABLE 2. Studies of Sexual Behavior in Adolescent Girls with Chronic Illness

Study Population	Sample Size	Age	Sexually Active (%)
Various diseases	36,284	13–18	45
Inner-city, various diseases	338	14–17	33
Spina bifida	35	13–19	3
Mentally retarded	87	11–23	39
Cystic fibrosis	16	12–17	0

of United States high school students, more than two-thirds of all students report having initiated sexual intercourse by the senior year of high school, with almost 18% reporting 4 or more lifetime partners.[6] At first intercourse, most girls use some form of contraception, but more than one-third do not.[7] Twelve percent of 15–19-year-old girls become pregnant each year.[8]

There are few large population-based studies of sexual behavior of adolescents with chronic illnesses (Table 2). Analysis of the Minnesota Adolescent Health Survey of over 30,000 7th–12th-graders showed that there were no differences between adolescent girls with chronic illness, both visible and invisible, and non-ill girls in terms of age at first intercourse, which on average was 14 years.[9] A significantly greater proportion of girls with visible chronic illnesses reported a history of STIs than the other two groups. In a study of over 300 inner-city adolescents with chronic illness and their healthy friends, adolescents with chronic illness were found to be just as likely to be sexually active as their friends.[10] However, girls with chronic illness initiated sexual activity at a significantly younger age (13.8 years) than their healthy friends (15.3 years). The average number of lifetime partners, pregnancy rates, contraception use, and sexually transmitted diseases were similar in both chronically ill and healthy girls.

Several studies of adolescents with specific chronic illnesses have been conducted. Cystic fibrosis is the most common genetic disease among Caucasians and often results in delayed puberty, including late menarche. In a small study of adolescent girls with cystic fibrosis, one-third were sexually active but all were over the age of 18 years, which may reflect the older age of menarche.[2] A study by Cromer et al. compared adolescents with myelomeningocele to those with cystic fibrosis and healthy controls.[11] This study found that adolescents with myelomeningocele were less likely to be sexually active than those with cystic fibrosis, who were similar to the control adolescents. Only one-fifth of the adolescents with myelomeningocele or cystic fibrosis had sought information from a physician regarding their sexuality.

Although conducted more than 20 years ago, a study by Dorner of sexual interest and activity in adolescents with spina bifida has some interesting findings not looked at in other studies.[12] Although 80% of the adolescents described relations with the opposite sex, only one of the 35 girls had sexual intercourse. Many of these adolescents had concerns about their childbearing capabilities. The girls with limited genital sensation were more concerned about childbearing than deriving pleasure from sexual intercourse. Instead, they described kissing and cuddling as satisfying ways to express sexuality. Chamberlain et al. examined sexual activity in mentally retarded female adolescents, most of whom were mildly-to-moderately retarded.[13] One-third of the moderately retarded girls and almost 10% of the severely retarded girls had been sexually active. Fewer than one-half had used contraception. One-quarter of the girls had been sexually assaulted.

These studies demonstrate that adolescents with chronic illnesses are at least thinking about their sexuality and many are sexually active. Handicapped adolescents may be self-conscious about their sexual performance and worried about their fertility. In addition, disabled adolescents may have fewer opportunities for peer interaction, and this alone may delay sexual debut. Sexual assault always remains an issue, especially for mentally retarded adolescent girls who are uniquely vulnerable to exploitation. Illnesses that delay puberty, such as cystic fibrosis, inflammatory bowel disease, and sickle cell anemia, also may be associated with older age at initiation of sexual intercourse. It is important to remember, however, that most chronic illnesses do not impair fertility in adolescent girls. Therefore, contraception is extremely important for sexually active adolescents with chronic illness.

CONTRACEPTION

To prevent unintended pregnancy, contraception should be discussed and prescribed for all sexually active girls with chronic illness. Some forms of contraception not only prevent pregnancy but also prevent sexually transmitted infections. Other contraceptives may actually improve the course of the chronic illness.

Hormonal Contraception

Hormonal contraception, in the form of the oral contraceptive pill (OCP), depo-medroxyprogesterone acetate injection (DMPA, Depo-Provera), or levonorgestrel implants (Norplant), is the most effective method of pregnancy prevention. However, hormonal contraception may not be suitable for adolescent girls who have certain medical conditions. In particular, since OCPs contain estrogen many practitioners hesitate to prescribe them to girls with conditions such as sickle cell disease, congenital heart disease, systemic lupus erythematosus, or diabetes mellitus because of fears of inducing a hypercoagulable state or worsening diabetic control. In some cases, there is also concern about using the progestin-only contraceptives Depo-Provera and Norplant, because the package inserts list the same risks of thrombophlebitis as those for OCPs despite the lack of evidence for such risks in clinical use. In practice, however, progestin-only hormonal contraceptives are quite safe for the majority of girls with chronic illness.

Diabetes Mellitus

Low-dose OCPs do not adversely affect glucose tolerance in diabetic girls. In addition, those containing third-generation progestins (norgestimate, desogestrel) promote a favorable lipid profile from the point of view of cardiovascular risk. The pills are estrogen-dominant because third-generation progestins are more specific for progesterone receptors and have less affinity for androgenic receptors. Progestin-only contraception is also a viable choice for girls with diabetes mellitus.

Sickle Cell Anemia

For girls with sickle cell anemia, Depo-Provera has been shown to reduce the frequency of vasoocclusive crises. Low-dose combinations of OCPs also may decrease the incidence and severity of sickling.[14] There is no evidence that OCPs increase the risk of thromboembolic events in girls with sickle cell anemia; however, OCPs should not be used in girls who have had these complications. Depo-Provera is also ideal for a girl with sickle cell anemia because the reduced amount of menstrual blood flow will decrease the risk for iron deficiency anemia.

Congenital Heart Disease

Many adolescents with surgically corrected congenital heart disease may safely use low-dose OCPs and progestin-only methods. OCPs are contraindicated, however, if a girl has pulmonary vascular disease, thromboembolic disease (or high risk due to an artificial aortic valve), or cerebrovascular disease. These girls should use barrier methods to prevent unintended pregnancy. OCPs are also contraindicated for girls with hypertension as a complication of chronic illness such as systemic lupus erythematosus, renal disease, or cardiac disease. Depo-Provera or Norplant may be used safely in these circumstances, especially if barrier methods have failed and the risk of unintended pregnancy is great.

Seizure Disorders

For girls with seizure disorders, OCPs have not been shown to increase the incidence of seizures.[15] In fact, Depo-Provera lowers the incidence of seizures in some girls. The major consideration for girls with seizure disorders, however, is the interaction of the hormonal contraception with anticonvulsant therapy. OCPs may be less effective for girls taking anticonvulsants such as phenobarbital, carbamazepine, and phenytoin, because they induce liver microsomal enzymes which, in turn, cause accelerated metabolism of the estrogen in the pill, resulting in lower effective doses. Breakthrough bleeding may be a good indicator of insufficient contraceptive effect. If such bleeding occurs, the estrogen dose in the OCP may need to be increased. Depo-Provera is an excellent contraceptive choice for girls on anticonvulsants because there are no adverse medication interactions.

It is important to determine if medications used to treat chronic illness have any interaction with hormonal contraceptives. Table 3 lists common chronic illnesses, the medications used to treat them, and potential interactions with the different hormonal contraceptives.

TABLE 3. Considerations in Choosing Contraception for Adolescents with Chronic Illness on Medication

Illness	Medicines	Interactions
Asthma	Theophylline	Decreased theophylline clearance with OCP
Seizure disorders	Dilantin Phenobarbital Tegretol Valproate	Decreased contraceptive effect of OCP
Heart valve replacement	Coumadin	Decreased levels with OCP
Depression	Tricyclics	Increased antidepressant levels with OCP
Tuberculosis	Rifampin	Decreased contraceptive effect of OCP
Systemic lupus erythematosus Multiple sclerosis	Steroids	Avoid intrauterine device

Barrier Methods

Barrier methods of contraception seem ideal because they prevent pregnancy and protect against sexually transmitted infections. The male condom is more effective than the female condom, diaphragm, or cervical cap for both pregnancy and STI prevention but not nearly as effective as hormonal contraception for pregnancy prevention. The only contraindication to male condom use is latex allergy, which is quite common in patients with myelomeningocele. Polyurethane condoms are available and may be used if latex allergy exists. Abnormal genital anatomy is a contraindication to use of the female condom, diaphragm, and cervical cap, because they may not fit well and thus will not provide optimal contraception. The intrauterine device is not usually prescribed for adolescent girls because of increased risk of pelvic inflammatory disease and resultant impaired fertility. However, it may be ideal for the older, monogamous girl who cannot use hormonal contraception and requires highly effective pregnancy prevention. Because of increased risk for a more prolonged course of a possible STI, the intrauterine device is not appropriate for the immunocompromised girl with HIV infection or the girl on immunosuppressive medications such as steroids or chemotherapy.

PREVENTING CONSEQUENCES OF SEXUALLY TRANSMITTED INFECTIONS

All sexually active adolescent girls should be advised to use condoms to prevent STIs even when they are also using hormonal contraceptives. However, for girls who are immunosuppressed, there is a high risk for a prolonged and more complicated course if they are infected with an STI. These girls should receive detailed instruction and frequent reinforcement regarding barrier contraceptive use. Genital infection with human papillomavirus is particularly virulent in girls who are immunocompromised, and they are at increased risk of developing cervical cancer. Such sexually active adolescents need frequent Pap smear and STI screening with close gynecologic follow-up and rapid treatment of any cervical dysplasias or infections.[16]

Although not a sexually transmitted infection, candidal vulvovaginitis is more common in the adolescent girl on immunosuppressive medications. Additionally, multiple courses of antibiotics for a girl with cancer or cystic fibrosis may also put her at risk for a more virulent candidal infection.

REPRODUCTIVE OUTCOMES

Genetic Considerations

Many chronic illnesses have proven genetic patterns of inheritance that allow prediction of risk of transmission. Table 4 lists the modes of inheritance for the most common genetic diseases. Screening is readily available for carriers of the gene for sickle cell anemia, beta thalassemia, cystic fibrosis, Duchenne's muscular dystrophy, and hemophilia, with others being developed at a rapidly progressing rate. If the adolescent has one of these heritable diseases or is a carrier, it is important for her to ascertain the status of her sexual partner so that the genetic risks of having an affected child may be determined. If the adolescent is a carrier of an autosomal recessive disorder and the partner is a carrier, there is a 25% chance the offspring will have the illness. If the adolescent has an autosomal dominant illness such as neurofibromatosis, there is a 50% chance of an affected offspring. For a sex-linked disorder such as hemophilia, girls are carriers but not affected with the disease. Female carriers have a 50% chance of having an affected male child or a female child who is a carrier. Discussing these genetic risks with sexually active girls may help to convince them to abstain from sexual intercourse or give them a reason to use effective contraception.

Teratogenicity of Medication

The sexually active adolescent girl with a chronic illness should be counseled about the necessity of carefully planning her pregnancies because she may be taking medication to treat her chronic illness that is potentially teratogenic to the developing fetus. Cancer chemotherapy and radiation are prime examples of teratogenic treatments. Fetal hydantoin syndrome is a well studied entity manifesting as craniofacial anomalies, limb defects, and growth and developmental retardation.[17] Table 5 lists common chronic illnesses and drugs used to treat them that are potentially teratogenic to the fetus.

It is essential to ensure effective contraception in the sexually active girl who is taking teratogenic medication. Before prescribing such medication, the

TABLE 4. Selected Genetic Diseases by Mode of Transmission

Autosomal Recessive	Autosomal Dominant	Sex-Linked
Sickle cell anemia	Neurofibromatosis	Hemophilia
Cystic fibrosis	Marfan syndrome	Duchenne and Becker muscular dystrophies
Tay-Sachs disease	Achondroplasia	
Beta-thalassemia		

TABLE 5. Chronic Illnesses and Commonly Used Medications that Are Harmful to the Fetus

Illness	Medication
Inflammatory bowel disease	Metronidazole, 6-mercaptopurine
Seizure disorders	Dilantin, valproate, trimethadione
Cystic fibrosis	Ciprofloxacin, aminoglycosides, tetracycline, metronidazole, sulfa
Systemic lupus erythematosus	Alkylating agents, antimetabolites
Cancer	Antimetabolites, alkylating agents, radiation, selected antibiotics
Rheumatoid arthritis	Nonsteroidal antiinflammatory agents, gold salts, penicillamine
Heart valve replacement	Coumadin

practitioner should take a sexual history and consider the possibility of early pregnancy. If the young woman desires pregnancy, some medicines such as coumadin, gold salts, penicillamine, and 6-mercaptopurine should be discontinued well before conception. The practitioner should be alert to the teratogenicity of the medication and weigh the benefits of treating the pregnant adolescent for her illness versus the risk of congenital fetal malformations. The *Physicians' Desk Reference* is extremely helpful in providing current information regarding prescription of medicines during pregnancy.

Pregnancy, Termination of Pregnancy, Childbirth

Most chronic illnesses do not impair fertility in young women. However, pregnancy may exacerbate the course of a chronic illness. In addition, some chronic illnesses create a high-risk pregnancy. If a girl with a chronic illness desires termination of pregnancy, she should be referred to a medical facility with practitioners who are comfortable with the high-risk environment.

Pregnancy may exacerbate severe asthma with concomitant potential for maternal mortality.[18] In severe asthma, fetal oxygenation may be compromised during an acute episode or in a girl with poorly controlled asthma. Sickle cell anemia is another chronic illness that may be exacerbated during pregnancy. Pregnancy increases the risk of stroke, pulmonary embolus, pneumonia, pyelonephritis, and endometritis in adolescents with sickle cell anemia.[19] Systemic lupus erythematosus and other autoimmune diseases such as inflammatory bowel disease may worsen or remit during pregnancy. Women with cystic fibrosis have a high risk of premature labor, maternal perinatal morbidity, and low fetal weight.[20]

Adolescents with congenital heart disease without pulmonary hypertension and those with mitral valve prolapse usually have uneventful pregnancies but must receive endocarditis prophylaxis with antibiotics during vaginal delivery, caesarean section, or for termination of pregnancy. The adolescent with pulmonary hypertension is at high risk for mortality during pregnancy and may also develop hypoxia, thromboembolism, and hypovolemia during delivery and therapeutic abortion. Therefore, these adolescents require intensive cardiorespiratory monitoring during these procedures.

CONCLUSION

With improvements in medical treatments, many girls with chronic illness are surviving to adolescence and engaging in high-risk sexual behaviors similar to those of their peers. The practitioner needs to address sexuality and the consequences of unprotected sexual intercourse with these young women. In addition, the physician needs to be aware of the multiple options available to the sexually active adolescent girl to prevent unintended pregnancy and sexually transmitted infections.

REFERENCES

1. Newacheck W, McManus MA, Fox HB: Prevalence and impact of chronic illness among adolescents. Am J Dis Child 145:1367–1373, 1991.
2. Neinstein LS, Stewart D, Wang C, et al: Menstrual dysfunction in cystic fibrosis. J Adolesc Health 4:153–157, 1983.
3. Sarafoglou K, Boulad F, Gillio A, et al: Gonadal function after bone marrow transplantation for acute leukemia during childhood. J Pediatr 130:210–216, 1997.
4. Byrne J, Mulvihill J, Myers MH, et al: Effects of treatment on fertility in long-term survivors of childhood or adolescent cancer. N Engl J Med 317:1315–1321, 1987.
5. Dein RA, Mennuti MT, Kovach P, et al: The reproductive potential of young men and women with Hodgkin's disease. Obstet Gynynecol Surv 39:474–481, 1984.
6. Ozer EM, Brindis CD, Millstein SG, et al: America's adolescents: Are they healthy? San Francisco, CA, University of California, San Francisco, National Adolescent Health Information Center, 1997.
7. Alan Guttmacher Institute: Sex and America's Teenagers. New York, Alan Guttmacher Institute, 1994.
8. Morris L, Warren CW, Aral SO: Measuring adolescent sexual behaviors and related health outcomes. Public Health Rep 108(Suppl 1):31–36, 1993.
9. Suris J, Resnick MD, Cassuto N, et al: Sexual behavior of adolescents with chronic disease and disability. J Adolesc Health 19:124–131, 1996.
10. Alderman EM, Lauby JL, Coupey SM: Problem behaviors in inner-city adolescents with chronic illness. J Dev Behav Pediatr 16:339–344, 1995.
11. Cromer BA, Enrile B, McCoy K, et al: Knowledge, attitudes and behavior related to sexuality in adolescents with chronic disability. Dev Med Child Neurol 32:602–610, 1990.
12. Dorner S: Sexual interest and activity in adolescents with spina bifida. J Child Psychol Psychiatry 18:229–237, 1977.
13. Chamberlain A, Rauh J, Passer A, et al: Issues in fertility control for mentally retarded female adolescents: I. Sexual activity, sexual abuse and contraception. Pediatrics 73(4):445–450, 1984.
14. Freie HMP: Sickle cell disease and hormonal contraception. Acta Obstet Gynecol Scand 62:211–217, 1983.
15. Mattson RH, Cramer JA, Darney PD, Naftolin F: Use of oral contraceptives by women with epilepsy. JAMA 256:238–240, 1986.
16. Coupey SM, Alderman EM: Sexual behavior and related health care for adolescents with chronic medical illness. Adolesc Med 3:317–329, 1992.
17. Dalessio DJ: Seizure disorders and pregnancy. N Engl J Med 312:559–563, 1983.
18. Shulman V, Alderman EM, Ewig JM, Bye MR: Asthma in the pregnant adolescent: A review. J Adolesc Health 18:168–176, 1996.
19. Morrison JC: Hemoglobinopathies and pregnancy. Clin Obstet Gynecol 22:819–842, 1979.
20. Cohen LF, DiSant'Aynese P, Friedlander J: Cystic fibrosis and pregnancy—a national study. Lancet 2:842–849, 1980.

CHAPTER 13

Contraceptive Counseling and Prescription

Walter D. Rosenfeld, M.D.
Susan M. Coupey, M.D.

Rates of sexual activity increase dramatically as girls move through the teenage years. In their early teens few girls have sexual intercourse, but by age 19 years, approximately 80% of young women have become sexually active. During middle adolescence, ages 15–17 years, a significant number of girls initiate sexual activity and are at risk for unintended pregnancy and sexually transmitted diseases (STDs); thus, routine contraceptive counseling is warranted. When and by whom should this counseling be done? If the group of primary care medical providers who are seeing adolescents for headaches, school physicals, and other health issues are not considering the potential need for contraception, they are going to miss a unique opportunity to protect the health of their patients and to prevent teenage pregnancy. Contraceptive counseling should not be considered the province of a few specialized providers.

It is essential that primary care providers try to open the door to communication with adolescents fairly early in their sexual development to get them thinking about the fact that they may need contraception now or in the future. A large majority of adolescent girls make their first medical visit for contraception more than one month after they have begun having sex. This fact is disturbing because a majority of pregnancies in teenagers occur within the first 6 months of initiating sexual intercourse and many occur within 1 month. Thus, if providers do not provide anticipatory guidance to young adolescents about pregnancy and STD prevention and wait instead until the girls request contraception, a whole group of teenagers at risk will miss the opportunity to learn about their contraceptive options from a knowledgeable and authoritative source. Most often, by the time adolescents become sexually active, they are at the peak of their fertility, so conception shortly after the onset of intercourse occurs quite frequently. Unfortunately, myths about fertility, such as "You can't get pregnant with your first intercourse" or "Adolescents are relatively infertile," persist despite evidence to the contrary.

TABLE 1. The Primary Care Provider and Contraceptive Counseling

- Be aware of the scope of the problem.
- Make your practice adolescent-friendly.
- Make good working liaisons with colleagues to use as referral sources.
- Be aware of the developmental factors contributing to adolescent pregnancy.
- Learn to communicate effectively with adolescent girls and their parents.

THE ROLE OF THE PRIMARY CARE PROVIDER

The Scope of the Problem

How can primary care providers help adolescent girls to prevent unintended pregnancy and STDs? The first task is to become aware that there is a problem (Table 1). Many providers and parents have the mistaken belief that teenage sexual activity and pregnancy happen in other practices or other communities; they do not believe that their own patients or their own children are having sex. However, national data indicate that among 15–19-year-old females, there is little difference in the percent who are sexually active by ethnicity, with 60% of African-Americans, 49% of Hispanics and 52% of whites in this age group reporting sexual activity. Similarly, in comparisons of young women reporting sexual activity in poor versus low-income versus higher-income groups, Roman Catholic versus Protestant religions, and urban versus rural residences, the differences range from a high of 60% to a low of 48%, which is not a very large range. This behavior crosses all social boundaries and is practiced by at least half of the 15–19-year-old female population.

In younger adolescent girls, aged 12–15 years, sexual intercourse is not normative and can be viewed as a risk-taking behavior. Risk behaviors tend to cluster within individuals. Data from the Centers for Disease Control and Prevention (CDC) Youth Risk Behavior Survey indicate the associations among several risk behaviors in young adolescents. Two-thirds of 14–15-year-olds who said that they regularly used alcohol, 69% of those who smoked cigarettes, and 87% of those who smoked marijuana were sexually active. These rates of sexual activity are much higher than those in the general population of 14–15-year-olds, which has a rate of sexual activity of about 25%. Therefore, when there is any positive history of risk taking in a young adolescent, a full inquiry about sexual activity should be made.

Making Your Practice Adolescent-Friendly

The second important task for health care providers is to be "user-friendly" by specifically targeting their practices toward adolescents. For example, there should be some literature in the waiting room that is of interest to young people to convey the message that their issues are important to the provider. The office staff should be trained in aspects of confidentiality so that they do not inadvertently breach it. A simple pamphlet can be put on display in the office advising parents and youth that the provider is interested in and knowledgeable about the special issues of teenagers. Examples such as concerns about sexuality, body image, eating disorders, and prevention and intervention for substance abuse should be cited to help communicate a clear message. Some pediatricians have used this mechanism to explain that, beginning when the patient is 11 or 12 years old, they will spend time alone with the adolescent, allowing her an opportunity to discuss sensitive matters in private. This explanation should convey the message that the practitioner is supportive of family communication but that on occasion, even in the best of circumstances, a young person will ask certain questions or reveal embarrassing personal information only when privacy and confidentiality are assured. The limitations of this confidential bond should be identified so that parents can be assured that immediately life-threatening information such as suicidal ideation will be exposed if it is uncovered.

Liaisons with Professional Colleagues

A third task for the provider is to develop good working liaisons with professional colleagues who can be used as a referral source. Problems related to sexuality, pregnancy, and contraception in adolescents often are accompanied by psychosocial issues that require consultation with a mental health professional and by complications that require referral to obstetrician/gynecologists, infectious disease specialists, or endocrinologists. It is important to remember, though, that the primary care provider for adolescents makes a major contribution by understanding the needs of teenagers and effectively communicating about and providing for those needs. Referral to another provider too early in the process of establishing a relationship with a teenager may be misinterpreted as disinterest, resulting in failure of the young person to return for follow-up of her problems.

FACTORS CONTRIBUTING TO ADOLESCENT PREGNANCY

Myths and Beliefs

Even though this chapter focuses on contraception, it is important to understand the broader picture, which includes the many contributing factors leading to pregnancy in adolescence. The solution to unintended pregnancy is much more complicated than simply providing contraception. There are a number of issues related to lack of knowledge and misinformation. Adolescents and their parents believe many myths about the risks and benefits of contraception, particularly hormonal contraception (Table 2). They may believe, for example, that the birth control pill causes cancer, that prolonged use of hormones decreases fertility, or that use of the pill creates a substantial risk of death from a blood clot. Belief in such myths interferes with adherence to

TABLE 2. Common Myths about Hormonal Contraception

- Health risks are as great as those of pregnancy and childbirth.
- The failure rate is high.
- They cause cancer.
- They cause heart attacks.
- Long-term use will decrease fertility.
- They cause birth defects.

contraception. In contrast, the many noncontraceptive benefits of hormonal contraceptives often are unknown.

Developmental Issues

Many adolescent girls have an insecure identity and low self-esteem. They are not self-confident enough to assert their wishes and desires related to pregnancy prevention. Their partners' influence may be critically important, and, unfortunately, many adolescent boys also are insecure in their masculine identity. As proof of masculinity, some boys want to know that they can impregnate a girl. Such young men may actively discourage their girlfriends from using birth control consistently. Parents too can give mixed messages to their daughters, appearing to be against both sex and contraception, so the daughters may actually believe that using contraception is more dangerous to their health than having sex. In addition, adolescents themselves are impulsive and lack future-planning skills, both of which may interfere with correct use of contraception. Many teens feel invulnerable, that nothing bad can happen to them, and that they can control their whole environment. Some girls seem to be actively trying to become pregnant, perhaps as an attempt to replace a loss or as a response to stress. To others, becoming a mother may represent a means to gain respect and status. In some communities, having a baby as a teenager does not have the same stigma as it does in the broader culture. For the impoverished adolescent, parenthood may reflect a lack of other alternatives. Unless the clinician takes a few moments to explore such issues, the brief, authoritative statement—"You must use birth control 100% of the time"—is often met with failure.

The reasons that adolescents do not use contraception consistently and correctly are varied and complex. Thus, when counseling an adolescent who has not used her birth control pills properly or is late for her depot-medroxyprogesterone acetate (DMPA, Depo-Provera) injection, the provider who focuses the inquiry superficially on why she forgot often misses the underlying reasons. The reason that the patient has not used her contraception properly is not usually sporadic forgetfulness. It is more likely that some personal, developmental, or cultural issues are interfering with her ability to adhere to an effective regimen.

COMMUNICATION AND COUNSELING TECHNIQUES

Provider–Patient–Parent Communication

Perhaps the most important task of the primary care provider is to communicate effectively with both adolescent girls and their parents (Table 3). It is tempting to take a paternalistic approach and simply tell patients what they should be doing or not doing. However, a more effective approach is to attempt to convince the young woman to become a partner with you in protecting her health. Statements such as "I am working for you, so you and I need to agree"; "It is important that you tell me what you think"; or "I'm here to give you information, so let me give you that information and then let's discuss

TABLE 3. Communication Techniques

- Resist taking a paternalistic approach.
- Attempt to engage the patient in a partnership.
- Act more like a coach than a lecturer.
- Reinforce positive behavior.
- Resist criticizing negative behavior.
- Be nonjudgmental but do provide guidance.

together what is going to be best for you" serve to introduce the concept of partnership and to help adolescent patients to feel empowered. With such an approach, young women understand that the provider will listen to them and respect their opinions.

A direct approach to addressing sexual behavior may not be effective with some adolescents. In such cases, it is helpful to remember the concept of the hook and the lure. Every practitioner has had patients who do not seem to listen to advice and who experience repeated health problems related to their sexual behavior. It is natural to become frustrated and at a loss about what to do. Sometimes it helps to change the subject and to engage the adolescent in a discussion of some other problem that, while it may seem trivial, is of great immediate concern to her (e.g., the three pimples on her forehead). After making a connection, offer to help her with appropriate treatment and schedule a new appointment about that problem. By doing this, one begins to establish a helping, trusting relationship; it provides an opportunity to communicate better with the patient and to begin to engage her in proble solving related to her sexual behavior.

Contraceptive Counseling

Effective counseling about sexuality and contraception is a process of guidance or coaching rather than lecturing. The provider needs to watch for verbal and nonverbal cues, encourage the adolescent to explain her point of view, ask specific questions in a nonjudgmental manner, and take into account the adolescent's beliefs, concerns, and past history when developing a treatment plan. It usually works best if the provider can find something positive that the adolescent is doing and build the counseling from there, rather than starting with criticism about something she is not doing (Table 4). For example, if the provider knows that the patient is sexually active and using no contraception but, upon further questioning, ascertains that she is trying to employ a type of

TABLE 4. Contraceptive Counseling

- Take the initiative to introduce the topic.
- Take a detailed sexual history in private without the parents present.
- Assure the patient of confidential care related to her sexuality.
- Include abstinence as an option.
- Provide information about emergency contraception.
- Encourage the patient to tell a parent about her contraceptive decision.
- Include a parent when giving instructions about use and side effects of hormonal contraceptives (if the patient gives permission).

rhythm method by not having sex in the middle of the month, the provider can praise her efforts at trying to prevent pregnancy and suggest a better method. It is tempting in this situation to lecture her about the inadequacies of the rhythm method in general and her interpretation of it in particular, but this approach only serves to make her feel inadequate and incompetent. To achieve good compliance, the provider must make the patient feel empowered and competent to carry out the treatment plan.

It is important and essential to discuss abstinence as part of contraceptive counseling. Letting girls know that the healthiest option is to delay sexual activity until they are older is appropriate. It also may be helpful to communicate that choosing abstinence after having initiated sexual intercourse is a logical and acceptable option. These messages should be worded carefully so as not to convey the impression that one is trying to impose his or her own moral judgment on the patient, for this perception may have the unwanted effect of undermining her trust, causing her to withhold the truth about her behavior. It is a fine line to balance and requires careful attention to language and tone of voice. Often, it helps to point out the statistics about how many teenagers are *not* sexually active. Rather than saying that 60% of 15–19 year olds are sexually active, one can say that 40% have not had intercourse. One out of every 5 young women waits until she is out of her teens before initiating sexual intercourse. Sharing this information with your patient validates her decision to remain abstinent and displays knowledge and expertise about adolescent behavior. Of interest, some studies show that teenagers think their peers are more sexually active than is reported by the peers themselves. Giving accurate information can help to counter such overestimates.

When counseling adolescents, the provider must find a way to establish a trusting relationship. Ensuring privacy for discussions of sexual matters is essential. Even when parents insist that their daughter tells them "everything" and the daughter agrees, it still is not appropriate to expect the adolescent to provide details of her sexual behavior in front of her parents. Most adolescents need assurances of confidentiality before they will trust a provider with sensitive information about their sexual practices, such as the number of partners they have had or whether they have engaged in oral or anal sex. Many girls, however, will discuss their contraceptive use with their mothers, and this behavior should be encouraged. It is perfectly appropriate and even desirable, if the adolescent allows it, to have the mother present when explaining the use and side effects of hormonal contraceptives. Good communication with the mother and the mother's knowledge of her daughter's contraceptive use are associated with better adherence to contraceptive regimens in adolescent girls.

CONTRACEPTIVE OPTIONS

It is helpful to acknowledge at the outset that there is no perfect option for contraception. In fact, there is no option that comes close to perfect. Every available choice has some drawbacks. One option, and it is important to articulate it as an option to your adolescent patients, is to get pregnant; another is to remain abstinent. The pros and cons of these latter two choices should be included in all decision-making discussions.

TABLE 5. Percentage of Women Experiencing an Accidental Pregnancy in the First Year of Continuous Use

Method	Lowest Expected	Typical Use
(No contraceptive)	(85)	(85)
Oral contraceptives, combined	0.1	3
Diaphragm with spermicidal cream or jelly	6	18
Spermicides alone (foams, creams, etc.)	6	18
Levonorgestrel implants (Norplant)	0.09	0.09
Depot-medroxyprogesterone acetate (Depo-Provera)	0.3	0.3
Condom without spermicides		
Female	5	21
Male	3	12
Periodic abstinence (all methods)	1–9	20
Female sterilization	0.4	0.4
Male sterilization	0.10	0.15

Adapted from Hatcher RA, Trussell J, Stewart F, et al: Contraceptive Technology, 16th revised ed. New York, Irvington, 1994.

Efficacy

The efficacy of different methods of contraception varies. Hormonal methods are the most effective reversible methods of contraception, with failure rates in the < 1–3% range (Table 5). Male condoms have a 12% failure rate in typical use when all ages are considered. It is likely, though, that condoms have a higher failure rate in typical use by adolescents. The question—"Do you use condoms?"—does not capture usage patterns. The question should be phrased, "Do you use condoms 100% of the time?" However, it is difficult to gain accurate information because adolescents want the provider to think well of them, so they may answer "yes" even though that answer may be stretching the truth somewhat. Even for the hormonal methods, typical use failure rates do not adequately describe the most common problem among adolescents, which is discontinuation of the method. Nevertheless, it is important to stress to young women and their parents that when used consistently and correctly, many of the available contraceptive methods are highly effective.

Oral Contraceptive Pills

Oral contraceptive pills (OCPs) are the most frequently requested method of contraception, and for most teenagers they are the most accepted method. Usually, the indication for OCP prescription is pregnancy prevention, although OCPs are an effective treatment for a number of gynecologic disorders common in adolescent girls, including polycystic ovary syndrome, irregular menses, and severe dysmenorrhea, as well as acne, a skin disorder prevalent in this age group. It is important to consider the contraindications as well as the major and minor side effects of OCPs. Generally, OCPs are very safe when used by young women. The risk of serious side effects is negligible, so much so that there is consideration at a national level of making "the pill" an "over-the-counter" medication.

Counseling about Risks and Benefits

There is a lot of misunderstanding even among health care professionals about the risks and benefits of OCPs. Frequently, the risks are overemphasized. When counseling a patient about having an appendectomy, surgeons do not begin by telling her that an artery can be lacerated during surgery and she can bleed to death. Instead, the surgeon explains why it is important that she have her appendix removed. The surgeon reassures the patient about the safety of the procedure and, lastly, discusses the complications. Unfortunately, when health care providers counsel about oral contraceptives, they often begin with all of the negatives, including all of the risks. This approach is frightening to a teenager who has no way of putting the information into an appropriate perspective. It is preferable to start by counseling about the efficacy of OCPs, which is very high, and the benefits, which are considerable for young women. Lastly, discuss the risks, putting them into perspective by comparing them with the risks of pregnancy and childbirth. It is important that a realistic balance of benefits and risks emerges so that the young woman walks away with a sense that OCPs are a safe and effective method of birth control that will also do a number of good things for her, even though there are some risks.

Noncontraceptive Benefits

The noncontraceptive benefits of oral contraceptives are substantial and important, including a 40% reduced risk of developing ovarian cancer and a 50% reduced risk of developing endometrial cancer later in life (Table 6). Young women who have a family history of ovarian cancer in first-degree relatives should seriously consider using OCPs. These data are unequivocal and have been reproduced in every major controlled clinical trial. The prevailing opinion about breast cancer and oral contraceptive use is that, most likely, there is no effect on the future risk of breast cancer and no reason to withhold OCPs from girls with a family history of breast cancer. Benign breast disease is reduced by about 30–60%. OCPs also reduce the risk of developing ovarian cysts and decrease menstrual symptoms, including menorrhagia and dysmenorrhea.

TABLE 6. Noncontraceptive Benefits of Hormonal Contraceptives

Protection Against	OCs*	Depo-Provera	Norplant
Acne	++	–	–
Anemia	++	++	+
Dysmenorrhea	++	++	+
Ovarian cysts	+	+	–
Breast cysts	+	?	–
Hirsutism	++	–	–
Pelvic inflammatory disease	++	++	+/–
Ectopic pregnancy	++	++	+
Sickle cell crisis	+/–	+	?
Ovarian cancer	+	?	–
Endometrial cancer	++	++	–

* Combined oral contraceptive pills containing ethinyl estradiol and desogestrel or norgestimate.

TABLE 7. Contraindications to Oral Contraceptive Use

- Undiagnosed vaginal bleeding
- History of thrombophlebitis or pulmonary embolism
- Hypercoagulable state
- Known or suspected pregnancy

Iron deficiency anemia is rare in women taking OCPs because of reduced menstrual blood flow. Risk of ectopic pregnancy is reduced by 99%. The risk of developing acute salpingitis or pelvic inflammatory disease, the leading cause of acquired infertility in women, is significantly reduced if the contraceptive pill is taken for 6 months or longer. This protection is a major benefit for adolescent and young women who have high rates of STDs.

CONTRAINDICATIONS

There are several contraindications to the use of OCPs. Undiagnosed vaginal bleeding is always listed as a contraindication (Table 7). This does not mean that the pill should not be used for management of dysfunctional uterine bleeding; it is the treatment of choice for this condition in adolescents. It just means that efforts must be made to exclude trauma, infection, ectopic pregnancy, or some other cause for the bleeding. Any history of thrombophlebitis or pulmonary embolism is a contraindication to OCP use, and such conditions do occur, albeit rarely, in adolescents. Similarly, any girl with a condition potentially associated with a hypercoagulable state such as systemic lupus erythematosus or antithrombin-III deficiency should not take OCPs. Although known or suspected pregnancy is a contraindication to OCP use, if a mistake is made and the patient does take OCPs during early pregnancy, there is essentially no risk to the fetus. Active liver disease is also a contraindication to OCP use, but a history of hepatitis in the past is not, so long as liver function tests are normal. Medications that induce hepatic microsomal enzymes, such as phenobarbital or rifampin, cause accelerated metabolism of the estrogen component of OCPs, thus lowering the effective dose. For girls taking such medications, the pill is not contraindicated, but it is much less likely to be effective in preventing pregnancy and is not a good contraceptive choice.

MORTALITY RISK

The number of deaths associated with control of fertility increases in a continuous line with age. Thus, the emphasis in counseling adolescents should be on the difference between the mortality risk in young women and older women. Among adolescents aged 15–19 years who are not using any method of birth control, 7/100,000 will die of complications related to pregnancy or childbirth as compared with 28/100,000 women aged 40–44 years (Table 8). Compare these death rates with the mortality rate in nonsmoking 15–19-year-old OCP users, which is 0.3/100,000, 23 times less. It is important to emphasize also that the mortality rate for 15–19-year-old smokers who take OCPs only rises to 2.2/100,000, which is still much less than the risk of death from pregnancy for this age group. Thus, smoking is not a contraindication to OCP use in adolescent girls. Of course, girls who smoke should be counseled to quit; it really is bad for their health! So if an adolescent patient is concerned that she

TABLE 8. Annual Number of Deaths Associated with Control of Fertility per 100,000 Nonsterile Women, by Fertility Control Method

Method of Control and Outcome	15–19	20–24	35–39	40–44
No fertility control methods*	7.0	7.4	25.7	28.2
Oral contraceptives, nonsmoker†	0.3	0.5	13.8	31.6
Oral contraceptives, smoker†	2.2	3.4	51.1	117.2
Intrauterine device†	0.8	0.8	1.4	1.4
Condom*	1.1	1.6	0.3	0.4
Diaphragm/spermicide*	1.9	1.2	2.2	2.8
Periodic abstinence*	2.5	1.6	2.9	3.6

* Deaths birth-related.
† Deaths method-related.
Adapted from Ory HW: Mortality associated with fertility and fertility control. Fam Plann Perspect 15:57–63, 1983.

might die from taking the pill, one can reassure her and inform her that she is much more likely to die if she is not using any contraception. In fact, she is more likely to die if she is sexually active and uses condoms or a diaphragm for contraception because they are less effective contraceptives and the risk of death from pregnancy-related complications is higher.

Side Effects

In practical terms, the biggest problem with adolescents' use of OCPs is not mortality but side effects. Common side effects include nausea, breast tenderness, breakthrough bleeding, and light menstrual flow (Table 9). The first three usually disappear after a few months of pill use, if the adolescent can be convinced to continue taking the pills. However, these "nuisance" side effects are among the main reasons adolescents give for discontinuing OCPs. Smoking is associated with a higher incidence of breakthrough bleeding while taking OCPs, so compliance with pill use may be particularly poor in adolescents who smoke. Light menstrual flow is usually considered a benefit, especially if the girls are counseled to expect a lighter flow. Many adolescents are absolutely convinced that they will gain weight on the pill. However, controlled studies with low-dose combination OCPs indicate no effect of pills on weight. Just as many women lose weight as gain weight while on OCPs, and the changes are related to diet, exercise, and other factors, not the medication. Uncommon pill side effects include amenorrhea and depression. When amenorrhea occurs, girls may become anxious about the possibility of pregnancy. When there has

TABLE 9. Side Effects of Oral Contraceptive Pills

Common	Uncommon	Rare*
Nausea	Amenorrhea	Hypertension
Breakthrough bleeding	Depression	Thrombophlebitis
Light menstrual flow		Pulmonary embolism
		Myocardial infarction

* More likely to occur in pregnant adolescents.

been noncompliance or when the patient has been taking another medication that can interfere with the metabolism of the hormones, a pregnancy test should be done. Otherwise, pill-related amenorrhea is easily treated with estrogen supplementation. If a young woman becomes clinically depressed, one should be aware that the pill may be etiologically related and consider discontinuation. Serious side effects of OCP use, including hypertension, thrombophlebitis, pulmonary embolism, and myocardial infarction, are exceedingly rare in the adolescent age range. Pregnancy, of course, is associated with high risk for the first three of these serious conditions. New studies on gallbladder disease and OCPs indicate that low-dose combination pills are not associated with an increased incidence of gallstones; however, pregnancy is a major risk factor for gallstones in adolescence. Clinicians clearly have a vital role to play in helping adolescent girls and their parents to put the risks and side effects of OCPs into appropriate perspective. That perspective is achieved most effectively when the health care provider takes a few moments to elicit the preexisting knowledge and to listen to the concerns expressed by patients.

Pelvic Examinations and OCPs

The Food and Drug Administration (FDA) recently made an important change regarding prescription of OCPs. It is now acceptable to prescribe birth control pills to a woman of any age *before* she has had a pelvic examination, but after a careful medical history and general physical examination to rule out any contraindications to pill use. This change is of great benefit to teenagers because, all too often, fear of the first pelvic examination stops them from seeking or receiving appropriate contraceptive care. Now when a young patient who is contemplating sexual activity says, "I can't stay today to have the pelvic, but I really want to go on the pill," the clinician can prescribe OCPs and have her come back later for the pelvic examination. For adolescents who are apprehensive about the gynecologic examination, clinicians can spend some time building a relationship with the patient and describing the process of the examination. They can start a teenager on the pill and have her return at a later time when she will be more prepared to undergo the examination process. Meanwhile, she will be protected from unintended pregnancy. Primary care providers who are not doing office gynecology themselves still can take a sexual history, determine the need for contraception, do a general physical examination, and prescribe OCPs. Then they can refer the patient to an adolescent medicine specialist or gynecologist for the pelvic examination.

Choosing an Oral Contraceptive Pill

Many different brands of OCPs are on the market, but there is very little difference among them in clinical practice (Table 10). Generally, it is sufficient to become familiar with three or four brands of low-dose combination OCPs to use in most situations. One important difference is whether the pills are in a triphasic formulation, which has three different progestin doses over the month, or a monophasic formulation, which contains the same hormone dose in all pills. The theoretical advantage of the triphasics is that the total

TABLE 10. Selected Examples of Combination Oral Contraceptive Pills

Brand Name	Estrogen	Progestin
Alesse	Ethinyl estradiol, 20 μg	Levonorgestrel, 0.1 mg
Desogen, Ortho-Cept	Ethinyl estradiol, 35μg	Desogestrel, 0.15 mg
Loestrin 1.5/30	Ethinyl estradiol, 30 μg	Norethindrone acetate, 1.5 mg
Lo/Ovral	Ethinyl estradiol, 30 μg	Norgestrel, 0.3 mg
Norinyl, Ortho-Novum	Ethinyl estradiol, 35 μg	Norethindrone, 1 mg
Ortho-Cyclen	Ethinyl estradiol, 35 μg	Norgestimate, 0.25 mg
Ortho Tri-Cyclen	Ethinyl estradiol, 35 μg	Norgestimate, 0.18–0.215–0.25 mg
Tri-Levlen, Triphasil	Ethinyl estradiol 30–40–30 μg	Levonorgestrel, 0.05–0.075–0.125 mg

monthly dose of progestin is slightly lower than in monophasic pills, whereas the estrogen dose is similar. However, differences are too small to be clinically significant. Some adolescents are confused by the different colors of pills in the triphasic packs and show better compliance with a monophasic formulation.

New Progestin Pills

A recent new development in OCPs has been the approval by the FDA of two new progestational agents, norgestimate and desogestrel, as components of low-dose combination pills. These third-generation progestins are more selective for the progesterone receptor and have less affinity for the androgen receptor than first- and second-generation progestins such as levonorgestrel and norethindrone. Thus combination pills containing the new progestins may have fewer androgenic side effects such as acne, hair loss, and atherogenic lipid changes. Indeed, one of the new progestin pills, Ortho Tri-Cyclen, has been approved by the FDA for treatment of acne, the first approved noncontraceptive indication for an OCP. These new progestin pills are indicated for adolescents with acne, hyperandrogenic states (e.g., polycystic ovary syndrome), dyslipidemias, as well as those with diabetes mellitus who are at increased risk of atherosclerosis. Most low-dose combination pills contain the same estrogen, ethinyl estradiol, in doses of 30 or 35 μg. However, there are 20-μg ethinyl estradiol pills for use when lower doses of estrogen are indicated. The progestin-only pill is not recommended for adolescents because it has a higher failure rate than combination pills, and a progestin-only injectable that is highly effective is now available for those patients who cannot tolerate estrogen. An excellent reference for more detail about all types of contraceptives is the book *Contraceptive Technology*.[12]

Use of OCPs as Emergency Contraception

In 1997, the FDA approved certain OCPs for emergency or postcoital contraceptive use (Table 11). Pills must be taken within 72 hours of unprotected intercourse. Used in this manner, emergency contraceptive pills reduce risk of pregnancy by 75%. Emergency contraception is indicated under conditions of rape or forced sex, when condoms break, when a regular OCP user misses two or more pills, or simply when sex was unplanned and protection was not used. Counseling about the availability of emergency contraception should be given

TABLE 11. Emergency Contraceptive Pills

Product	Dose
Ovral	2 tablets now, then 2 tablets in 12 hours
Lo/Ovral, Nordette, or Levlen	4 tables now, then 4 tablets in 12 hours
Triphasil or Tri-Levlen (yellow tablets only)	4 tablets now, then 4 tablets in 12 hours
Levonorgestrel 0.75 mg	1 tablet now, then 1 tablet in 12 hours

to all adolescents whether or not they are sexually active. Many girls do not use contraception the first time they have sex. These girls can benefit from emergency contraception if they know about it. Some providers prescribe a package of pills for girls to keep on hand and use in the event that they experience an unprotected sexual event. A prepackaged kit, PREVEN®, is available containing instruction, a home pregnancy test, and 4 tablets containing a total of 200 μg of ethinyl estradiol and 2 mg of norgestrel. In 1999, a progestin-only emergency contraceptive pill was approved by the FDA. It contains levonorgestrel 0.75 mg and is marketed under the brand name Plan B. Progestin-only emergency contraception is as effective as older regimens with less nausea reported by users.

Depot-Medroxyprogesterone Acetate

The long-acting, progestin-only, injectable contraceptive, depot-medroxyprogesterone acetate (DMPA, Depo-Provera, "the shot") is an excellent choice for some adolescents and young women. Like oral contraceptive pills, DMPA inhibits ovulation. After a 150-mg contraceptive injection, ovulation is suppressed for at least 12 weeks. DMPA also causes thickening of the cervical mucus, thus decreasing sperm penetration. DMPA is a highly effective method with pregnancy rates below 1% per year. Return to fertility after discontinuing DMPA may be slower than with other hormonal contraceptives. However, full fertility is restored within a year of stopping the medication. This delayed return to fertility may actually be a benefit for adolescents who rarely discontinue a method in order to plan a pregnancy.

Noncontraceptive Benefits

Like OCPs, DMPA has a number of important benefits besides contraception. Protection from endometrial cancer is similar to that seen with the pill, and it is likely that DMPA provides protection from ovarian cancer as well. Although this drug was initially kept out of the U.S. market because of worry that it might cause breast cancer, recent large studies have put that fear to rest. Because of decreased menstrual flow, risk of iron deficiency anemia is considerably reduced. DMPA is also associated with decreased risk of pelvic inflammatory disease and thus helps to protect the fertility of adolescents. This contraceptive method is good for girls with certain chronic illnesses. DMPA has been shown to decrease the number and frequency of crises in sickle cell disease and is the contraceptive of choice in this condition. Also it is an excellent method to use for girls with seizure disorders who may be taking medication that reduces the efficacy of OCPs because of the accelerated hepatic metabolism of estrogen. DMPA itself has anticonvulsant properties and is well tolerated by young women with epilepsy.

Menstrual Changes

With continued use of DMPA, the endometrium becomes atrophic, so many users develop amenorrhea. Amenorrhea is reported by 57% of DMPA users at the end of 1 year and 68% after two years. Initially, however, irregular bleeding and spotting are common. Heavy bleeding may occur, although rarely. The regular menstrual cycle is disrupted in virtually all DMPA users. It is extremely important to spend time counseling adolescent patients about these menstrual changes before the first injection. If not prepared, many girls will become anxious and think that there is something wrong with them. They should be told about the possibility that they will stop having periods. It also should be emphasized that not having periods while on "the shot" does not indicate pregnancy and is not dangerous to health. Exploring what the patient believes about the meaning and function of menstruation and correcting misapprehensions are important parts of counseling. It is also important to discuss the positive effects of amenorrhea with the patient; most girls experience amenorrhea as a benefit of DMPA once they are reassured. However, adolescent patients do not tolerate excessive bleeding well. If heavy bleeding does occur, rapid treatment helps to prevent discontinuation of the method. The provider should keep in mind that excessive bleeding while using DMPA is often associated with STDs, particularly chlamydia infection, which must be diagnosed and treated. Once infection is excluded, bleeding can be managed with nonsteroidal antiinflammatory drugs (e.g., ibuprofen, naproxen sodium) or with the addition of a low-dose estrogen pill (e.g., 0.975 mg of conjugated estrogens or low-dose combination OCPs) for a week or two.

Side Effects

Besides irregular menstrual bleeding, which is not a side effect but an expected result of DMPA contraception, weight gain is the problem that causes the most distress for patients. Although not all patients gain weight, many do; the average gain is about 5 pounds in the first year with a subsequent 3-pound annual weight gain. The mechanism of the weight gain is via appetite stimulation related to the androgenic effects of the progestin. Thus, counseling patients to monitor their eating behavior after starting Depo-Provera and to make appropriate diet modifications as necessary is important. Occasionally, an adolescent gains weight very rapidly after DMPA injection, and this is a valid reason to discontinue the method. Other androgen-related side effects such as alopecia and worsening of acne are less common but do occur.

One potential side effect of DMPA that is worrisome for the adolescent age group is osteopenia. The medication causes profound hypothalamic suppression with resultant ovarian suppression leading to a relative estrogen deficiency. Estrogen levels in DMPA users are in the lower end of the range for the follicular phase of the menstrual cycle. Under such conditions of low estrogen secretion, mineralization of bones may be suboptimal. Some studies in adult women have documented mild osteopenia with DMPA use that is reversible upon discontinuation of the method. However, as adolescence is the period when peak bone mineralization takes place, there is concern that long-term DMPA use at this critical time may have irreversible effects. Part of the dietary counseling of adolescent DMPA users should focus on ensuring that they consume enough calcium-rich foods and/or take a calcium supplement. Investigations are currently underway to determine the long-term significance of this potential osteopenic effect and whether interventions such as adding back small doses of estrogen may be useful.

Initiating DMPA Use

Almost all pregnancies that occur in patients using DMPA are diagnosed shortly after beginning the medication because the patient was pregnant at the time of her first injection. Providers must be very careful to rule out existing pregnancy before injecting the first dose and before any subsequent dose injected more than 14 weeks after the previous one. In general, the initial dose of Depo-Provera should be given during a menstrual period and after a sensitive pregnancy test performed on the same day is negative. The medication can also be injected immediately after a termination of pregnancy and after childbirth, even if the mother is breast feeding. Patients should be scheduled to return for subsequent injections every 12–13 weeks. If a patient has gone more than 14 weeks since her last injection and has a negative pregnancy test, she can be placed on OCPs for two weeks, retested for pregnancy and, if negative, injected with DMPA. This regimen ensures that the injection is not given during the two-week window of time after fertilization but before the pregnancy test is positive.

Levonorgestrel Implants

Levonorgestrel implants (Norplant System) is a long-acting, progestin-only, highly effective, reversible contraceptive method. It is consists of six silastic capsules containing levonorgestrel that are implanted in a fan-like pattern under the skin of the upper arm. In most patients they are not visible, but they are palpable. The progestin slowly leaches out of the capsules, and, when insertion is done at the time of active menstrual bleeding, the contraceptive effect begins after 24 hours and lasts for 5 years. Norplant is highly effective with a failure rate of less than 0.5%, comparable to failure rates of tubal ligation. Continuation rates in the adolescent age group are higher than with other contraceptive methods. Norplant is the only contraceptive method that has been shown to effectively prevent second pregnancies in adolescent mothers because the young women are less likely to discontinue the method. Studies in adult women report continuation rates of 85% in the first year and at least 50% after three years. The fact that this method cannot be discontinued without surgically removing the capsules is a major advantage for adolescents. The need for surgical removal is also one of the disadvantages of this method; sometimes removal can be difficult, particularly if the capsules have been implanted too deeply under the skin. When the capsules are removed, return to full fertility is immediate. Other disadvantages of the method include the high initial cost and the insertion procedure, which frightens many adolescents.

The mechanism of contraceptive action of Norplant is different from that of DMPA. Unlike suppression of ovulation with OCPs and DMPA, suppression with

Norplant is variable. Especially in the later years of use, many women using Norplant ovulate regularly and have regular menstrual periods but still are protected from pregnancy. Norplant causes thickening of the cervical mucus, thus impeding sperm migration, and fosters changes in the endometrium that make it less receptive to implantation of a fertilized ovum. Because ovulation occurs with this method, there is some risk of developing ovarian cysts or ectopic pregnancy, whereas with OCPs and DMPA these risks are virtually nonexistent.

Noncontraceptive Benefits

Noncontraceptive benefits of Norplant are not as numerous as those with OCPs and DMPA. Reduction in risk of gynecologic cancers, salpingitis, acne, and ovarian cysts is less likely with this method because of the variable suppression of the hypothalamic–pituitary–ovarian axis. Norplant use is associated with a decrease in dysmenorrhea. Estrogen levels remain relatively normal, and risk of developing osteopenia or osteoporosis is much less of a concern with this method than with DMPA.

Menstrual Changes

The effect of Norplant on menstrual patterns is variable. However, the majority of women who use Norplant have a change in their menstrual cycle. Unlike with DMPA, the change is less likely to be a decrease in menstrual frequency or flow and more likely to be breakthrough bleeding or excess bleeding. In the first year of Norplant use, 28% of women have prolonged bleeding, 9% have amenorrhea, and 15% have irregular or frequent onset of bleeding. Adolescents may be more likely than adult women to experience amenorrhea during the first year after implantation. The frequent irregular bleeding common in the first year of Norplant use is less well tolerated by adolescents than the amenorrhea that more often occurs with DMPA use.

Side Effects

Weight gain in the range of 1–2 pounds per year may be associated with Norplant. As with DMPA, this gain is related to appetite stimulation by the anabolic effect of the progestin. Some adolescents using Norplant complain about emotional changes related to this contraceptive method, and it is recommended that Norplant be removed if clinically significant depression occurs. Alterations in serum lipids do occur with Norplant, but the clinical significance is unknown. Total cholesterol levels are decreased, and clinical trials have reported both increases and decreases in HDL-cholesterol levels. Another potential disadvantage of Norplant is that because it lasts for 5 years, adolescents may be less likely to return for follow-up Pap smears and STD screening. However, the few published studies indicate that follow-up rates were not different between OCP and Norplant users or between adult and adolescent Norplant users. Unfortunately, follow-up rates were poor in all contraceptive users studied.

Barrier Contraception

Barrier methods of contraception, particularly male condoms, have an important role to play in pregnancy prevention because of their role in reducing

STD transmission. However, the likelihood of less than 100% compliance, with substantial unintended pregnancy rates must be considered when these methods are used alone. Available methods include male and female condoms, diaphragm, and cervical cap.

Over 100 different types of male condoms are available, including those made of latex, polyurethane, and skin. Pregnancy rates for consistent and correct condom use are as low as 2%, with a range from 12–30% for typical use. Latex condoms reduce the risk of transmission of human immunodeficiency virus (HIV), herpes simplex virus (HSV), hepatitis B virus (HBV), cytomegalovirus, *Chlamydia trachomatis,* and *Neisseria gonorrhoeae*. Natural skin condoms are not as effective barriers to virus transmission as are latex condoms and are not recommended for protection against HIV. Polyurethane condoms have not yet been sufficiently tested to determine efficacy, but indications are that they may slip or break more readily than latex condoms. Condoms are inexpensive, easily available, safe, and effective if used with every sexual act. Latex condoms rarely cause allergy, and for those patients who experience allergy, polyurethane condoms can be used. Important points to be made in counseling adolescents about condom use are (1) use a condom with every sexual act, (2) roll the condom onto the erect penis leaving a space at the tip to collect sperm, and (3) remove the penis from the vagina while still erect and while holding the base of the condom (Table 12). In addition, it is important to remind adolescents that oil-based lubricants and storage in hot environments cause latex condoms to weaken and deteriorate.

The female condom has been available since 1994 and consists of a polyurethane sheath connected by an inner and outer ring. The inner ring is closed and is inserted into the vagina to be held in place against the pubic bone. The outer ring is open and extends onto the vulva. The female condom protects the external genitalia as well as the vagina and cervix and can be inserted up to 8 hours before use. The pregnancy rate for consistent and correct use of the female condom is 5%, with a range from 18–25% for typical use. Disadvantages include a relatively high cost ($3.00 each versus $1.00 each for male condoms) and the visible outer ring, which may not be appealing to the partner.

Diaphragms and cervical caps are molded rubber cups that must be fitted by a health care provider. The diaphragm fits over the cervix and anterior wall of the vagina, whereas the cervical cap is smaller and fits only over the cervix. Pregnancy rates for consistent and correct use are about 6%, with typical-use failure rates for the diaphragm ranging from 16–18%. Many adolescents find these methods difficult to use, and they have few advantages over the male or female condom. Diaphragms and cervical caps are contraindicated in patients

TABLE 12. Instructions for Correct Condom Use

1. Use a new condom with each intercourse.
2. Avoid damage by fingernails or teeth.
3. Put on erect penis before any genital contact with partner.
4. Ensure that no air is trapped in the tip.
5. Ensure adequate lubrication during intercourse.
6. Use only water-based lubricants.
7. Hold condom and withdraw while penis is still erect.

with a history of toxic shock syndrome or allergy to latex or spermicidal agents. Use of the diaphragm for contraception is associated with recurrent urinary tract infections.

The challenge to health care providers working with adolescent girls is to address the myriad difficulties associated with use of a coitus-dependent contraceptive method. Most providers recommend the use of male condoms to protect against STDs even when the young woman is also using a hormonal method of contraception. Providers should counsel girls about correct condom use and help them to think about how they might negotiate condom use with their partners. Adolescents are more likely to use condoms if they receive comprehensive sexuality education, talk about STDs with their partners, believe that condoms can prevent HIV infection, perceive peer support for condom use, have discussed condom use with a clinician, and have easy access to condoms.

CONCLUSION

Adolescents in our culture receive mixed messages from adults, who often are highly critical of teenage behavior. But consider what young people are exposed to in magazines, newspapers, television, and movies. Explicit sexuality is everywhere, and pregnancy or contraception is rarely addressed. There seem to be few unhealthy consequences of sexual activity portrayed by the media. Health care providers try to provide more realistic sexuality and contraceptive education, but patients are exposed every day to the influence of the media while health care visits may occur only once or twice a year. Nevertheless, despite the limited opportunities, the health care provider can have a disproportionate influence on adolescent patients if they believe in the provider's expertise and trust that he or she has their best interests at heart.

SUGGESTED READING

1. Allan Guttmacher Institute: Sex and America's Teenagers. New York, Allan Guttmacher Institute, 1994.
2. Berenson AB, Weimann CM: Patient satisfaction and side effects with levonorgestrel implant (Norplant) use in adolescents 18 years of age or younger. Pediatrics 92:257–260, 1993.
3. Centers for Disease Control and Prevention: Update: Barrier protection against HIV infection and other sexually transmitted diseases. MMWR 42:589–591, 1993.
4. Centers for Disease Control and Prevention: Youth Risk Behavior Surveillance—United States, 1995. MMWR 45:1, 1996.
5. Collins DC: Sex hormone receptor binding, progestin selectivity and new oral contraceptives. Am J Obstet Gynecol 170:1508–1513, 1994.
6. Committee on Adolescent Health Care: Safety of oral contraceptives for teenagers. ACOG Committee Opinion, 1991.
7. Coupey SM: Improving contraceptive compliance in your adolescent patient. Dialogues in Contraception 3:6–9, 1991.
8. Cromer BA, Smith RD, Blair JM, et al: A prospective study of adolescents who choose among levonorgestrel implant (Norplant), medroxyprogesterone acetate (Depo-Provera), or the combined oral contraceptive pill as contraception. Pediatrics 94:687–694, 1994.
9. Cundy T, Evans M, Roberts H, et al: Bone density in women receiving Depo medroxyprogesterone acetate for contraception. BMJ 303:13–16, 1991.
10. Gold MA, Coupey SM: Young women's attitudes towards new contraceptive methods. J Pediatr Adolesc Gynecol 11:17–24, 1998.

11. Grimes DA, Wallach M (eds): Modern Contraception. Totowa, NJ, Emron, 1997.
12. Hatcher RA, Trussell J, Stewart F, et al: Contraceptive Technology, 16th revised ed. New York, Irvington, 1994.
13. Neal W, Coupey SM: New contraceptive options for adolescents. Compr Ther 24:439–445, 1997.
14. Polaneczky M, Slap G, Forke C, et al: The use of levonorgestrel implants (Norplant) for contraception in adolescent mothers. N Engl J Med 331:1201–1206, 1994.
15. Redmond GP, Olson WH, Lippman JS, et al: Norgestimate and ethinyl estradiol in the treatment of acne vulgaris: A randomized placebo controlled trial. Am J Obstet Gynecol 89:615–622, 1997.
16. Trussell J, Leveque J, Koenig J, et al: The economic value of contraception: A comparison of 15 methods. Am J Public Health 85:494–503, 1995.

CHAPTER 14

Overweight, Underweight, and Dieting

Ann L. Engelland, M.D.

Issues related to weight are a part of nearly every adolescent's life. Clinical experience shows that for many, these concerns are paramount. A 1996 survey[1] of 9- and 10-year-old American girls showed that as many as 40% of them are already, at this young age, "trying to lose weight." Even though a recent study suggested that in the older adolescent, the prevalence of problematic eating, dieting, and body image–related behavior may have begun to abate,[2] nearly two-thirds of girls continued to report body dissatisfaction and a desire to lose weight. In a 1997 survey of New York metropolitan girls, aged 10–19 years, almost all were concerned about their weight, now or in the future.[3]

Table 1 illustrates a useful paradigm for thinking about adolescent weight issues. Adolescents may be of "normal" weight, overweight, or underweight. In the course of evaluating each patient, it is useful to define her weight status objectively, then to define her weight status according to her own perception, and finally to get a picture of whether she is a dieter or not.

Throughout this chapter, ten girls are portrayed who exemplify the three weight categories and and typical perceptions about weight and dieting status. Their fictitious names and probable diagnoses are listed on the right side of Table 1. The vast majority of adolescent girls are of normal weight. However, *many normal-weight adolescents like Betty and Norma present with unusual eating habits*—sometimes merely unwise, but sometimes unhealthy, imprudent, or even dangerous.

In this discussion, overweight girls are divided into *obese* and *fat* categories. *Obese girls* are overweight according to accepted, objective, medical standards, and *fat girls* think of themselves as overweight and/or perceive themselves as fat *whether they are or not according to objective measures or opinions*. Adolescent behavior, which exposes them to high risk that will dictate different medical approaches to management, hinges upon their own subjective perceptions as much as on any objective measurement of weight status. For this reason this chapter devotes special attention to the *fat* girls exemplified by Rachel and Terry.

TABLE 1. A Paradigm for Understanding Adolescent Weight Issues

Weight Status		Dieting (+/–) Example from Text	Diagnosis
Normal weight		+ Betty	Vegetarian
		– Norma	Imprudent
Overweight	Objectively "obese"	+ Sandra	Exogenous obesity
		– Roxanne	Exogenous obesity, possibly depressed
	Subjectively "fat"	+ Rachel	Inappropriate dieting
		– Terry	Possibly depressed
Underweight	Weight loss	+ Anna	Anorexia
		– Doreen	Hyperthyroid
	No weight loss	+ Olga	At risk for anorexia nervosa, amenorrhea
		– Cindy	"Skinny"

+ = dieter; – = nondieter.

The paradigm of Table 1 further subdivides girls into dieters and nondieters. In 1991, as many as 12% of Minnesota female adolescents were found to be chronic dieters.[4] Dieters span the gamut from emotionally healthy to pathologically eating-disordered. For purposes of this discussion, dieting is broadly defined as any attempt to restrict caloric intake, to narrow the range of foods, to exercise excessively, or to overuse medications. Dieters also include those observing a vegetarian regimen, who present other nutritional issues. Table 2 lists this range of dieting behaviors.

Finally, in an era of prevalent eating disorders, underweight girls also need to be screened for dieting behaviors. They may have experienced weight loss or failure to gain weight and may carry underlying medical or psychological diagnoses. Other underweight girls like Cindy are merely "skinny."

All adolescents deserve a good nutritional and psychological screen in order to sort out medical and psychological risk from benign adolescent behavior. In a busy clinical setting, there are seven major questions that the primary care provider needs to keep in mind when evaluating a patient from a nutritional point of view:

1. Is this young woman ***overweight***?
2. Is this young woman ***underweight***?
3. Is she ***dieting***? Is it warranted? Is it safe? Is it healthy?
4. Which ***medical issues*** cause concern?
5. Which ***psychological issues*** need consideration?
6. Are ***referrals*** to subspecialists necessary?
7. What ***advice*** can be given now?

DEFINING OVERWEIGHT

There are a number of methods for defining excess body fat (i.e., obesity). The American Medical Association's *Guidelines for Adolescent Preventive Services*[5] and other experts now recommend that the body mass index (BMI) is the most practical and reliable screening method in the clinical setting. BMI is a calculated number:

$$\text{BMI} = \frac{\text{weight (kg)}}{\text{height (meters)}^2}$$

This is highly correlated to skin-fold thickness, which remains the gold standard. Figure 1 shows the BMI for different heights and weights in feet and inches. This method translates cumbersome calculations from metric measurements. Once BMI is established from Figure 1, it can be plotted on Figure 2, which shows BMI for age and the ranges that define *overweight* and *at risk of overweight*. The key number to remember for defining overweight is a BMI over 27.

DEFINING UNDERWEIGHT

Excessive weight loss and underweight are usually defined as less than 85–90% of average weight for height. Standard growth charts such as Figure 3 reflect national data. For example, if a 14-year-old girl is 160 cm, her average weight is 110 pounds. So, if she weighs less than 100 pounds (110 – [110 × 0.9]) she is considered underweight. Of course, in addition to being impractical, this method does not take different body types and muscle mass into consideration. Nevertheless, it remains the standard most often quoted. An easier way of assessing underweight is to refer to BMI graphs (see Figs. 1 and 2). Simply stated, if BMI for age is less than 15%, the adolescent is at risk for being underweight. A BMI less than 18 needs investigation.

TAKING A DIET HISTORY

There are a number of techniques for gaining an objective assessment of diet. The 24-hour recall is the most commonly cited. However, even in an abridged format, it may not be practical for a busy clinician to administer, read, score, and evaluate such a questionnaire in the course of an office visit.

Following are nine categories of questions which form the backbone of a quick screening diet history of an adolescent: first, introduce the topic with something like, "I am going to ask you a few questions about your eating habits." As the girl responds, the provider is able to home in on her high-risk areas. The following are risk areas to keep in mind:

- Calcium
- Iron
- Calories
- Unhealthy habits (meal times, snacks, exercise, diets)
- Unhealthy foods (fat, "junk," artificial)
- Unhealthy body image or unrealistic expectations

	Stature m (in)																				
Weight kg (lb)	1.24 (49)	1.27 (50)	1.30 (51)	1.32 (52)	1.35 (53)	1.37 (54)	1.40 (55)	1.42 (56)	1.45 (57)	1.47 (58)	1.50 (59)	1.52 (60)	1.55 (61)	1.57 (62)	1.60 (63)	1.63 (64)	1.65 (65)	1.68 (66)	1.70 (67)	1.73 (68)	1.75 (69)
20 (45)	13	13	12	12	11	11	10	10	10	9	9	9	8								
23 (50)	15	14	13	13	12	12	12	11	11	10	10	10	9	9	9	9	8				
25 (55)	16	15	15	14	14	13	13	12	12	12	11	11	10	10	10	9	9	9			
27 (60)	18	17	16	16	15	15	14	13	13	13	12	12	11	11	11	10	10	10	9	9	
29 (65)	19	18	17	17	16	16	15	15	14	14	13	13	12	12	12	11	11	10	10	10	10
32 (70)	21	20	19	18	17	17	16	16	15	15	14	14	13	13	12	12	12	11	11	11	10
34 (75)	22	21	20	20	19	18	17	17	16	16	15	15	14	14	13	13	12	12	12	11	11
36 (80)	24	22	21	21	20	19	19	18	17	17	16	16	15	15	14	14	13	13	13	12	12
39 (85)	25	24	23	22	21	21	20	19	18	18	17	17	16	16	15	15	14	14	13	13	13
41 (90)	27	25	24	23	22	22	21	20	19	19	18	18	17	17	16	15	15	14	14	14	13
43 (95)	28	27	25	25	24	23	22	21	20	20	19	19	18	17	17	16	16	15	15	14	14
45 (100)	29	28	27	26	25	24	23	22	22	21	20	20	19	18	18	17	17	16	16	15	15
48 (105)	31	30	28	27	26	25	24	24	23	22	21	21	20	19	19	18	17	17	16	16	16
50 (110)	32	31	30	29	27	27	25	25	24	23	22	22	21	20	19	19	18	18	17	17	16
52 (115)	34	32	31	30	29	28	27	26	25	24	23	23	22	21	20	20	19	18	18	17	17
54 (120)	35	34	32	31	30	29	28	27	26	25	24	24	23	22	21	20	20	19	19	18	18
57 (125)	37	35	34	33	31	30	29	28	27	26	25	25	24	23	22	21	21	20	20	19	19
59 (130)	38	37	35	34	32	31	30	29	28	27	26	26	25	24	23	22	22	21	20	20	19
61 (135)	40	38	36	35	34	33	31	30	29	28	27	27	25	25	24	23	22	22	21	20	20
64 (140)	41	39	38	36	35	34	32	31	30	29	28	27	26	26	25	24	23	22	22	21	21
66 (145)	43	41	39	38	36	35	34	33	31	30	29	28	27	27	26	25	24	23	23	22	21
68 (150)	44	42	40	39	37	36	35	34	32	31	30	29	28	28	27	26	25	24	24	23	22
70 (155)	46	44	42	40	39	37	36	35	33	33	31	30	29	29	27	26	26	25	24	23	23
73 (160)	47	45	43	42	40	39	37	36	35	34	32	31	30	29	28	27	27	26	25	24	24
77 (170)	50	48	46	44	42	41	39	38	37	36	34	33	32	31	30	29	28	27	27	26	25
79 (175)		49	47	46	44	42	40	39	38	37	35	34	33	32	31	30	29	28	27	27	26
82 (180)		51	48	47	45	44	42	40	39	38	36	35	34	33	32	31	30	29	28	27	27
84 (185)			50	48	46	45	43	42	40	39	37	36	35	34	33	32	31	30	29	28	27
86 (190)				49	47	46	44	43	41	40	39	37	36	35	34	32	32	31	30	29	28
88 (195)				51	49	47	45	44	42	41	39	38	37	36	35	33	32	31	31	30	29

FIGURE 1. Body mass index for selected weight and stature.

1. "Did you eat breakfast today? Do you usually eat breakfast? Typically, what do you have? If you don't eat breakfast, what are the reasons?"

What you are looking for: There are many excuses for not eating breakfast. They range from not having time, to not feeling hungry, to bad habits. Poor family or personal organization, lack of education about the importance of energy for brain function, and poor appetite in the morning can all be addressed through this question.

2. "Do you drink milk? Do you eat cheese, pizza, yogurt, ice cream, calcium-fortified orange juice?"

What you are looking for: This question not only sorts out the girl who may have inadequate calcium intake, but also may be the first opportunity for her to describe what is easily recognizable as lactose intolerance. She may be open to suggestions about ways to increase the calcium in her diet. Recommend

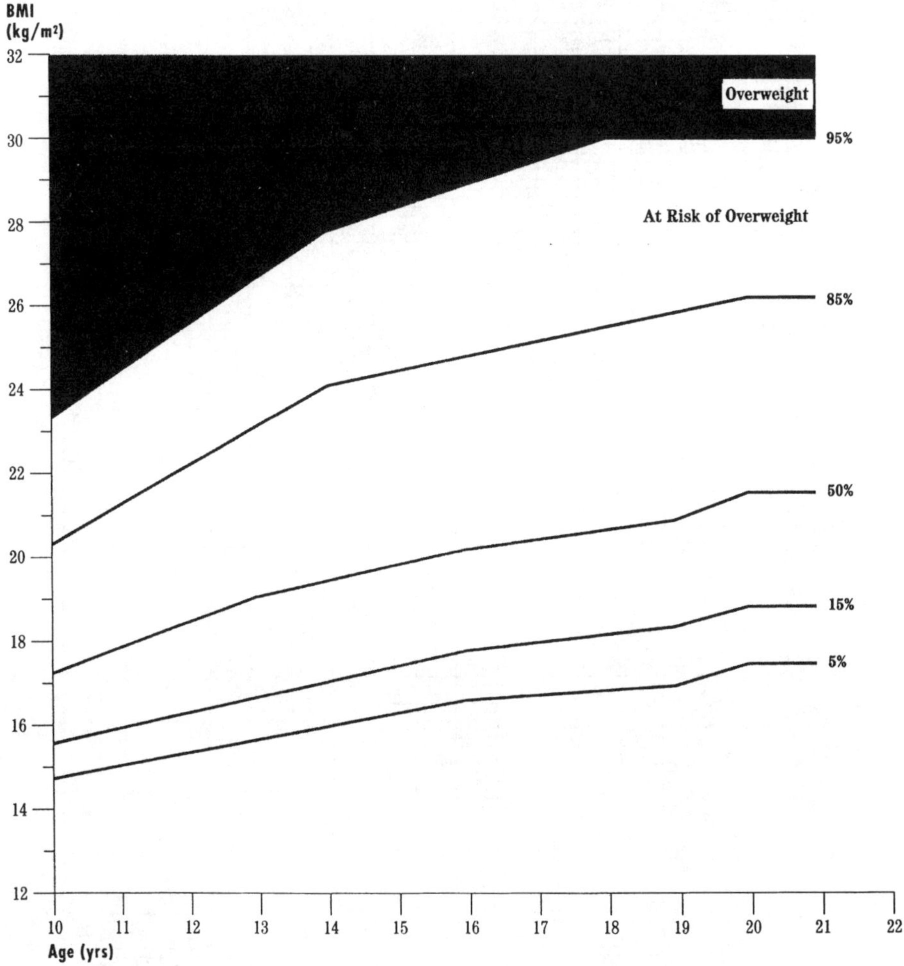

FIGURE 2. Height, weight and body mass index (BMI) by age (female).

Tums (4–5 per day), Lactaid milk, or lactase tablets if she is averse to dairy products.

3. "Do you eat red meat? Does that mean no pepperoni, no meat balls, no hamburgers? Do you eat chicken, fish, tuna, eggs, cheese?

What you are looking for: These questions discover the vegetarian. It is important to find out where on the spectrum of "vegetarian behavior" the girl is located. The more *restricted* she wishes to be, the more *educated* she needs to be. Adequate iron ingestion is important for menstruating teenagers. If they have no red meat in the diet, other sources should be sought (nuts, greens, eggs). Inquire about sources of information, cooperation from family, and length of time on the diet. Children who are committed to a strict vegetarian lifestyle may need a referral to a nutritionist.

4. "What do you drink when you are thirsty?" Assess for soda, milk, water.

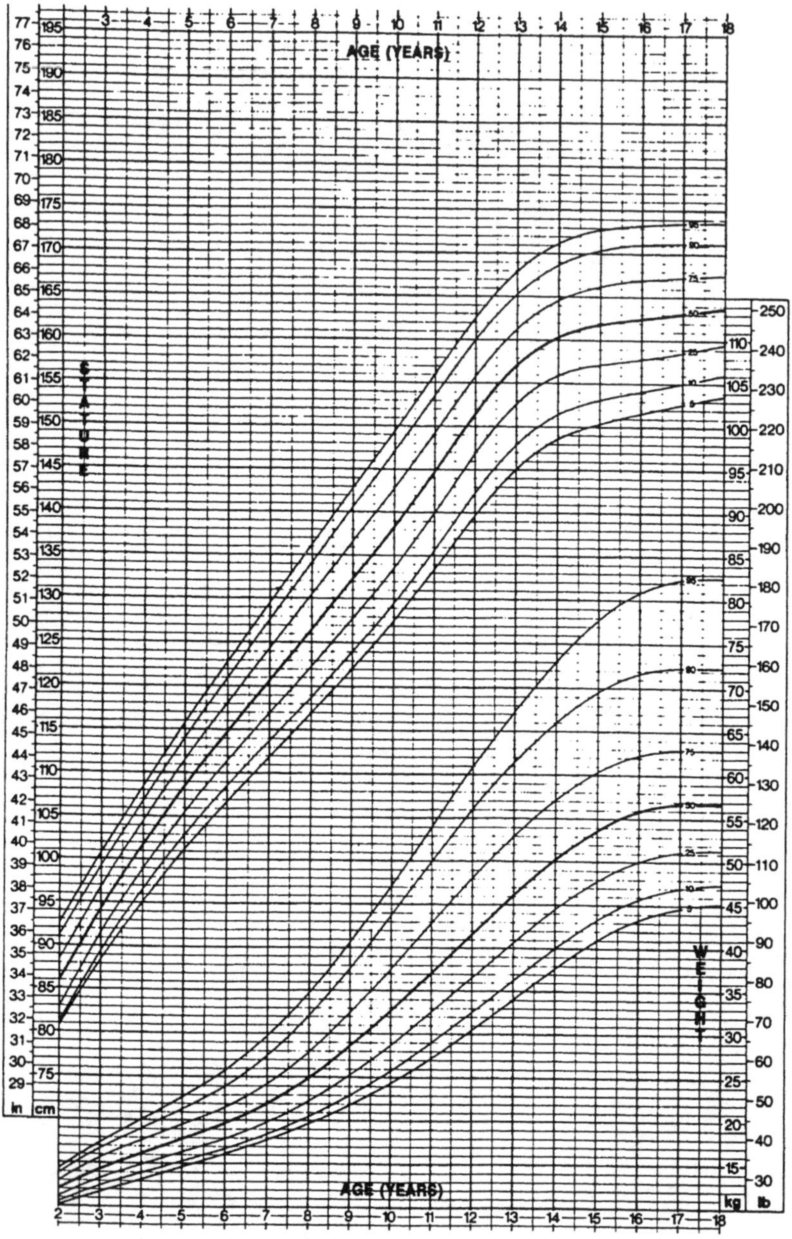

FIGURE 3. Growth chart for girls, 2–18 years of age. (From National Center for Health Statistics, NCHS growth charts, 1976, Monthly Vital Statistics Report 25(3), Suppl. (HRA) 76–1120. Rockville, MD, National Center for Health Statistics, 1976, with permission.)

What you are looking for: Excess calories. Children often quench their thirst with 400–500 calories a day. Watch also for artificial sweeteners, "junk" drinks, excess electrolyte-rich drinks. Point out the calories in orange juice, Gatorade, and other similar drinks.

5. "Tell me about snacks."

What you are looking for: Since snacking is often tantamount to small meals, encourage healthy and complete snacks. Discover if the girl's school schedule is too hectic to allow for meals, thereby promoting snacking behavior. Help her to adjust the food in her backpack to fill nutritional and hunger needs. Talk about "free foods," very low or calorie-free foods, which she can indulge in at any time (e.g., popcorn, Italian ice, pretzels, apples, water, tea, carrot sticks—she can generate her own list with a bit of help).

6. "How do you feel about your weight? Is weight an issue for you? Do you ever diet? What have you tried? Did it work?"

What you are looking for: If a girl has tried dieting, it is important to find out the goal of the diet, what other weight and appetite control measures have been tried (excess exercise, diet pills, starvation, liquid diets, Weight Watcher's, weight loss camps, health food store supplements). Family cooperation or resistance to dieting should be assessed. Whether allies or underminers of her efforts, they inevitably play a pivotal role. Some girls respond best to a referral to a nutritionist simply because they view the professional as an arbiter in conflict-laden family situations.

7. "You say you feel fat. What part of you feels fat? What part of you would you most like to change?"

What you are looking for: Girls who want to change their faces or "everything" are usually beyond the "norm" of adolescent body culture and may lack seriously in self-esteem. They may be experimenting in high-risk dieting techniques.

8. "What sports and exercise are you involved in?" Include dancing in front of the mirror, home exercise equipment, and walking to and from school.

What you are looking for: Encourage any amount of exercise. Screen for the extremes: the "couch potato" and the super athlete. The super athlete needs a screen for adequate calories, amenorrhea, stress fractures, eating-disorder–type thinking.

9. "Do you know what an eating disorder is? Do you know what anorexia nervosa and bulimia mean? "Do you know anyone who has these problems?"

What you are looking for: The answers to these questions will give you a glimpse at the sophistication of the girl, her sources of information, and her personal involvement with eating disorders. The answers may provide hints at her diagnosis.

THE ADOLESCENT OF NORMAL WEIGHT

Dieting

Betty, 14 years old, 5′2′′, 115 lbs., BMI 21 (normal for height and age), has been a lacto-ovovegetarian for 8 months. She is committed to continuing her diet, and her family has gone along with it. Her main source of iron is eggs. However, upon questioning it is clear that she has inadequate calcium in her diet.

Not Dieting

Norma, 17 years old, 5′9′′, 135 lbs., BMI 20 (Normal for height and age), has a stressful academic life. She has no time for breakfast and consumes, by her own admission, too much junk food, soda, and caffeine. She is active in soccer nearly all year round. She is not on any type of diet.

TABLE 2. Dieting Behavior

Restriction of calories
Restriction of range of foods (vegetarian, macrobiotic, lactose-free)
Excess exercise aimed at weight loss
Pharmacologic adjuncts (laxatives, diuretics, amphetamines)
Purging

No evaluation of an adolescent is complete without an exploration of dieting and eating behavior, even in an apparently healthy and normal-weight young woman. As defined in Table 2, dieting encompasses many different behaviors, some of which can be of potential risk to the patient. For instance, large numbers of adolescents experiment with vegetarian lifestyles and diets. They are motivated by a number of issues, ranging from ethical ones to a desire to lose weight. The more restricted these girls wish to be with respect to protein sources, the more they are at risk. The clinician should pay special attention to caloric intake, iron, calcium, and protein. Except in the most rigorous vegetarian, however, micronutrients (e.g., zinc, magnesium) are usually not a problem.

Vegetarians should be queried about motivation and support from other family members. Parents may undermine a girl's effort at a more healthful, vegetarian diet because they themselves lack information. On the other hand, the entire family usually can benefit from a reduction in meats and fats and more experimentation with grains, fruits, and vegetables. There are many on-line sources through the Internet and many books written especially for adolescents on becoming vegetarian.[6]

By late adolescence, many girls have decided that they are lactose-intolerant. They may think of themselves as allergic to milk based on limited, albeit unpleasant, experience. Some have completely eliminated dairy products, and therefore most calcium, from their diets. The clinician may suggest smaller aliquots of milk or milk products, recommend antacids containing calcium as a supplement, or prescribe lactase tablets with some written guidelines on how to use them.

Many normal-weight adolescents like Norma have hectic lifestyles, and they are notoriously erratic eaters. Fast food, high-fat food, and unusual mealtimes with an emphasis on snacks as important sources of calories characterize their habits. The wise clinician works with and around these habits rather than trying to make changes that fit a more adult model of eating. Suggesting salad pizza rather than cheese pizza, for instance, encourages healthier eating without altering lifestyle.

THE OVERWEIGHT ADOLESCENT

The Obese Adolescent

Dieting

Sandra, 18 years old, 5′6′′, 190 lbs., BMI 31 (overweight by all standards), has tried dieting off and on for 3 years or so. Her weight ping-pongs. Most recently she has tried Weight Watchers and has lost 15 pounds in 4 months. Her mother, who is also overweight, is supportive and is on a diet with her. Sandra has realistic goals and is optimistic about her prospects.

Not Dieting

Roxanne, 14 years old, 5′4′′, 175 lbs., BMI 30 (overweight for age and height), is not active. Her hobbies include writing poetry and watching television. There is no exercise she enjoys because she is overweight. Although she has been overweight most of her life, it has become much worse in the past 3 years. She tried a diet once, but it did not work; she gained it all back. Because "weight problems run in the family," she is feeling discouraged.

Obese adolescents may present with medical issues. Obese children may be divided into two groups, those with endogenous obesity and those with exogenous obesity.[8] Those with exogenous obesity are the vast majority, and for reasons which are multifactorial they gain weight more readily and/or have an imbalance in caloric intake and expenditure. Table 3 shows the causes of endogenous obesity. All are rare but often require complex management for associated problems. Almost all are associated with growth failure and thus are easy to spot.

Every dieting, obese adolescent presents the clinician with a challenge. After taking a brief diet history as outlined above, the clinician needs to decide whether the girl's approach to weight loss is safe and healthy. Various methods of obesity management exist, including nutritional/dietary counseling, behavior modification, exercise, pharmacotherapy, and even surgery. However, few methods are successful in the long term if they exclude behavior modification. Group programs for adolescents such as Shapedown and Weight Watchers claim the greatest success. Most nutritionists now counsel moderation, food exchanges, and portion control. Much recent advice is based on the food pyramid of the United States Department of Agriculture. A version of it that has been modified for adolescents is shown in Figure 4.

The dieting, obese adolescent should be screened for cholesterol, lipids, electrolytes, blood sugar, and blood pressure. Although these data help to rule out unusual medical etiologies and complications of obesity, they also can be used as benchmarks to follow as the girl is successful with weight loss. An objective drop in cholesterol or blood pressure after weight loss may encourage the girl and even be viewed as a reward.

The adolescent committed to weight loss should see a nutritionist for guidance. Many girls who develop anorexia nervosa begin their long course with a *warranted* weight loss. So, at the very least, a dieting adolescent should be reevaluated every few months.

Any overweight, dieting adolescent needs to be congratulated and encouraged. In addition to medical screening, she should be evaluated for concomitant

TABLE 3. Differential Diagnosis of Endogenous Obesity

Diagnosis	Features
Hypothyroidism	Short, plump, dull, constipated
Hypercortisolism	Short, obese, moon-faced, striae
Froelich's syndrome	Secondary to hypothalamic tumor, polyphagia
Laurence-Moon-Biedl syndrome	+/– short, mental retardation, polydactyly, hypogonadism
Prader-Willi syndrome	Short, small hands, mental retardation, hypogonadism

How to adapt the

Food Guide Pyramid

to meet nutritional needs in Adolescence

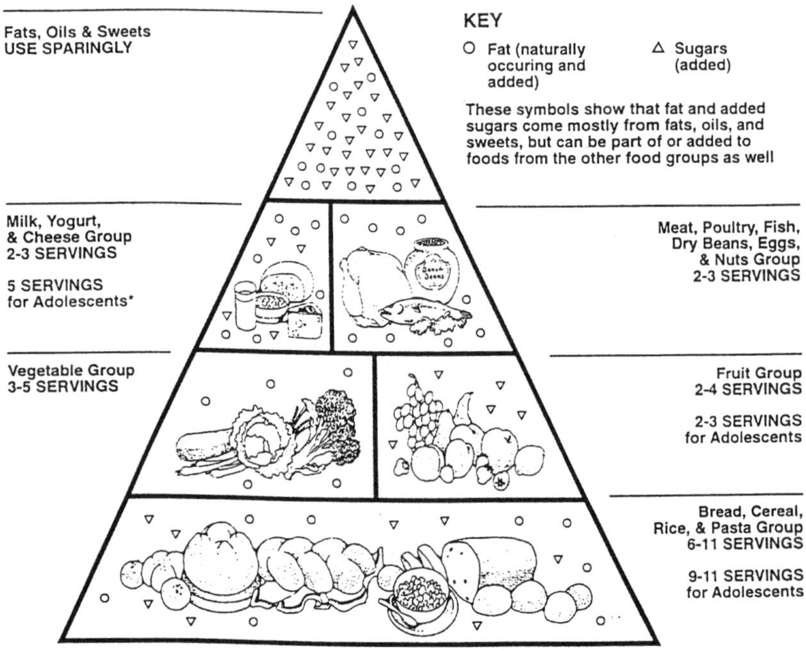

*5 dairy servings provide 1500mg Calcium

WHAT COUNTS AS ONE SERVING?

Breads, cereals, rice, and pasta: 1 slice of bread; ½ cup of cooked rice or pasta; ½ cup of cooked cereal; 1 ounce ready-to-eat cereal
Vegetables: ½ cup of chopped raw or cooked vegetables; 1 cup of leafy raw vegetables
Fruits: 1 piece of fruit or melon wedge; ¾ cup of juice; ½ cup of canned fruit; ¼ cup of dried fruit
Milk, yogurt, and cheese: 1 cup of milk or yogurt; 1 ½ to 2 ounces of cheese
Meat, poultry, fish, dry beans, eggs, and nuts: 2½ to 3 ounces of cooled lean meat, poultry or fish. [Count ½ cup of cooked beans, or 1 egg, or 2 tablespoons of peanut butter as 1 ounce of lean meat (about ⅓ serving).]

FIGURE 4. The Food Guide Pyramid. (From Skiba A, Loghmani E, Orr DP: Nutritional screening and guidance for adolescents. Adolesc Health Update 9(2), 1997, with permission.)

psychosocial issues. Poor self-esteem, depression, or anxiety may have been a part of a girl's make-up for a long time. Sometimes a diet is the first step toward self-improvement, and this may be the perfect time for psychological or nutritional referral.

It is important not to let any personal prejudice or preconceived ideas stand in the way of a full sexual history in the overweight adolescent. Many are sexually mature, healthy, and active. However, some may be acting out their depression or self-esteem issues in the sexual sphere.

Referral may be necessary for nutritional guidance, psychological or social work support, group counseling, weight loss programs, or, in rare cases, medical evaluation. It is useful to keep a roster of providers who are skilled in treating and enjoy working with adolescents.

Assessment for psychosocial issues is critical in girls who like Roxanne have a long history of being overweight and have had no success in controlling the problem. Poor self-esteem, depression, or even abuse may be causes or consequences of obesity. As with the dieter, medical screening for lipids, blood pressure, endocrine abnormalities, or endogenous obesity should be done. Occasionally, an abnormal laboratory value can motivate a girl to begin a diet or a healthier lifestyle.

Losing weight is not easy. Care should be taken not to harangue about weight loss. Exploring a history of dieting and family history with a sympathetic ear and listening for "hooks" with which to gently motivate and counsel is most effective. For instance, through inquiries about what the girl drinks when thirsty, a daily intake of several hundred calories can be revealed. Simple, practical tips (like substituting seltzer or diet soda or water) may be very helpful to these girls. By engaging in a brief discussion, the clinician can assess a girl's sophistication about nutrition. Some do not know what "calorie" or "fat gram" or "carbohydrate" means. Frequently basic education is required before the girl can begin to make changes. A referral to a good, supportive nutritionist is most helpful if she seems at all motivated.

It should be kept in mind that social, cultural, and family norms sometimes favor heavy women. The provider needs to be equally sensitive to the obese girl for whom weight is *not* a problem.

The Fat Adolescent

Dieting

Rachel, 16 years old, 5′1′′, 105 lbs. BMI 20 (normal by objective standards). She is in a popular clique and began dieting when another girl of similar build began to lose weight and got lots of compliments. This made her begin to feel pressure to lose weight also and to change her body shape. Her family is slightly chubby. She has tried fasting off and on for a few months. She has thought of dabbling in the "heavy" techniques, like pills and purging, but has not done so yet.

Not Dieting

Terry, 16 years old, 5′10′′, 157 lbs. BMI 24 (normal by objective standards). Terry is discouraged, she has tried diets. She still feels "fat" in spite of being told she does not need to lose weight. She especially dislikes her thighs and dreads swim class at school. She won't look in mirrors, and wears extra baggy clothes. She feels large and unattractive and has shunned any intimacy in her life.

These girls do not look as if they need to lose weight, but they feel "fat" and may have begun to diet to improve body image. A good exploration of the adolescent's dieting behaviors (see Tables 2 and 5) often alerts the clinician to pathological behaviors that she has embarked upon in response to a distorted self-image. In this situation, the most skillful screening for eating disorders needs to take place.

Sometimes girls like Terry have become discouraged from dieting and have given up trying even though they still think of themselves as "fat." As with the girl who merely dabbles in casual dieting, some cognitive reorientation and encouragement of good eating habits and exercise are useful here. The clinician's role is to encourage healthy behavior and to point out objective measures (BMI, strength) as well as academic, social, or athletic achievements. Emphasis on cardiovascular and emotional fitness is more productive in counseling these girls than engaging in a discussion of "fatness." However, "feeling fat" may be a disguise for adolescent depression. Screening and referral, if necessary, for psychological or psychiatric evaluation certainly is appropriate.

Most dieting adolescent girls are simply misinformed or feel fat and go on a diet. Many of these girls are victims of unrealistic social norms for weight and body size. They sometimes respond to simple cognitive education such as showing the growth chart, explaining caloric requirements, or pointing out the normal size and shape range of beautiful, successful, and happy people. Follow-up is critical. If there is a lot of conflict between the parents and these girls, a referral for nutrition counseling or, at the very least, a follow-up visit within a short period of time is warranted.

The "innocent" or "casual" dieter usually does not present with medical risk. However, dieters like Rachel need to be prevented from sliding down the slippery slope toward a true eating disorder. In the course of screening, one should inquire about use of laxatives, diuretics, purgatives, and diet pills. These riskier behaviors may have dramatic, even lethal side effects if left undetected and untreated.

THE UNDERWEIGHT TEENAGER

The Underweight Adolescent with No Recent Weight Loss

Not Dieting

Cindy, 16 years old, 5'8'', 115 lbs., BMI 17 (underweight), has been tall, "skinny," and active all her life. She first menstruated last year. Although she is always told she looks anorexic, she has never dieted. She has even tried unsuccessfully to gain weight. She is considered very healthy. Her mother is also lean and active.

The girls in this group have not *lost weight,* but have always been thin or "skinny." A skinny girl may simply have an ectomorphic body habitus. Often a family history, a menstrual history, and thorough physical examination evaluating for secondary sex characteristics help to determine the health of such a patient.

Some thin girls are late bloomers. On average, late bloomers are taller and thinner. They have a remarkable family history of late onset of pubertal development and menarche. If this information is available, it is useful in evaluating and making predictions for such a patient. She often needs reassurance about her pubertal development, reproductive potential, and growth potential. An evaluation of sexual maturity rating, also known as Tanner staging, and growth parameters can be very helpful in completing the evaluation.

The Underweight Adolescent with Recent Weight Loss

Not Dieting

Doreen, 17 years old, 5'4'', 100 lbs., BMI 17 (underweight), recently lost 10 pounds without making an effort. She also has had difficulty sleeping, has experienced

TABLE 4. Differential Diagnosis of Weight Loss

Biological or Medical Causes	Biopsychosocial Causes	Psychological Causes
Malabsorption or inflammatory bowel disease	Anorexia nervosa	Depression
Hyperthyroidism	Bulimia nervosa	Psychosis
Malignancy	A combination of anorexia nervosa and bulimia	Obsessive compulsive disorder
Diabetes mellitus		
Chronic infections, e.g., tuberculosis, human immunodeficiency virus (HIV)		

some heart palpitations, and feels warm most of the time. She has been eating more than usual. She exercises a lot and is a good student.

If weight loss has been *unintentional*, a complete history, physical, and appropriate laboratory tests aimed at the five most common diagnoses of Table 4 should be undertaken. These diagnoses are inflammatory bowel disease, hyperthyroidism, occult malignancy (e.g., lymphoma), diabetes mellitus, and chronic infection (tuberculosis or HIV). A social history often raises enough red flags to clarify the need for referral and evaluation for depression or psychosis.

The Underweight Adolescent Who Is Dieting

With Weight Loss

Anna, 17 years old, 5'3'', 92 lbs., BMI 16 (underweight by objective standards), lost her brother in a car accident several years ago. She has difficulty controlling many aspects of her life, including her weight and eating habits. Her parents have not really noticed or commented on her recent 20-pound weight loss. One of the cafeteria personnel at school noticed her eating habits and notified her guidance counselor.

Without Weight Loss

Olga, 16 years old, 5', 90 lbs., BMI 18 (underweight by objective measures), is a gymnast competing at the national level. She does not claim to diet, but she is extremely careful, under her coach's supervision, about her intake. She has maintained her weight at 90 pounds for the past 15 months. She does not use diet pills, although she has tried diuretics in the past. She has not had her first period yet. Her grades in school are passing, but they are not important to her.

DIAGNOSING EATING DISORDERS

For the busy clinician faced with an underweight teen, the critical task is to determine whether a medical and/or psychological condition exists. In a *dieting and underweight* patient or in one who reports *weight loss,* an answer must be found. Each of three girls—Doreen, Anna and Olga—is at risk in different ways. Table 4 illustrates the differential diagnosis of weight loss. Girls who are intentionally losing weight and in whom the clinician suspects an eating disorder fall into one of three categories:[9]

- A girl probably *does not have an eating disorder* if she has
  no signs or symptoms of malnutrition,
  nutritionally sound dietary habits,
  a goal weight of at least 85% of average weight for height and age,

a normal body image and a good self concept,
not been vomiting, using laxatives or purgatives,
and consumes more than 1000 cal/day.

- A girl *may be dieting excessively* if she has
  some of the features of an eating disorder,
  an idiosyncratic approach,
  uneducated or unrealistic goals,
  and has no distortion of her body image.
- A girl *may have an eating disorder* if she has
  symptoms or signs of malnutrition,
  inadequate dietary habits or severely restricted diet,
  a goal weight less than 85% of average or *no goal weight,*
  a distorted body image,
  and has been vomiting, exercising excessively, or abusing laxatives.

ROLE OF THE PRIMARY CARE PROVIDER IN EATING DISORDERS: WHEN TO REFER

Table 5 lists the key features of eating disorders and the useful questions to ask when a clinician is considering the diagnosis. Although a confirmed diagnosis should probably be made by a professional who deals with eating disorders on a frequent basis, the primary care provider can and should do a significant amount of preliminary screening and laboratory work to define the most appropriate channels of referral. Initial appropriate labs are shown in Table 6.

TABLE 5. Diagnosing Eating Disorders

Diagnostic Features	Questions
Anorexia nervosa	
Fear of fat or weight gain, even though underweight	Do you think you are too thin? Do you count fat grams? How often do you weigh yourself?
Inability to maintain weight or make expected weight gain	How much exercise do you do? Do you feel cold?
Disturbed body image, denial of seriousness of low weight	What would be a weight goal for you? What would be an ideal weight? Do you think your thighs are fat? Do you use any pills to help you to lose weight?
Amenorrhea	When was your last period? When was your first? Have you ever had a stress fracture?
Bulimia nervosa	
Recurrent episodes of binge eating	Do you ever eat so much that you feel "gross" or embarrassed? Describe a binge.
Feelings of loss of control	Do you eat secretly? Do you sometimes feel you cannot stop eating?
Vomiting or other methods to prevent weight gain	Do you ever throw up intentionally? How often? Do you ever feel you need to do something to get rid of the uncomfortable feeling after a binge? What have you tried?

TABLE 6. Initial Laboratory Tests for Suspected Eating Disorders

Complete blood count (differential), erythrocyte sedimentation rate, urinalysis Electrolytes Calcium, phosphorus
EKG
Thyroid function tests

Evaluation of amenorrhea, especially if longer than 12 months
  Pelvic examination
  Pregnancy test
  Follicle-stimulating hormone, luteinizing hormone, prolactin

MRI for neurologic symptoms or increased prolactin

Often the primary care provider needs to stay involved on a regular, ongoing basis to determine the extent of the medical issues. Furthermore, in a managed care environment, the patient may not have ready access to other providers who are experts in the field, and the primary provider therefore has a very active role.

Table 7 lists some of the responsibilities of the primary care provider. Above all, the initial provider who makes a diagnosis of an eating disorder or even suspects one is obligated at the first visit to *convince himself or herself and the patient and her family* that there is medical risk. Every effort should be made not to lose the patient to follow-up. The patient is often resistant, but an aggressive attempt to keep her coming for weight checks, even if she refuses therapy at first, is of critical importance. These girls can lose 20 or 30 pounds in a short time and slip into deeply pathological behavior, which becomes harder and harder to treat.

A key responsibility of the primary care provider is to establish criteria and thresholds for hospitalization. Table 8 outlines some of the indications for hospitalization. Because other team members (social workers, psychologists, psychiatrists, nutritionists, nurse practitioners) may not be fully comfortable or trained in medical management, the primary care provider is responsible for monitoring the medical complications and for managing their treatment.

TABLE 7. Primary Care Treatment of Anorexia Nervosa

Medical and nutritional assessment of weight loss, including lab studies
Establishing weight gain goal (target, 85% of average; rate of gain, 1–2 lb/week)

Providing guidelines for daily activities:
  Eating schedule
  Exercise
  After-school activities
  Sports and recreation

Establishing follow-up visits to maintain therapeutic relationship with the family and the patient
Consultation with and referral to specialists; then coordination with specialists
Establishing criteria for hospitalization and communicating them to the patient, family, and other therapists

Adapted from Kreipe RE, Uphoff M: Treatment and outcomes of adolescents with anorexia nervosa. Adolesc Med 3:519–540, 1992, with permission.

TABLE 8. Indications for Hospitalization in Eating Disorders

Severe malnutrition: weight < 75% of ideal body weight
EKG abnormalities: hypokalemia, prolonged QTc, dysrhythmia
Physiologic complications and instability Electrolyte disturbances Bradycardia Hypotension Hypothermia Orthostatic changes Dehydration
Syncope, seizures, pancreatitis, cardiac failure
Failure of outpatient management, especially to gain or maintain weight as defined by team approach at the outset
Psychiatric emergencies: psychosis, severe depression, obsessive compulsive disorder, suicidal ideation
Refusal to eat
Uncontrollable binging and purging

Adapted from Fisher M, Golden NH, Katzman DK, et al: Eating disorders in adolescents: A review. J Adolesc Health 16:420–437, 1995, with permission.

CONCLUSION

Eating, dieting, and body image are issues for every adolescent girl. Some girls are at medical risk. Some are at psychological risk. Fortunately, many are both psychologically and medically healthy. However, all need guidance, often in the form of very simple advice. The primary care provider is in a unique position to screen for problems and to intervene with sound medical, psychological, and practical advice.

REFERENCES

1. Schreiber GB, Robins M, Striegel-Moore R, et al: Weight modification efforts reported by black and white preadolescent girls. Pediatrics 98:63–70, 1996.
2. Heatherton TF, Nichols P, Mahamedi F, et al: Body weight, dieting, and eating disorder symptoms among college students, 1982 to 1992. Am J Psychiatry 152:1623–1629, 1995.
3. The Commonwealth Fund Survey of the Health of Adolescent Girls, November 1997.
4. Story M, Rosenwinklel K, et al: Demographic and risk factors associated with chronic dieting in adolescents. Am J Dis Child 145:994–998, 1991.
5. Elster A, Kuznets N: AMA Guidelines for Adolescent Preventive Services. Baltimore, Williams & Wilkins, 1994, p 48.
6. Krizmanic J: A Teen's Guide to Going Vegetarian. New York, Viking, 1994.
7. Coupey SM, Boeck MA: The Underweight and Overweight Adolescent. Norwalk, CT, Appleton-Century-Crofts, 1984.
8. Kreipe RE, Comerci GD: Assessment of Weight Loss in the Adolescent. Ross Monograph, 1988.

CHAPTER 15

Depression and Suicide

Catherine Monk, Ph.D.
Alec L. Miller, Psy.D.

As someone working with adolescents, the practitioner is accustomed to—and likely enjoys—the spectrum of demeanors and dress that he or she faces in daily practice: bravado, petulance, passivity, reticence, melancholy, inhibition, and exhibitionism permeate the waiting room in the way that the smell of teens' favored McDonald's fries can saturate the office. The clothes are usually hugely oversized and loud or tight and provocative. Often, a teenager's presentation dramatically changes from one appointment to the next or within a single visit. This is, after all, adolescence, the developmental period when strong emotions and experimental styles are expected. The biological, cognitive, social, and emotional changes associated with adolescence lead to profound challenges and difficulties, yet the majority of teenagers muddle through without falling ill. This chapter focuses on identifying adolescents who are not making it and are evidencing psychopathology, which puts them at risk for suicide.

FACTS ABOUT SUICIDE

Adolescent Suicide, A National Health Crisis

- In the otherwise healthy age group of 15–24-year-olds, suicide is the third leading cause of death after accidents and homicides, killing on average 13 young people per day per year.[1]
- Approximately 2,000 adolescents between 15 and 19 years old take their own lives annually; about 330 children between 10 and 14 years old end their own lives, as do 3,000 20–24-year-olds.[2]
- The suicide rate for young males is, on average, 3–5 times higher than for females, but young women make 3–10 times as many suicide attempts as young men.[3]

Is There Warning Before Suicide? The Role of the Primary Care Doctor

The vast majority of young people who kill themselves give a variety of verbal and nonverbal clues about their plans to die, but, sadly, most often these signs go unnoticed. One study of adolescent suicide completers found that over 83% made suicidal threats to others the week prior to their death.[4] Adolescents experiencing emotional problems, including suicidality, seek more medical treatment than their emotionally healthy peers. They present with somatic complaints but are often looking—without necessarily knowing it or announcing it—for another kind of help.[5] One report of medical doctors' knowledge of their patients' wishes to die found that while 41% of Finland's annual number of suicide completers had seen their doctor in the 4 weeks before they died, less than one-half of them discussed their suicide intent during the appointment.[6]

How can the busy primary care physician identify and help such adolescents? Knowing common risk factors as well as when, what, and how to ask adolescents about their mental health may aid in the prevention and intervention of teen suicide as well as get other troubled adolescents the psychological treatment they need. Thus, the primary care doctor is in a unique position to "eyeball" the emotional functioning of adolescents and to play a critical role in combating this health crisis.

The following section briefly reviews the constellation of disorders associated with adolescent suicide. Second, it describes the common predisposing factors leading to suicide and the kind of communications that can signal the intent to die. Third, it focuses on the particular symptom picture of adolescent depression and how to conduct a brief suicide assessment. This information enables the practitioner to more rapidly diagnose adolescent depression, assess the current stressors, and make triage decisions regarding the level of suicidality and the need for immediate psychiatric treatment. Finally, it offers suggestions for helping adolescents to open up about their emotional lives and discusses treatment and referral options.

PSYCHIATRIC ILLNESS AND SUICIDE

The Comorbidity of Adolescent Psychiatric Disorders and Suicide

For adolescents, comorbidity of psychiatric illness is the rule rather than the exception. Most frequently, major depressive disorder is present comorbidly with dysthymic disorder, anxiety disorders, disruptive behavior disorders (such as conduct disorder) and substance abuse. Studies have found that between 40 and 70% of depressed adolescents have comorbid psychiatric disorders, and at least 20–50% meet criteria for two or more comorbid diagnoses.[7]

Suicidal behavior is the "cardinal symptom of psychiatric disorder."[8] Although most adolescents with mental disorders are not suicidal, the majority of adolescents who attempt or complete suicide are suffering from psychiatric disorders, and the frequency and lethality of suicide attempts increase with the degree of comorbidity.[9] Greater than 90% of adolescents who kill themselves meet criteria for a psychiatric diagnosis at the time of their death. The most common diagnoses are mood disorder alone or in combination with conduct disorder and/or substance abuse.[10]

How Common Are Mood Disorders and Suicidal Ideation in Adolescents?

Population studies of major depressive disorder have reported prevalence rates for adolescents that range from 0.4–8.3%. For dysthymia, point prevalence rates from 1.6–8.0% have been found. The lifetime prevalence rate of major depression in adolescents has been estimated to range from 15–20%. As these numbers are comparable to lifetime rates of adult depression, they suggest that depression in adults often begins in adolescence.[7]

However, the rate of suicidal ideation is higher in adolescents compared with adults.[11] Studies of nonclinical samples (e.g., high school students) repeatedly have found that between 25 and 80% thought a lot about suicide in the past year without making an attempt. Sixteen percent of high school students developed a suicide plan. Of these students, 8–10% reported having made a suicide attempt, 5% sustained an injury, and 2–3% sought medical attention for the injury.[12]

The Increase in Adolescent Depression and Suicide

Surveys of adolescent mental illness show an alarming increase in mood disorders and death by suicide. Recent investigations have found that individuals born in the latter part of the 20th century are at greater risk for developing major depressive disorder and dysthymia.[7] Other reports have shown that the youth suicide rate reached its lowest point in this century in the mid-1950s (2.3 per 100,000 for adolescents aged 15–19 years and 5.6 per 100,000 for adolescents aged 20–24 years), increased to a peak at 18.2 per 100,000 in 1977, and more recently has hovered below that value at about 13 deaths per 100,000 for the combined ages of 15–24 years.[1,13] However, despite the recent leveling off, in the 30-year period between 1957 and 1987 the overall suicide rate for young people aged 15–24 years more than tripled (an increase of 222%!).[9]

According to some statistics, the reasons for the increased rates of adolescent depression are either environmental factors or the interrelation of environmental factors and genes, because the genetic makeup of the population has not changed substantially.[7] In a domino fashion, some relate the rise in suicides to increased incidences of affective disorders and substance abuse,[13] while others attribute the once-climbing adolescent suicide numbers to changes in demographics. As the portion of the U.S. population in the 15–24-year-old age bracket grew so did the suicide rate for that group. In other words, there is demographic evidence that the rate of adolescent suicide is associated with the relative percentage of youth coming of age.[9,13]

The Specific Vulnerability of Female Adolescents

Today, young women experience higher rates of depression than their male counterparts, and in young women who killed themselves, it has been found that fully two-thirds of them suffered from a mood disorder.[14] Young women also have significantly higher incidences of suicidal ideation and,[11,15] as previously mentioned, make more suicide attempts.[3] The typical teen suicide attempter is a young women who ingests pills.[9] Follow-up studies of female teen suicide attempters show that the rate of completed suicide is from 1–4% greater than the general population and that frequencies of subsequent attempts by males and females who tried before range as high as 50% over a 3-year period.[9] Approximately 50% of female suicide completers made a previous attempt.[11]

PREDISPOSING CONDITIONS AND PRECIPITATING FACTORS LEADING TO SUICIDE

Depression and past suicide attempts are the two greatest risk factors for future suicide attempts.[11] However, other socioenvironmental circumstances have been found to be associated with teen suicide as well as to add significantly to teenagers' suicide risk independent of psychiatric illness.[16] Knowing these factors can help the interviewer to know what to look for in a potentially suicidal teen and aid in the assessment process.

This section delineates the *distal* and *proximal* factors contributing to suicidality. Distal factors are the indirect factors, such as psychopathology, which can be understood as necessary, but not sufficient for suicidal behavior. Distal factors most often have been part of the adolescent's life for a long time. Proximal factors refer to more direct, present-day stressors precipitating suicidality. These factors are neither necessary nor sufficient to lead to suicide but combined with distal factors provide the context in which most teenage suicidal behavior takes place. First, research-based distal and proximal factors are summarized in Table 1. The clinically based distal and proximal factors also are worth noting.

Research-based Distal Factors

Psychological autopsy reports based on adolescent suicide completers have shown that they often come from nonintact families in which the adolescent has poor communication with the mother and father. In addition, the mother often has a mood disorder; the father often has a history of trouble with the law; and there have been attempts and/or completions of suicide in the extended family.[16]

Other research-based distal factors include psychopathology. In one of the few studies to break down results by gender, it was found that in female suicide victims, approximately 68% had depressive symptoms, 12% had substance abuse problems, 36% had conduct disorders, and 28% had anxiety disorders.[10] Psychoses, as evidenced by command auditory hallucinations telling the adolescent to kill herself and bizarre delusions, also can be associated with suicide. Finally, some research has found borderline personality disorder in combination with major depression leads to elevated levels of suicidality,[17] and other work has found bulima[18] and learning disabilities[19] in the histories of suicide completers.

Research-based Proximal Factors

In evaluations of the precipitating factors in adolescent suicide, research has found four common stressful events: interpersonal loss, such as a break-up

TABLE 1. Research-based Risk Factors for Adolescent Suicide

Proximal Factors/Stressful Events	Distal Factors
Interperson loss, such as break-up with boyfriend or girlfriend	Non-intact family
Discipline crisis such as suspension from school or appearance in juvenile court	Poor communication with mother and father
Difficulties in school, or neither working, being in school, or going to college	Mother having a mood disorder
Depression related to friend's suicide	Past suicide attempt
	Father having trouble with the law
	Attempts and completion of suicide in family
	Psychopathology:
	Affective disorders (major depressive disorder and bipolar disorder)
	Substance abuse
	Conduct disorder
	Anxiety disorder
	Borderline personality disorder
	Eating disorder
	Psychoses
	Learning disability
Additional Less Common Stressors	**Additional Less Common Distal Factors**
Humiliation	Poor interpersonal relationships
Rejection	Cognitive/academic difficulties
Guilt	Poor school performance/underachievement
Embarrassment	History of sexual assault
	Loss of a parent
	Presence of firearm in the home

with a boyfriend; disciplinary crisis, such as suspension from school or appearance in juvenile court; difficulties in school, or neither working, being in school, nor going to college;[16] and depression related to a friend's suicide.[11]

Additional, Less Common Distal and Proximal Factors

Adolescents who take their own lives often have specific deficits which are manifested in poor interpersonal relationships and cognitive/academic difficulties. Particularly, poor school performance and underachievement have been observed in this group of adolescents. A history of sexual assault, which is more common among women, has been associated with an increased lifetime rate of attempted suicide. When the trauma occurs before the woman is 16 years old, the odds of attempting suicide are 3–4 times greater than when the assault occurs after age 16.[20] The loss of a parent before the adolescent is 12 years old also has been associated with increased suicide attempts.[11]

Acute stressors, which pose the threat of loss to the teenager, such as rejection by a boyfriend, or which induce in the adolescent the feelings of failure, guilt, or humiliation, have been found to be precipitating causes in teen suicide attempts.

An adolescent who presents at the office with one proximal factor (recent stressor) and one distal factor is carrying a combination of factors that may predispose her to attempt suicide. With this type of adolescent, it is particularly important to find out more information about her level of emotional functioning.

The following brief clinical vignette serves as an illustration of the utility of considering predisposing factors associated with suicide:

> Emily, a carefully groomed yet slightly awkward 17-year-old, was referred to the Adolescent Depression and Suicide Program following her ingestion of 16 Tylenol pills, which had resulted in an overnight stay in a local hospital. Emily, who had never before been in the care of a mental health professional, came from an intact Irish-Catholic family and had always been a good student who was also involved in numerous activities, from the swim team to year book, all while holding down an office job two days a week after school. Usually perky, cheerful, obedient, active, popular—she appears to have an adolescence far from a tumultuous one. Yet during her initial interview, she described wanting to die on the night she ingested the pills, and she met criteria for major depressive disorder.

Of course, hindsight is 20–20, and a young woman of Emily's caliber and ambition may have worked particularly hard to hide her problems. What can one learn from her story? As it turns out, Emily's grades had dropped for the first time the semester before her suicide attempt, and she was feeling very humiliated by her sense of failure. Her school performance was one of the most overt manifestations of her depression. Furthermore, both a close friend as well as an aunt had recently moved away, and she felt unable to attract the boyfriend she really wanted.

Except for her depression, which she worked hard to hide, Emily did not seem to have any of the other distal factors associated with suicide. However, she felt deep humiliation about her school performance and experienced the precipitous loss of two close people in her life, as well as the experience of loss in not getting the boyfriend she wanted. Careful attention to the *marked* change in her school functioning may have led to uncovering her depression. This, in addition to learning about the current stressors she was facing, may have prevented Emily from trying to take her life.

In general, most important to an initial assessment of adolescents is allowing oneself to ask questions, even when the adolescents themselves have not verbally given an easy entry. Considering the association of suicidal ideation and attempts with psychiatric symptomatology and the comorbidity of depression and other disorders, any signs of mental illness, particularly in the context of the distal and proximal factors associated with adolescent suicide, should suggest the need for a careful evaluation of depression and suicidal ideation.

ASSESSING DEPRESSION IN TEENAGERS

The *Diagnostic and Statistical Manual of Mental Disorders (DSM-IV)*[21] lists the research-based criteria for diagnosis of major depression and dysthymia. Although the criteria for both major depression and dysthymia are straightforward, atypical features of each are seen in adolescents. The specific symptoms for each diagnosis, including the atypical adolescent features, are listed in Tables 3 and 4, respectively.

TABLE 2. DSM-IV Criteria for Major Depression* and Common Manifestations of Adolescent Depression[21]

DSM-IV Criteria	Adolescent Attributes of Depression
Depressed mood most of the day, nearly every day	Down, sad, irritable
Diminished interest or pleasure in all or most activities	Bored
Significant weight loss or gain not due to intentional dieting	
Insomnia or hypersomnia nearly every day	
Noticeable psychomotor agitation or retardation	
Loss of energy or tiredness	
Feeling worthless, low self-esteem, or excessive guilt	Rejection sensitivity
Problems thinking and concentrating, or feeling indecisive	School grades decline
Recurrent thoughts of death, suicidal ideation	

* To meet diagnostic criteria for major depression, the person has to have had five or more of symptoms for the same 2-week period, and at least one of the symptoms has to be depressed mood or loss of interest or pleasure.

For depressed adolescents, mood is not always experienced as depression and is not always labeled as such. Frequently, they deny feeling depressed but state that they feel down, sad, or irritable, and they agree that they've been told they are "copping an attitude lately." Or they may say that they feel bored, which appears to be another way of describing anhedonia or loss of interest. The sense of worthlessness for adolescents often is experienced in the context of rejection and is manifested as "rejection sensitivity," as in "It really hurt when my friend took the other bus home 'cause I felt like I'm stupid and nothing." Finally, adolescents who are seriously depressed do not usually act or look depressed consistently. Consider the case of Sue:

> Sue, a 15-year-old cheerleader, had made one previous suicide attempt before her recent ingestion of her mother's blood pressure pills. Despite having had her stomach pumped and being released from the hospital just hours before her first therapy session, Sue began the session by commenting exuberantly on her therapist's shoes and answering that "things are OK." Gaunt, with bags under her eyes and a tense, frightened expression, Sue seemed to move between an isolating preoccupation with her own self-denigrating thoughts and abrupt gestures of friendliness.

Sue's erratic behavior is common for depressed adolescents. In contrast with manifestations of adult depression, seriously depressed adolescents may be seen laughing with their friends and still spend hours grooming themselves. Before doing a thorough assessment, it is important not to dismiss the possibility of

TABLE 3. DSM-IV Criteria for Dysthymia[21]*

Depressed mood, most of the day, for more days than not for the past year

While depressed, person has two or more of the following:

- Poor appetite or overeating
- Insomnia or hypersomnia
- Low energy or fatigue
- Low self-esteem
- Poor concentration, decision making
- Feelings of hopelessness

* To meet diagnostic criteria for dysthymia, a person needs to have been depressed most of the day for the past year.

depression or dysthymia just because the adolescent exhibits positive emotions and some investment in her appearance.

If the practitioner believes he or she has uncovered sufficient evidence to suspect depression, it is obviously important to consider suicidal ideation before deciding on a treatment plan.

ASSESSING ADOLESCENT SUICIDE

Since 25–80% of teenagers have been found to experience suicidal ideation,[12] giving an adolescent a chance to acknowledge her wishes to die can often be a relief for her.

What to Find Out from the Adolescent

To assess suicidality, the practitioner should ascertain past suicidal ideation and attempts, current suicidal thinking, the content of suicidal plans, and the level of impulsivity as well as depression.[5] Suggestions for getting the information in these four domains are outlined in Table 4.

In general, the practitioner should find out specifically what is thought and how often it is thought. Does the girl wish she were dead once or twice a day, or does she get absorbed in imagining killing herself? For how long has she had these thoughts? The practitioner wants to know if she has a specific plan and, if so, exactly what it is and how realistic it is (e.g., does she have access to a gun or pills at home?) The practitioner also should gain a sense of how impulsive the adolescent is and if she is involved in abusing substances. He or she should inquire about what the adolescent does when she is upset and whether she

TABLE 4. Assessing Adolescent Suicidality

Past suicidal ideation and attempts
- Have you ever thought of killing yourself? If yes,
  - When was the last time?
  - For how long have you been thinking of killing yourself?
  - Do you think seriously about killing yourself?
- Have you ever tried to kill yourself? If yes,
  - What did you do to try to kill yourself?
  - Did you need medical attention? What kind?

Current suicidal thinking and content plan
- Are you currently thinking about killing yourself? If yes,
  - How often are you thinking this?
  - Do you have a plan?
  - Do you intend to do this?
  - Is there a reason *not* to kill yourself? Do you have a reason to live?
  - Do you think you could stop yourself from trying to kill yourself?
  - How badly do you think you want to die?
  - Do you have a means to carry this out?

Level of impulsivity and depression
- Do you ever do things you regret, maybe when you are angry?
- Are you using drugs, drinking? How often?
- Are you down and sad? (If yes, assess specifically for depression)

does anything she regrets, such as destroy property or run away. How about when she is drunk? How often is she getting drunk or high?

After discussing the adolescent's thoughts about suicide, the practitioner should be concerned if he or she finds any of the following factors:[5]

- She strongly wants to die
- She does not feel she can control her impulse (or the practitioner does not believe she can)
- She is depressed
- She has a history of past suicide attempts
- She has a realistic plan
- She has a history of being impulsive
- She is using and/or abusing substances

Indirect Suicidal Communications—"Red Flags"

Imminent suicidal behavior is often signaled by verbal and/or behavioral messages. These communications are summarized in Table 5.

Although adolescents write suicide notes less often than adults, they still communicate their suicidal thoughts in school essays, poems, diaries, journals, and artwork. In these mediums they may show a preoccupation with themes of death, dying, the afterlife, and suicide. A report of such work by the girl's parent or the girl herself should be considered a serious communication and be explored immediately. Sometimes adolescents demonstrate their suicidal thoughts by trying to engage others in abstract discussions of death and dying or in reports of dreams about death. Another form of suicidal communication is termination behaviors, in which the adolescent writes a will, gives away favored possessions, and makes preparations for death. Although these behaviors are rare in adolescence, they are clear markers when they occur. Finally, as previously suggested, any acute or marked behavioral change, such as an adolescent girl rapidly changing from shy to gregarious or from a good to a poor student, requires further evaluation.[9]

Protective Factors

Any assessment of risk also must include contraindications to self-harm behavior. The availability of both internal (cognitive) and external (interpersonal) resources for coping successfully with stress should be determined. In examining cognitive resources, the practitioner should evaluate what kind of problem-solving strategies the adolescent has and how rational or irrational she is in coping with her current crises. When examining interpersonal resources,

TABLE 5. Red Flag Communications

Preoccupation with themes of death and dying in school essays, poems, diaries, journals, and artwork
Trying to engage others in discussions of death and dying
Termination behaviors such as giving away favored possessions
Acute and marked behavioral change

the practitioner wants to know if she has people in her life with whom she talks and from whom she receives emotional support. Long-term alliances reduce teenagers' intolerable feelings of aloneness and suggest they may have the capacity to draw on others in times of need.

In addition, it can be useful to learn if the adolescent has a future time perspective. Is she thinking about life after high school? Does she have a future goal? Such a view suggests an interest in living and also can be used in helping the adolescent to get through her current sense of wanting to die. Does she have any religious convictions or other beliefs that she feels would prevent her from taking her own life? Is there someone in her life whom she would hurt greatly by such an act, and, therefore, she will not do it? Finally, a nonhostile, nonrejecting attitude toward the interviewer is also suggestive of an ability to work with others to get through the current crisis.

If the interview yields significant suicidal ideation in the context of depression or other proximal and/or distal factors, which cause concern about the adolescent's safety, then the following is the suggested plan.

TRIAGE FOR THE SUICIDAL ADOLESCENT

There are two primary options for a suicidal teen: emergency room evaluation or referral to outpatient treatment. However, because choosing the latter means sending home someone who is suicidal, one also can use the discussion of options for the adolescent as an opportunity for further assessment.

Empathize with how bad the adolescent feels, tell her directly about the two options being weighed, and monitor her reactions. Is there relief at the mention of going to a hospital? Fear? In weighing all this information, one can again ask her if she feels she can keep herself safe until she sees someone she can talk to. Obviously, if she says no, there is no longer a question of what the next step should be. But even if she says yes, one wants to work to challenge this assertion. Is she being passive, saying whatever it takes to get out of the office, or does she seem convinced of her statement and emotionally engaged with the practitioner while saying it?

Can She Keep to a Contract?

The practitioner can believe the patient is treatable as an outpatient if she accepts a verbal or written contract and, again, assess the quality of her commitment. Generally, people ask the adolescent to agree that she will not try to hurt herself for an agreed-upon period of time (e.g., a week) and that, if she feels that she is going to, she promises to tell someone (e.g., the practitioner or her mother) before doing this. Is she willing to involve her mother or father (or someone else) in this contract?

Social Supports

Find out how involved people are at home, how much the adolescent will be home (or anywhere) alone, and if she feels someone at home can help her until she gets help. Again, will she let these people become involved in the discussion of her current suicidality? Is there someone to involve? (This is important so that the practitioner and the patient do not feel as though the practitioner is the only visible support.)

Offer Assistance (by Pager) during the Crisis

If the practitioner is able to offer himself or herself as available by pager until the adolescent is in outpatient treatment, it helps to assess her reaction to this offer. Does she nod diligently or seem to soften and feel grateful that someone is there for her? Pour on the details, like "You can page me at 2 a.m." What is her response? Does she flinch? Often, knowing someone is concerned and available can help the adolescent to feel some hopefulness. Often she will use the pager number as a source of comfort, without actually paging the doctor, until she is in her own treatment.

However, in some instances the adolescent will be unable to convince the practitioner that she can control herself, stick to a contract, and use the pager, or that she has people in her life to help her. *Trust intuition*. Perhaps she is at too much risk to be anywhere but at a hospital right now. At this point, consulting with a psychiatrist or psychologist can help the practitioner to think through the best options for this young woman.

If the practitioner decides it is appropriate to send home a mildly suicidal adolescent (who does not have a plan or intent to die) with a referral for follow-up treatment, he or she can tell the adolescent that she can go to any hospital emergency room at any hour of the day or night if she feels suicidal or needs to talk with someone. Numbers for local crisis hotlines also are helpful.

REFERRAL OPTIONS

Several treatment approaches have been demonstrated empirically to be effective in the treatment of depressed adolescents. These include cognitive and behavior psychotherapy, both in individual and group modalities,[23] and interpersonal psychotherapy.[24] Miller and colleagues have begun to adapt dialectical behavior therapy, an empirically validated treatment for suicidal and parasuicidal adults, to treatment of suicidal adolescents. The preliminary pilot data have been promising. The treatment targets emotion dysregulation, confusion about self, impulsivity, and interpersonal problems by teaching various behavioral skills for each problem area.[25]

To date, no psychiatric medication has been shown empirically to be effective with suicidal adolescents. Results have been equivocal in studies in which adolescents take tricyclic antidepressants and selective serotonin reuptake inhibitors.[26] A double-blind, placebo-controlled study with a small number of adolescents failed to find significant differences in the effectiveness of fluoxetine and placebo.[27] Even a double-blind, placebo-controlled study based on a larger sample found improvement only on one outcome measure.[28]

Unfortunately, despite the obvious need for treatment, as many as 50% of adolescent suicide attempters do not receive any follow-up mental health care.[29] And, of those who do, up to 77% do not attend or fail to complete treatment.[30] Treating suicidal and depressed adolescents through the primary care practice is thus contraindicated on two fronts: (1) the data do not support antidepressant medication for this population and (2) the infrequency and brevity of primary care meetings do not give the treatment-resistant, hard-to-engage adolescent the kind of contact and support she needs, at minimum, to stay on the medication, let alone make progress in the areas of interpersonal and coping skills.

IDEAS FOR TALKING WITH ADOLESCENTS ABOUT THEIR EMOTIONAL LIVES

The practitioner routinely asks patients questions about their lives. As he or she well knows, the rule of thumb for getting information from adolescents is to ask directly and, in various ways, ferret out the necessary information. This is perhaps especially true for mental health concerns, which can be shameful and scary. Keen and encompassing observation of the patient helps one *not* take monosyllabic answers at face value. Most often adolescents will not announce that they feel depressed and, when asked how they are doing, will say "fine" even when they are not. However, if asked more detailed questions, they will reveal more about themselves; if an alliance is there, they will respond.

Ideas for Building an Alliance with Adolescents

With adolescents in the era of managed care, practitioners have a problem: they need to build an alliance with highly sensitive people who are suspicious of adults, and they need to do it quickly. One way they can start the process is to demonstrate to the young woman in the office that they can be straightforward. As discussed in chapter 6, issues of confidentiality are paramount. If practitioners are worried about an adolescent and want to get her to open up, they may state or remind her of their policy regarding confidentiality: what they are required by law to disclose and to whom. Also, they may tell her what information, if any, they routinely disclose and to whom. Practitioners must be very clear; they do not want to get into a situation in which they feel obligated to tell the adolescent's parents something they did not warn her about in advance. Yes, they can write off a failed alliance as one lost relationship, but for the distrustful and injured girl, it can be concrete evidence of why she should never again open up to anyone. If practitioners learn something important that they are neither legally nor ethically obligated to disclose but believe that disclosure to the parents will better serve the adolescent, they can negotiate with her for "permission" to tell. Being straight with her, letting her know where they stand, is a good starting point. They are in a better position to ask her to be straight with them.

Work Collaboratively

The practitioner also may try an approach of working collaboratively with the adolescent. That is, he or she can adopt a stance of "we've got a problem here" (e.g., "you are depressed and I'm worried about you"); "What should we do about it? Do you want to think it through with me?" The practitioner must try to get the patient involved in an assessment of her situation.

A technique for establishing this collaborative tone, as well as gaining the necessary history needed for medical practice and psychological screening, is to involve the adolescent in the construction of a family genogram. Rather than placing her in the passive role while one writes (a role the adolescent associates with her position as a child and would just as soon prefer to jettison from her mind), working with her collaboratively, even from session to session, on the representational—albeit crude—picture of her family genogram (using squares for men and circles for women) can facilitate an alliance with her and establish a productive tone for the relationship.

Getting Adolescents to Self-Disclose

To get her to talk about what is happening, the practitioner may try observing out loud what he or she sees and offering possible understandings of it by generalizing and normalizing it (e.g., "You look pretty down. Teenagers who look like you do usually have something going on, something pretty upsetting."). By taking a leap with an open-ended tone, one offers possibilities for what he or she is seeing: "You aren't looking at me as we talk. When people do that, something must be up. Are you feeling down or uncomfortable?" Such an approach continues a collaborative tone and hopefully will yield important diagnostic information.

CONCLUSION

Adolescent girls are challenged by various biological, cognitive, social, and emotional changes. While most young women survive unscathed, others exhibit varying levels of psychopathology, including suicidality. Many of these suicidal adolescents give verbal and nonverbal clues before their attempts to end their lives, but, sadly, most of them go unnoticed. All of us who work with adolescents need to take responsibility for being more cognizant of these clues. The primary care physician is often the first health professional these adolescents see when they are in physical *and* emotional distress. Thus, the primary care physician can be in the position of making life and death clinical determinations regarding these emotionally troubled youth.

The primary care physician should be able to diagnose adolescent depression, assess current stressors, evaluate verbal and nonverbal communications, and make triage decisions regarding the level of suicidality and the need for psychiatric treatment.

REFERENCES

1. McIntosh JL: U.S.A. Suicide: 1995 Official Final Data. Washington, DC, American Association of Suicidology, 1997.
2. Centers for Disease Control and Prevention: National Center for Injury Prevention and Control: Division of Violence Prevention: Suicide Mortality Data (1989–1995). Atlanta, GA, Centers for Disease Control and Prevention, 1997.
3. Brent DA, Perper JA, Moritz G, et al: Stressful life events, psychopathology, and adolescent suicide: A case control study. Suicide Life Threat Behav 23:179–187, 1993.
4. Brent DA, Perper JA, Goldstein CE, et al: Risk factors for adolescent suicide. Arch Gen Psychiatry 45:581–588, 1988.

5. Restifo KS: Identifying the suicidal adolescent in primary care settings. Prim Psychiatry 4:26–34, 1997.
6. Isometsa ET, Heikkinen ME, Marttunen MJ, et al: The last appointment before suicide: Is suicide intent communicated? Am J Psychiatry 152:919–922, 1995.
7. Birmaher B, Ryan ND, Williamson DE, et al: Childhood and adolescent depression: A review of the past ten years: Part I. J Am Acad Child Adolesc Psychiatry 35:1427–1439, 1996.
8. Crumley FE: The adolescent suicide attempt: A cardinal symptom of a serious psychiatric disorder. Am J Psychother 36:158–165, 1982.
9. Berman ALJ: Adolescent Suicide Assessment and Intervention. Washington, DC, American Psychological Association, 1991.
10. Shaffer D, Gould MS, Fisher P, et al: Psychiatric diagnosis in child and adolescent suicide. Arch Gen Psychiatry 53:339–348, 1996.
11. Lewinsohn PM, Rohde P, Seeley JR: Adolescent suicide ideation and attempts: Prevalence, risk factors, and clinical implications. Clin Psychol Sci Pract 3:25–46, 1996.
12. Centers for Disease Control and Prevention: Attempted suicide among high school students—United States, 1990. MMWR 40:633–635, 1991.
13. Clark DC: Suicidal behavior in childhood and adolescence: Recent studies and clinical implications. Psychiatr Ann 23:271–283, 1993.
14. Marttunen MJ, Henriksson MM, Aro HM, et al: Suicide among female adolescents: Characteristics and comparison with males in the age group 13 to 22 years. J Am Acad Child Adolesc Psychiatry 34:1297–1307, 1995.
15. Compas BE, Oppedisano H, Connor JK, et al: Gender differences in depressive symptoms in adolescence: Comparison of national samples of clinically referred and nonreferred youth. J Consult Clin Psychol 65:617–626, 1997.
16. Gould MS, Fisher P, Parides M, et al: Psychosocial risk factors of child and adolescent completed suicide. Arch Psychiatry 53:1155–1162, 1996.
17. Clarkin JF, Friedman RC, Hurt SW, et al: Affective and character pathology of suicidal adolescent and young adult patients. J Clin Psychiatry 45:19–22, 1984.
18. Favaro S, Santonastaso P: Suicidality in eating disorders: Clinical and psychological correlates. Acta Psychiatr Scand 95:508–514, 1997.
19. Peck ML: Crisis intervention treatment with chronically and acutely suicidal adolescents. In Peck NL, Farberow NL, Litman RE (eds): Youth Suicide. New York, Springer, 1985, pp 112–122.
20. Davidson JR, Hughes DC, George LK, Blazer DG: The association of assault and attempted suicide within the community. Arch Gen Psychiatry 53:550–555, 1996.
21. American Psychiatric Association: Diagnostic and Statistical Manual of Mental Disorders, 4th ed. Washington, DC, American Psychiatric Association, 1994.
22. Wetzler S, Asnis GM, Hyman RB, et al: Characteristics of suicidality among adolescents. Suicide Life Threat Behav 26:37–45, 1996.
23. Lewinsohn PM, Clarke GN, Hops H, Andrews JP: Behavioral treatment for depressed adolescents. Behav Ther 21:385–401, 1990.
24. Mufson L, Moreau D, Weissman MM, et al: Modification of interpersonal psychotherapy with depressed adolescents (IPT-A): Phase I and phase II studies. J Am Acad Child Adolesc Psychiatry 33:695–705, 1994.
25. Miller AL, Rathus JH, Linehan MM, et al: Dialectical behavior therapy adopted for suicidal adolescents. J Pract Psychiatry Behav Health 3:78–86, 1997.
26. Birmaher B, Ryan ND, Williamson DE, et al: Childhood and adolescent depression: A review of the past ten years. Part II. J Am Acad Child Adolesc Psychiatry 35:1575–1583, 1996.
27. Simeon J, Dinicola V, Ferguson H: Adolescent depression: A placebo-controlled fluoxetine treatment and follow-up. Progr Neuropsychol Pharmacol Biol Psychiatry 14:791–795, 1990.
28. Emslie GJ, Rush AJ, Weinberg WA, et al: A double-blind, randomized, placebo-controlled trial of fluoxetine in children and adolescents with depression. Arch Gen Psychiatry 54:1031–1037, 1997.
29. Spirito A, Brown L, Overholser J, Fritz G: Attempted suicide in adolescence: A review and critique of the literature. Clin Psychol Rev 9:335–363, 1989.
30. Trautman P, Stewart N, Morishima A: Are adolescent suicide attempters non-compliant with outpatient care? J Am Acad Child Adolesc Psychiatry 32:89–94, 1993.

CHAPTER **16**

Tobacco, Alcohol, and Other Drugs

Richard B. Heyman, M.D.

The use of tobacco, alcohol, and other drugs by adolescent females is an issue that every practitioner must address, and demographic surveys as well as sociological phenomena of the 1990s suggest that this problem is only getting worse. Given that most women who will ever use tobacco, alcohol, or other drugs begin as teenagers (90% of those who will ever smoke regularly, for example, begin before age 19) and that nearly 90% will see a doctor at least every two years, prevention of substance abuse should be a goal of every care provider.[1]

DEMOGRAPHICS AND SCOPE OF THE PROBLEM

Most survey data, including the University of Michigan's Monitoring the Future,[2] reflect the fact that while historically the use of alcohol, marijuana, and other illegal drugs has been more prevalent among adolescent boys, there is steady growth in use by girls. The 1998 National Household Survey on Drug Abuse, for example, revealed that 10.3% of boys and 9.5% of girls aged 12–17 years had used an illegal substance within the previous month. Some 45% of women aged 17 and up used alcohol in the preceding month, compared with 59% of men. Tobacco use by teenage girls is rising, and the percentage of boys and girls who are smoking is now essentially even.[3]

While there are cultural, societal, racial, and ethnic differences in specific patterns, substance abuse is seen throughout the adolescent population. As tobacco, alcohol, and other drugs are portrayed more pervasively in the media and targeted advertising becomes more sophisticated, cultural differences in many areas are gradually disappearing.

In their classic studies of drug use progression, Yamaguchi and Kandel[4] demonstrated how drugs are used and that the pattern of such use differs for boys and girls. Alcohol appears to be the critical gateway drug for boys (they use earlier and heavier, with more intent to become intoxicated); nicotine seems to serve this function for girls, who tend to progress to alcohol and other drugs at a later age.[5] Thus, smoking serves as a critical marker for girls who may later develop problems with other substances of abuse—a fact which young people understand and acknowledge.[6]

The use of tobacco, alcohol, and other drugs by adolescent girls raises a number of specific concerns for the clinician, because girls who are engaging in these potentially risky behaviors are statistically more likely to engage in others. Furthermore, use of substances by young women who are taking contraceptive medications or who are pregnant or postpartum has specific health effects on both the woman and her child. Some of these issues are addressed in this chapter.

THE CHOICE TO USE TOBACCO, ALCOHOL, AND OTHER DRUGS

The choice about whether or not to use tobacco, alcohol, and other drugs is one of the most critical ones young people have to make. It is, unfortunately, a choice that must be made on an ongoing basis because the opportunity to change one's mind presents itself repeatedly and inexorably throughout adolescence. A major role of the health care provider is to help influence young people to choose not to use these substances, and the prevention message is one that should be reiterated at every possible opportunity.

Statistics suggest that some degree of experimentation with tobacco, alcohol, and even marijuana is the norm for American adolescents today. The problem, however, is that while young adolescents see themselves as all-powerful and in control of their experimentation, the mind-altering effects of these chemicals frequently lead to a pattern of increasing use and dependence.

Many writers and researchers have looked at the important issue of why young people turn to tobacco, alcohol, and other drugs,[7] and there is general agreement that the answer is multifactorial. Certainly the environment in which a teenager grows up is critical, and it is clear that family substance abuse and affiliation with a peer group that uses are critical risk factors. The personality of the individual is also of major importance. Young adolescents with low self-esteem and low sense of self-efficacy are at special risk. Girls especially are more prone to conform to peer standards and are extremely sensitive to media messages about behavioral and appearance norms.[8] Enjoyment of risky activities, willingness to engage in rebellious behavior, absence of attachment to traditional institutions (such as family outings, school activities, religious affiliation), and lack of commitment to goal-oriented future plans are individual characteristics that place adolescents at great risk as well.

Jessor's so-called "problem behavior theory" suggests that these factors tend to cluster and create an environment in which "problem behaviors" become dominant and, in fact, serve a very specific purpose. Thus, girls who are prematurely sexually active, involved in antisocial behaviors and delinquency, having problems with school and truancy, and just generally rebellious and noncompliant are at greater risk for involvement with tobacco, alcohol, and other drugs. All these behaviors have a perceived value to the adolescent, commonly that of helping to establish identity, being part of a peer group, achieving personal goals, and appearing more adult-like. The clinician dealing with such young people must be aware of this phenomenon, because caring for these girls implies the need to develop prevention activities and interventions for the behavior complex rather than for each behavior separately.

There are interesting correlations between young people's perceptions of themselves and their proclivity toward substance abuse. For example, perceived athletic competence is a major protective factor for boys, although not for girls. Those who see themselves as academically challenged are more likely to use drugs, and for girls higher levels of involvement with and social support from classmates is actually associated with increased likelihood of tobacco, alcohol, and marijuana use.[9]

Helping parents to identify protective factors may be critical in encouraging young people to choose not to use tobacco, alcohol, and other drugs or to engage in other risk behaviors. Young people who have goals, positive self-esteem, a sense of attachment to family and community, and a commitment to their own future are young people who are at lower risk for using. One key to prevention is helping them to identify these parameters, validating their importance, and pointing out the consequences of abandoning them.

ADOLESCENT GROWTH AND DEVELOPMENT AND THEIR ROLE IN TOBACCO, ALCOHOL, AND OTHER DRUG USE

Adolescence is a time of major psychosocial development. While a thorough discussion of this topic is beyond the scope of this chapter, it is important to recognize the gradual transition from concrete to formal operational thinking that takes place during the second decade of life. Young adolescents are consumed with their sense of power and may choose to experiment with tobacco, alcohol, and other drugs with the firm belief that they are "just experimenting," can use when and if they wish, and are in total control of whether or not they use.

The biologic changes of puberty complicate matters even further. Most girls enter puberty sometime between their tenth and eleventh birthdays. Those who experience earlier onset of puberty may be subject to increased stress levels because they perceive themselves as different. Early maturing girls appear much older than their peers, and because of appearances, they may experience increased social pressure to achieve the developmental tasks of adolescence faster, to socialize with older adolescents who in turn are doing things more appropriate for their chronological age, and to engage in risk behaviors.[10]

Media messages that identify smoking and drinking with girls who are sexy, popular, thin, and rebellious convey cigarette and beer use as normative and functional. Impressionable young girls who appear older than their stated age may be especially vulnerable to such images.

While no single model of prevention addresses all of these concerns, attempts to reduce risk factors and promote protective factors appear to hold the most promise for reducing use in this population (Tables 1 and 2). The care provider should allow ample time to thoroughly explore these areas of concern.

TABLE 1. Risk Factors for Substance Abuse in Teenagers

Community environment

Living in an economically depressed area with
- High unemployment and inadequate housing
- High prevalence of crime and illegal drug use

Minority status involving
- Race discrimination
- Culture devalued in American society
- Cultural and language barriers to getting adequate health care and other social services
- Low educational levels and low achievement expectations from society

Family environment
- Alcohol and other drug dependency of parent(s)
- Parental abuse and neglect of children
- Antisocial or mentally ill parents
- High levels of family stress, including financial strain, violence
- Large, overcrowded family
- Unemployed or underemployed parents with little education
- Single parent without family/other support
- Inadequate parenting and little parent/child contact
- Frequent family moves

Constitutional vulnerability of the child
- Child of an alcohol or other drug abuser
- Less than 2 years between the child and older/younger siblings
- Birth defects, including possible neurologic and neurochemical dysfunction
- Physical, mental health, or learning problems

Early behavior problems
- Aggressiveness combined with shyness
- Emotional problems, hypersensitivity, difficult temperament
- Inability to express feelings appropriately
- Inability to cope with stress
- Problems with relationships
- Cognitive problems

Adolescent personality traits and issues
- Lack of self-confidence with low self-esteem and fragile ego
- Inability to form positive close relationships
- Vulnerability to negative peer pressure
- Lack of bonding to society (family, school, and community)
- Rebelliousness and nonconformity, with resistance to authority
- Strong need for independence
- Present versus future orientation
- School failure and dropout
- Unemployed or underemployed
- Delinquency and violent acts
- Early unprotected sexual activity, teen pregnancy/parenthood
- Mental health problems, suicidality

From U.S. Department of Health and Human Services Public Health Service, Substance Abuse and Mental Health Services Administration: Making prevention work. DHHS Publication No. SMA95–120, 1995, with permission.

THE ROLE OF THE CARE PROVIDER IN DEALING WITH TOBACCO, ALCOHOL, AND OTHER DRUGS

Efforts to prevent the use of tobacco, alcohol, and other drugs as well as other related risk behaviors should begin at an early age. Certainly, by the time

TABLE 2. Protective Factors for Substance Abuse in Teenagers

Community environment
- Middle or upper class with low unemployment
- Adequate housing in pleasant neighborhood with low prevalence of crime
- Good schools that promote learning, participation, and responsibility
- High-quality health care and easy access to social services
- Flexible social services providers who put clients' needs first

Family environment
- Adequate family income
- Stable, nurturing family with little marital conflict
- Parents who promote learning
- Fewer than 4 children in family with 2 or more years between birth of each child
- Few chronic stressful life events
- Multigenerational kinship network
- Nonkin support network, e.g., supportive role models, dependable child care
- Warm, close relationships with parents and other adults
- Family stability and cohesiveness
- Plenty of attention during first year of life
- Clear behavior guidelines

Constitutional strengths
- Adequate early sensorimotor and language development
- High intelligence with good physical health
- No emotional or temperamental impairments

Personality of the child
- Affectionate, endearing, easy temperament
- Autonomous yet adaptable and flexible
- Positive outlook with good sense of self-efficacy
- Self-discipline with adequate internal locus of control
- Problem-solving skills and social adeptness
- Tolerance of people and situations

From U.S. Department of Health and Human Services Public Health Service, Substance Abuse and Mental Health Services Administration: Making prevention work. DHHS Publication No. SMA95–120, 1995, with permission.

the adolescent reaches middle school, the clinician should be talking directly to the preteen as well as her parents at every visit. Discussions may center on risk and protective factors, with emphasis placed on those that have particular relevance to the family involved. The care provider should be well informed about issues related to tobacco, alcohol, and other drug use so that, if there are problems in this area, he or she will be seen as a resource.[12]

Adolescents should be seen in private at virtually every visit. Many clinicians recommend separating parent and child as early as age 10 years, and it is important to do so at routine "illness" visits as well as at scheduled health checks. Only in this way can a girl complaining of sore throat be asked about smoking or can one complaining of abdominal pain be asked about about sexual activity. The issue of confidentiality and its limits should be reiterated at every visit so that as the preteen gets older she will feel comfortable trusting the relationship that has developed with her care provider.

Many clinicians are uncomfortable inquiring about sensitive topics such as substance abuse. Several principles may be kept in mind that should ease this discomfort. First, uncovered problems do not have to be solved at the same visit. Giving patients and families permission to talk about sensitive topics may enable that discussion to take place at a later date if it is too difficult for them to raise those issues at the time of the visit. Finally, referring such problems for evaluation is appropriate.

While open-ended questioning is perhaps the most effective method of eliciting information, structured interviews and even printed questionnaires are available to help clinicians obtain information. Starting an interview with general questions about lifestyle and leisure activity preference helps to set a pleasantly uncritical tone. Many care providers find that proceeding with indirect questions about friends ("Do your friends drink/smoke/use drugs?") is a less threatening way to launch into the more difficult part of an interview. Placing questions in the passive mode ("Has anyone ever offered you or encouraged you to use cigarettes, alcohol, or other drugs?") may make a young person more comfortable discussing the issue. Simply asking what a patient likes to do when she is just "hanging out" with her friends may yield information that suggests problems in this area.

Brief tools are useful in assessing levels of tobacco, alcohol, and other drug use once the problem has been identified, although their statistical reliability has been validated less thoroughly in children than in adults. The so-called "CAGE" questions, for example, ask if a person has ever felt the need to CUT DOWN use of alcohol or drugs, been ANNOYED by criticism about such use, felt GUILTY about using, or felt the need for an EARLY morning dose to "get going." Any positive answer suggests that tobacco, alcohol, and other drug use is a problem for the young woman.

Parents should be alerted to some common signs of tobacco, alcohol, and other drug use so that they are prepared to seek advice and consultation if they are suspicious. While early signs of substance abuse may be subtle, patterns tend to develop, and more compulsive use can usually be detected by an alert clinician and parent (Table 3).

Suspicion of substance use or the presence of suggestive signs and symptoms warrants a comprehensive evaluation by a clinician trained in this area. Evaluations by clinical interview usually allow the care provider to determine a level of use and thereby suggest appropriate intervention. Statistics suggest that most adolescents experiment with tobacco and alcohol; in fact, as many as

TABLE 3. Behavioral Signs of Substance Abuse

1. Excessive irritability, fatigue, alienation, isolation, and moodiness
2. Decline in school performance or change in attendance
3. Withdrawal from interests, hobbies, extracurricular activities, and sports
4. Change in peer group with new friends visiting home
5. Unexplained phone calls and hang-ups
6. Unaccounted for absences from home
7. Fighting, lying, and stealing—with conning, defensive behavior
8. Recurrent physical complaints (cough, red eyes, sore throat, dizziness, headache)
9. Decline in physical appearance, hygiene
10. Adopting of new dress, hair styles, tattoos, body piercing
11. Encounters with school authorities or the law
12. Unusual home symptoms, including strange odors, missing money or alcohol
13. Finding of drug paraphernalia or obvious intoxication
14. Breaking of curfews and other home rules

45% of 1996 high school seniors report having tried marijuana.[2] Some experts[13] suggest that this phase of "learning the mood swing" is, in fact, normative adolescent behavior and, while not to be ignored, may warrant nothing more than counsel and advice about to the dangers of developing more compulsive use.

Adolescents who develop a pattern of increasing use of more potent drugs on a more frequent basis may enter a phase of actually "seeking the mood swing." Although there are objective definitions of substance abuse and dependence, it is the impact on the adolescent's ability to function in social, academic, and family settings that defines when a problem must be addressed. Clearly those who move on to preoccupation with drugs and eventually needing them to feel normal require formal intervention in a clinical setting designed to deal with chemically dependent young people.

The evaluation of the substance-abusing adolescent must involve a comprehensive investigation of other risk behaviors as well. Young women who use drugs are more likely to have experienced childhood sexual abuse,[14] to have engaged in antisocial behavior and delinquency, and to be involved in unsafe sexual activity. Depression, anxiety, and other mood disorders are far more common among adolescent girls who use tobacco, alcohol, and other drugs, and there also is a strong statistical association between girls who engage in unhealthy eating and weight loss practices.[15] Suicidality is more common among girls who are heavy users of substances.

Of note, although in males substance abuse is most often associated with conduct disorders and problems of impulsivity, in girls it is found more often among those who are socially isolated and depressed. The possibility of comorbidity must be explored in every girl found to be using alcohol and other drugs, and referral and treatment options must take this phenomenon into account.

TOBACCO

Girls who use tobacco experience the same short-term and long-term health consequences as boys. Smoking has become the leading cause of cancer deaths among women in America, having surpassed breast cancer a decade ago. One-quarter of teenage girls now smoke. Although many of them claim to be just experimenting, most become addicted to nicotine, and the quit rate among women is as dismal as that for men.[16] Although the use of smokeless tobacco is much less common among girls than among boys, the dangers of such products must be stressed because they are not a safe alternative to smoking.

Although many of the reasons that girls and boys take up smoking are similar, there are some remarkably consistent differences. Adolescent girl smokers tend to be socially competent and outgoing, with high levels of self-esteem and willingness to engage in rebellious behavior. Boys, on the other hand, tend to be more insecure, less outgoing, and more in need of a fixture to demonstrate their "adultness."[17]

The onslaught of targeted advertising and promotion of cigarettes to girls has been a major factor in the increase in their uptake of the habit. As early as the 1920s, the tobacco industry began to advertise to women's concerns, touting the appetite-suppressive effect of cigarettes and the resulting thinness and sexiness one might achieve. More recently, the tobacco companies have introduced terms such as "fresh," "thin," "slim," and "natural" into their marketing ploys and portrayed their products as being used pervasively by girls who are sexy, tough, independent, and popular.[18] Cigar manufacturers have recruited highly paid female models to promote their products as offering instant sophistication. Other "benefits" of smoking for women may include the perception that it gives them more energy, provides something "to do" with their hands, provides pleasure and relaxation, and makes them feel part of the crowd. The perceived value of smoking is significant for many young girls, especially those who have no plans to go on to college.[19]

Smoking and exposure to environmental tobacco smoke have a number of significant health effects. Short-term effects include increased incidence of upper respiratory and ear infections, pharyngitis, stained teeth, phlegm production, and persistent cough, in addition to foul-smelling breath, decreased exercise tolerance, and the damage inevitably done to clothes. Long-term effects, which concrete-thinking preadolescents disregard as problems related only to adults, include chronic bronchitis, emphysema, and lung and bladder cancer.

Women who are exposed to tobacco smoke show elevated levels of nicotine in cervical lavages, and smoking is strongly associated with cervical dysplasia as well as increased invasiveness and aggressiveness of endometrial cancer.[20] Perhaps because of the antiestrogen effect of nicotine or its effect on the hypothalamus, adolescent women who smoke have an increased incidence of secondary amenorrhea as well as other menstrual disorders, infertility, and early menopause. Sexual activity, vaginal discharge, suspicion of sexually transmitted infection, undiagnosed abdominal pain, and possibility of pregnancy are common reasons for initiating gynecologic care in adolescent women. Smoking should be another equally valid indication.

ALCOHOL

The landmark study of Frezza et al.[21] has provided a scientific basis for the observation that alcohol seems to have more devastating effects on women than on men. Women have lower levels of gastric alcohol dehydrogenase than men; thus a given amount of alcohol causes a higher blood-alcohol level for a longer time. This phenomenon is greatly exaggerated in alcoholic women who have virtually no metabolism of ethanol in the stomach. Furthermore, alcohol consumed by girls is generally distributed in a smaller total body volume, thereby further increasing concentrations.

Teenagers do not generally engage in "social drinking"—that is, one does not find groups of teenagers standing around, conversing, and nursing a beer. Adolescents drink to get drunk and tend to consume large amounts of alcohol very quickly. Some 62% of high school seniors in 1996 reported that they had been drunk at some point in their lives.[2]

Such heavy drinking has significant psychosocial effects on adolescent girls. Society generally condones heavy drinking in men, as portrayed in advertising and the media; thus becoming intoxicated may be seen as a boy's rite of passage. Society's condemnation of this behavior in women may lead to increased incidence of "closet drinking" as well as have a major effect on self-esteem.[22] Combined with the female tendency to internalize problems and the consequent predisposition to depression, this chemical depressant can exacerbate preexisting mental health problems.

Adolescent girls going to college represent another group at great risk for excessive alcohol consumption. Many women perceive that alcohol provides certain benefits, such as increased comfort in social situations. Clinicians must counsel these girls carefully, for women who enter college with low levels of concern for the effects of alcohol on their cognitive and behavioral patterns appear to be at high risk for heavy drinking.[23]

Heavy drinking, which again may be subject to a stricter interpretation in women because of the metabolic aspects alluded to earlier, carries with it the obvious health risks associated with intoxication. There is suggestive evidence that women are drinking and driving more aggressively. Falls and other accidents are more common (studies show that as many as one-third of emergency room visits for adults are associated with alcohol), and the problem of unwanted and unresisted sexual activity is a significant danger for women.

Finally, although complications of chronic alcohol consumption generally are not seen in teenagers, young people with a strong family history of alcoholism are at increased risk for the disease and its complications. Cirrhosis, alcoholic hepatitis, and esophageal varices are problems that are dose-responsive; there is a definite association between chronic excessive alcohol use and breast cancer in women, as well.

MARIJUANA

Marijuana remains the most popular illegal drug used by adolescents. The Monitoring the Future survey reveals that in 1996 nearly one-third of high school senior girls had used marijuana within the previous 12 months. This number has risen steadily in the last decade, although it does not approach the near 50% level of the late 1970s.

Of great concern is the persistent perception of marijuana's harmlessness. The marijuana of today bears little relationship to its cannabinoid-poor relative of the 70s, having concentrations of active ingredients that are some fivefold higher. This increase in concentration is critical in the change in usage patterns observed in teens today—from the "harmless giggle" of 20 years ago to the high-potency/high-reward dependence so characteristic of today. Girls who are compulsive users of marijuana may develop unhealthy relationships with their dealers or take to dealing themselves to pay for their habit.

Recent referenda in Arizona and California have led to the "medicalization" of marijuana, claiming that it has unique effects for various conditions ranging from the treatment of glaucoma to the nausea associated with cancer chemotherapy and that it is medically safe. A recent workshop conducted by the National Institutes of Health failed to identify any conditions for which smoked marijuana was a first-line therapy and suggested that additional research was needed.

Smoked marijuana has a number of effects on adolescent girls, causing respiratory infections, cough, and the exacerbation of asthma. There are also effects on human T-cell function, and the intensity at which the products of combustion are drawn into the lungs may have long-term effects that cause chronic lung conditions and cancer. A single dose of marijuana taken following ovulation suppresses luteinizing hormone levels by as much as 30% and may be a significant cause of infertility.

The target organ for marijuana is, of course, the brain. The recent identification of cannabinoid receptor sites in the brain and the development of an antagonist suggest that the potential for addiction is real. It is known that marijuana users experience acutely the loss of motor coordination and impairment of reaction time. Memory is impaired, and there are many experts who feel that chronic marijuana users develop an apathetic and lackadaisical state of mind commonly referred to as the "amotivational syndrome." Whether this condition is real or not is perhaps not important: girls who use marijuana on a regular basis do not do well in school, are not able to maintain relationships with family, and are unable to function at a job.

OTHER DRUGS AND SOME SPECIFIC EFFECTS ON YOUNG WOMEN

Cocaine

Powdered cocaine (usually inhaled or "snorted" as the hydrochloride salt) and its freebase congener (commonly called "crack") are used by a subset of adolescents who generally are heavily involved with drugs. While fewer than 2% of high school seniors use the drug, this statistic fails to represent its actual usage because most regular cocaine users are, in fact, not attending school. Major effects of cocaine include intense mood swings from exhilaration to despair and the overwhelming addictiveness of the drug, to which women may be especially susceptible.

Research from the National Institute on Drug Abuse suggests that women's hormonal changes, most notable during the luteal phase when progesterone levels are especially high, create thickening of nasal mucus, which impedes absorption and necessitates greater amounts to achieve a given effect. Women also may have high levels of the cholinesterase enzymes that break down cocaine, causing briefer chemical effects and increased drive for repeat dosing. This need for repeated doses of cocaine is a common factor driving young women into prostitution.

Sedatives, Tranquilizers, and Hallucinogens

Prescription and illegal drugs in these classes are commonly used by depressed girls who may self-medicate with such products in an attempt to feel better, but inadvertently exacerbate their mood swings. They are commonly used to mediate the effect of stimulants such as amphetamines.

Of particular concern is the use of drugs in these classes as "date rape" pills. Short-acting benzodiazepines are especially popular for this purpose because they are tasteless and may leave the victim with no memory of events during or preceding the assault.

Amphetamines and Amphetamine-like Over-the-Counter Products

Amphetamines are very popular drugs among girls attempting to lose weight, providing appetite suppression and the perception of increased energy. The ease with which methamphetamine is synthesized makes it readily available on the street, and methylphenidate (Ritalin) has become increasingly available as more young people are treated for attentional problems.

Over-the-counter medications also are abused by people who are attempting to suppress their appetite. Most of these products are ephedrine congeners, and overuse of products such as phenylpropanolamine and pseudoephedrine has been associated with cerebral hemorrhage as well as cardiac problems.

SPECIAL POPULATIONS

Users of Contraceptives

Much has been written about the relationship among combination oral contraceptive use, smoking, and cardiovascular disease in adult women. While smoking is not a contraindication to oral contraceptive use, pill users certainly should be given encouragement to quit, and nicotine replacement therapy is appropriate for women who desire assistance in smoking cessation. Nonetheless, oral contraceptive use by smokers is clearly less hazardous than pregnancy.

Perhaps because of its effect of increasing estrogen catabolism, cigarette smoking adversely affects cycle control among oral contraceptive users. This effect not only increases the chance of contraceptive failure, but also creates the concern that users may discontinue the pill because of unwanted spotting.[24]

No conclusive evidence suggests that smoking increases the risks associated with progesterone-only contraception such as injectable medroxyprogesterone (Depo-Provera) or levonorgestrel implants (Norplant). Given the predisposition to engage in risk behavior that many sexually active, drug-using teens exhibit, these methods may be the first choice for pregnancy prevention.

The Female Athlete

Performance-enhancing drugs are an increasing problem as girls engage in more elite competitive sports. The use of androgenic steroids, for example, carries the same risk of liver damage for women as it does for men. Additional problems include menstrual irregularities, growth of increased body hair, and exacerbation of acne.

Beta blockers are commonly used by women who need steadiness of hand and body. Archers, musicians, gymnasts, dancers, and billiards players may use products such as propranolol to help eliminate intention tremors and inhibit anxiety. Dangers of such use include hypotension, bradycardia, and depression.

Clearly, the short-term effects of inhaled products such as tobacco and marijuana have immediate effects upon stamina and mucus production and may be responsible for exercise-induced coughing and bronchospasm. The identification of these properties may be a useful deterrent to use of such products during the athletic season.

The Female with an Eating Disorder

Eating disorders, including anorexia nervosa and bulimia, are discussed elsewhere in this book. There is a high incidence of a comorbid substance abuse disorder among women with disordered eating behavior. Nicotine is a potent appetite suppressant, and smoking clearly exacerbates the menstrual irregularities associated with anorexia. The successful marketing of "thin" and "long" cigarettes to girls may make the habit more appealing to those who are concerned with body image.

The Female with School Problems

As with other mental health disorders, attention deficit disorder is significantly associated with substance use among adolescent girls. Poor school performance also is associated with increased likelihood of substance abuse and is a factor independent of the peer group with which a girl associates. Lack of participation in extracurricular activities and sports leaves a void that is frequently filled by tobacco, alcohol, and other drug use. Those who are having academic problems and thus are barred from such participation may find themselves with time on their hands and begin associating with similar students who use substances.

Many drugs have significant effects on learning ability. Nicotine appears to actually enhance short-term memory, whereas marijuana is commonly associated with a mellowness, absence, and a lack of commitment frequently alluded to as the "amotivational syndrome." Girls who have difficulty completing their school work experience school failure—a major cause of poor self-esteem, truancy, dropout, and other risk behaviors.

The Pregnant and Postpartum Female

The effects of tobacco, alcohol, and certain other drugs on the developing fetus are well known, and details are beyond the scope of this chapter. Alcohol causes a complex of birth defects of varying severity. So-called "fetal alcohol syndrome" is characterized by mental retardation and a variety of fairly specific facial and lip anomalies. Hearing and visual loss are also common. Milder forms, commonly called alcohol-related neurodevelopmental disorder and alcohol-related brain damage, may be associated with neurologic, learning, and behavioral disorders. Heavy bursts of consumption to the point of intoxication appear to be more dangerous than occasional drinks, but it must be stressed that there is no known "safe dose" of alcohol; all women must be cautioned not to drink during pregnancy.

Cigarette smoking affects the growth of the fetus, and there appears to be a linear dose-response relationship. On average, women who smoke throughout pregnancy can expect a 5% reduction in the size of their infant. There are no specific physical abnormalities related to smoking, and there is no effect on gestation, although the likelihood of ectopic pregnancy among smokers is increased twofold compared with nonsmokers. Although marijuana use during pregnancy has not been studied extensively, there appears to be an increase in minor physical abnormalities and shortening of gestation in the offspring of users, but no effect on infant size.[25]

Postnatal exposure to environmental smoke is a health hazard to the infant, increasing the likelihood of sudden infant death, as well as upper respiratory and ear infections, bronchitis, and asthma. These health effects may provide a significant motivation to quit for young smoking mothers, and the astute clinician should use this window of opportunity to offer strong advice about cessation.

Teenagers using cocaine, heroin, and other narcotics predictably have offspring with all the problems associated with in-utero exposure. Cocaine, for example, is associated with preterm labor and low birth weight. Heroin addicts receiving prenatal care are frequently maintained on methadone to prevent preterm labor. Lack of prenatal care, caused by denial, fear of repercussions if pregnancy is acknowledged, or lack of recognition of the pregnancy, only exacerbates these problems in infants of adolescents. Pregnancy may provide a motivation to quit in some adolescent women.

The Adolescent Girl with Mental Health Problems

A frequent clinical dilemma occurs when one encounters an angry, rebellious, truculent adolescent girl who clearly is dealing with self-esteem issues and is using drugs. Depressed adolescents may use drugs (such as stimulants or alcohol) to feel better. Conversely, some drug-using adolescents develop psychiatric disturbances such as depression, hallucinations, paranoid delusions, and symptoms consistent with psychosis. Finally, mental health problems and substance abuse problems may occur comorbidly. Accurate diagnosis depends on establishing the chronological relationship of mental health symptoms to substance abuse, the severity of such symptoms, and their persistence during times of abstinence.

It is critical for the clinician to identify patients with coexisting mental health and substance abuse problems, for appropriate treatment depends on accurate diagnosis. An older school of thought essentially insisted on considering substance abuse as the primary diagnosis when it existed and designed treatment programs to be free of all mind-altering substances. Current thinking recognizes that because of the high incidence of anxiety and depression among adolescent female substance abusers, psychopharmacologic therapy may be appropriate while these patients are being treated for their chemical dependency.

Adolescent Daughters of Alcohol- and Substance-Abusing Parents

It is estimated that one in five American children grows up in the home of a substance-abusing parent. There is clearly a genetic component to familial alcoholism—an estimated 18% of the female offspring of an alcoholic parent are likely to become alcoholic themselves by age 20 years—suggesting that the combination of genetics plus the stress of living with an impaired parent may be overwhelming to this population of girls.

Adolescent girls living in substance-abusing families suffer from a higher incidence of mental health problems. Parents may be emotionally unavailable, role modeling may be nonexistent, and the nurturing environment so critical to children's emotional health may simply be absent. In addition, there is a higher incidence of physical, emotional, and sexual abuse. Teenage girls who grow up in such homes have a higher incidence of psychosomatic as well as genuine physical complaints. The clinician should be alert to such problems and include the possibility of family substance abuse in the differential diagnosis of the patient who comes in repeatedly with difficult-to-diagnose problems or no evidence of disease.

SUMMARY

The use of tobacco, alcohol, and other drugs by adolescent females usually takes place in association with other risk behaviors. Girls who choose to use these substances almost invariably consort with others who have made similar choices, and the likelihood of engaging in unsafe sexual practices, having trouble at school, pursuing delinquent behavior, and being in trouble with the law is statistically much greater. Clinicians caring for adolescent girls should put these behaviors in context, and the identification of any one of them should lead to careful assessment for the others.

REFERENCES

1. Kaufman N: Smoking and young women: The physician's role in stopping an equal opportunity killer. JAMA 271:629–630, 1994.
2. Johnston LD, O'Malley PM, Bachman JG: Monitoring the Future: Questionnaire Responses from the Nation's Students. Ann Arbor, MI, Institute for Social Research, University of Michigan, 1996.
3. U.S. Department of Health and Human Services Public Health Service, Substance Abuse and Mental Health Services Administration: National Household Survey on Drug Abuse, 1998. Washington, DC, Department of Health and Human Services, 1999.
4. Yamaguchi K, Kandel DB: Patterns of drug use from adolescence to young adulthood: II. Sequences of progression. Am J Public Health 74:668–672, 1994.
5. Martin C, Milich R, Martin W, et al: Gender differences in adolescent psychiatric outpatient substance abuse: Associated behaviors and feelings. J Am Acad Child Adolesc Psychiatry 36:486–494, 1997.
6. Center on Addiction and Substance Abuse at Columbia University: National Survey of American Attitudes on Substance Abuse. New York, 1995.
7. Jessor R: Risk behavior in adolescence: A psychosocial framework for understanding and action. J Adolesc Health 12:597–605, 1991.
8. Botvin G, Botvin E: Adolescent tobacco, alcohol and drug abuse: Prevention strategies, empirical findings and assessment issues. J Dev Behav Pediatrics 13:290–301, 1992.
9. Lifrak P, McKay J, Rostain A, et al: Relationship of perceived competencies, perceived social support and gender to substance use in young adolescents. J Am Acad Child Adolesc Psychiatry 36:933–940, 1997.
10. Tschann J, Adler N, Irwin C, et al: Initiation of substance abuse in early adolescence: The roles of pubertal timing and emotional distress. Health Psychol 13:326–333, 1994.
11. U.S. Department of Health and Human Services Public Health Service, Substance Abuse and Mental Health Services Administration: Making prevention work. DHHS Publication No. SMA95-120, 1995.

12. Heyman R: Tobacco: Prevention and cessation strategies. Adolesc Health Update 9(3), 1997.
13. Macdonald D: Drugs, Drinking and Adolescents. Chicago, Yearbook, 1984.
14. Pearce E, Lovejoy F: Detecting a history of childhood sexual experiences among women substance abusers. J Subst Abuse Treat 12:283–287, 1995.
15. Neumark-Sztainer D, Story M, French S: Covariations of unhealthy weight loss behaviors and other high-risk behaviors among adolescents. Arch Pediatr Adolesc Med 150:304–308, 1996.
16. Fiore M, Bailey WC, Cohen SJ, et al: Smoking Cessation: Clinical Practice Guideline No. 18. Rockville, MD, U.S. Department of Health and Human Services, Public Health Service, Agency for Health Care Policy and Research, AHCPR Publication No. 96-0692, 1996.
17. Waldron I: Patterns and causes of gender differences in smoking. Soc Sci Med 32:989–1005, 1991.
18. Pierce J, Lee L, Gilpin E: Smoking initiation by adolescent girls 1944 through 1988: An association with targeted advertising. JAMA 271:608–612, 1994.
19. French S, Perry C: Smoking among adolescent girls: Prevalence and etiology. J Am Med Womens Assoc 51:25–30, 1996.
20. Critchlow C, Wolner-Hansenn P, Eschenbach D, et al: Determinants of cervical ectopia and cervicitis: Age, oral contraception, specific cervical infection, smoking and douching. Am J Obstet Gynecol 173:534–543, 1995.
21. Frezza M, di Padova C, Pozzato G, et al: High blood alcohol levels in women: The role of decreased gastric alcohol dehydrogenase activity and first pass metabolism. N Engl J Med 322:95–99, 1990.
22. Thomas B: The effectiveness of selected risk factors in mediating gender differences in drinking and its problems. J Adolesc Health 17:91–98, 1995.
23. Werner M, Walker L, Greene J: Relationship of alcohol expectancies to problem drinking among college women. J Adolesc Health 16:191–199, 1995.
24. Rosenberg M, Waugh M: Smoking and cycle control among oral contraceptive users. Am J Obstet Gynecol 174:628–632, 1996.
25. Cornelius M, Taylor P, Geva D, Day N: Prenatal tobacco and marijuana use among adolescents: Effects on offspring gestational age, growth and morphology. Pediatrics 95:738–743, 1995.

CHAPTER 17

Breast Disorders

Paritosh Kaul, M.D.
Susan M. Coupey, M.D.

The breast plays an important role for the adolescent girl in her awareness of her sexuality. It is an organ for nourishment of the young, yet today it is a symbol of womanhood, femininity, and sexual attractiveness. Although a breast mass in this age group is most often benign, it is a source of anxiety for the patient and her parents. The physician taking care of young women often faces concerns about breast development or breast lumps. This chapter reviews the embryology and timing of breast development as well as discusses the breast examination and pathologic conditions of the adolescent breast.

STRUCTURE AND DEVELOPMENT

Breasts are milk-producing sweat glands. They lie over the anterior chest wall between the second rib and sixth intercostal space. Each breast contains 15–20 lobes arranged in a radial pattern (Fig. 1). Each lobe consists of many lobules, which in turn consist of 10–100 alveoli. These alveoli are the structural units of the breast.

The breast develops in the sixth week of intrauterine life as an ectodermal thickening along mammary ridges, which extend bilaterally from the axilla to the groin (Fig. 2). This is known as the "nipple line" or "milk line." The areola develops during the fifth fetal month. At birth, only main mammary ducts are present. The glands develop during puberty.

The growth of the breast is dependent on hormones, which act primarily during two developmental periods, puberty and pregnancy. At puberty, increased estrogen secretion from the ovaries causes the size and pigmentation of the areola to increase and stimulates the growth of breast tissue underneath. In addition, at this time estrogen stimulates an overall increase in adipose tissue and stromal growth in the breast. The circulating estrogen binds to the receptors in the breast, causing its physiologic effects.

Progesterone, a hormone secreted during the luteal phase of an ovulatory menstrual cycle and in large amounts during pregnancy, influences growth of the alveolar components of the lobule. This hormone initiates lobular growth and alveolar budding. It also contributes to alveolar secretory development.

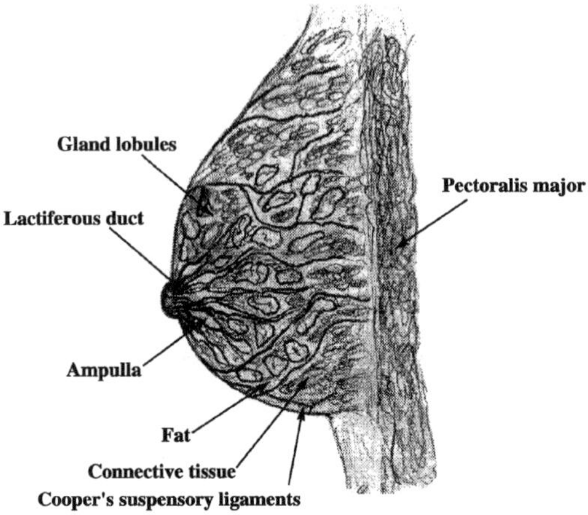

FIGURE 1. Diagram of structure of breast. (From Greydanus DE, Patel DR, Baxter TL: The breast and sports: Issues for the clinician. Adolesc Med 9:535, 1998, with permission.)

Prolactin, secreted by the lactotroph cells of the anterior pituitary gland in increased amounts during pregnancy and lactation, stimulates the growth of milk-secreting cells of the alveolar lining. The final differentiation of the alveolar cell occurs in the presence of prolactin. Although prolactin is necessary for the final differentiation of the secreting cells, this effect is only possible after these cells have been exposed to two hormones, insulin and cortisol. The physiologic effects of estrogen on the breast occur when estrogen binds to its receptor. This binding of the estrogen and its receptor occurs only in the presence of prolactin. Optimal breast development requires estrogen, progesterone, insulin, cortisol, thyroxine, prolactin, and growth hormone. If there is a deficiency of any of these hormones, increased secretion of prolactin, as occurs with lactation, can compensate for the hormonal deficiencies and complete the development of the breast.

Sexual Maturity Rating (SMR)

Sexual maturity rating (SMR), also called Tanner staging, is used to classify the stage of breast development in adolescents. This rating system was developed

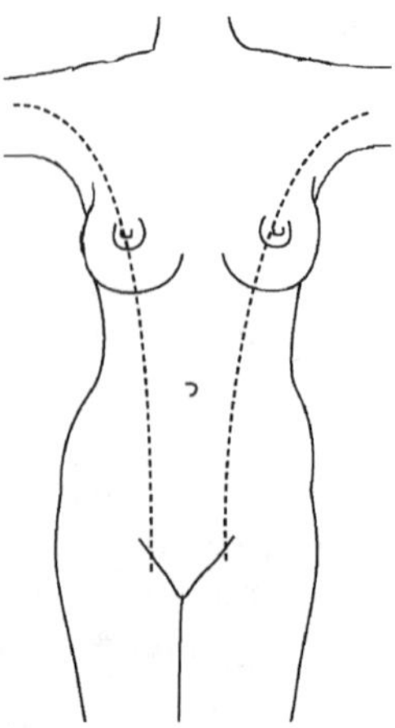

FIGURE 2. Nipple lines along embryonic mammary ridges. (From Greydanus DE, Patel DR, Baxter TL: The breast and sports: Issues for the clinician. Adolesc Med 9:534, 1998, with permission.)

TABLE 1. Sexual Maturity Rating (SMR)

SMR	Breast	Areola
1	Prepubertal	Conforms to chest wall
2	Breast bud	Areola widens
3	Breast mound enlargement	Areola enlarges
4	Breast mound elevation	Raised areola
5	Adult breast	Papilla projects above areola

in 1962 by Tanner, a British anthropologist. A description of the five steps is shown in Table 1 (also see photo, chapter 1).

Thelarche is the term used to describe the onset of breast development corresponding with SMR 2. The average age at thelarche for girls in the United States is 9.8 years, with a range from 8–13 years for 99% of the population. Thelarche is usually the first sign of puberty in girls.

Premature and Delayed Thelarche

Premature thelarche is defined as breast development beginning before the eighth birthday. Premature thelarche should be differentiated from true precocious puberty. The latter may indicate a serious underlying cause. The two conditions may be differentiated by bone age, which should be normal in premature thelarche and advanced in precocious puberty. Serum estradiol levels should be between 70 and 220 pg/ml in premature thelarche, whereas they are higher in precocious puberty.

Delayed breast development is defined as no breast budding by the thirteenth birthday. Whether delayed thelarche occurs alone or in conjunction with delayed puberty, it requires a full evaluation. Particular attention should be given to the girl's height and weight, overall growth pattern, symptoms of chronic illness or eating disorders, and endocrinologic evaluation. Delayed thelarche may be associated with systemic disorders like malnutrition, Crohn's disease, radiation therapy, congenital adrenal hyperplasia, gonadal dysgenesis, hypogonadotrophic hypogonadism, and 17-alpha hydroxylase deficiency.

EXAMINATION OF THE BREAST

The examination of the breast should be part of the routine health maintenance visit for every adolescent girl. Some clinicians defer examination of the breast out of sensitivity to the girl's modesty. However, making it part of the routine visit demystifies the issue and helps the adolescent to accept her breasts as part of her body. At the age of 8 or 9 years when thelarche occurs, examination of the breast can serve as a forum for anticipatory guidance related to puberty and menstruation for both the patient and the parents. During the routine breast examination, the clinician also may instruct the patient regarding self-examination. In addition, the appearance of breast budding should be a cue to the clinician to examine carefully the musculoskeletal system, especially the spine for scoliosis, because the girl will begin her adolescent growth spurt within a year.

Breast Self-Examination

Instructing all adolescents to perform breast self-examination is controversial. The incidence of breast cancer in this age group is extremely low, and insistence on frequent self-examination may serve only to increase anxiety. Heightened anxiety and attention to the breast may result in increased health care visits and surgical intervention. The time that the clinician spends giving a detailed explanation of the technique of breast self-examination may be better used in counseling about decreasing high-risk behavior, which accounts for much morbidity in the adolescent years.

On the other hand, adolescents are highly conscious of their developing breasts, and breast self-examination helps to teach responsibility towards the body. The technique that is taught may be modified somewhat to make it less onerous, and the clinician should not be too insistent that the girl must do this every month (Fig. 3). Such insistence only sets up many patients for failure. Even if a girl does not remember to examine her breasts after every menstrual period, learning the technique of breast self-examination initiates a habit that can be reinforced as the young woman ages. The process of breast self-examination also enhances the adolescent's level of comfort with the clinical examination and provides an excellent opportunity for discussions of women's health issues.

CONGENITAL ANOMALIES OF THE BREAST

Polythelia is the existence of accessory nipples and areolae anywhere along the "milk line" and is seen in 1–2% of adolescent girls (Fig. 4). It has been linked to urologic and cardiovascular defects. Supernumerary breasts, polymastia, and nipples may be unilateral, bilateral, and/or familial. They usually require no treatment unless surgical excision is necessary for cosmetic reasons.

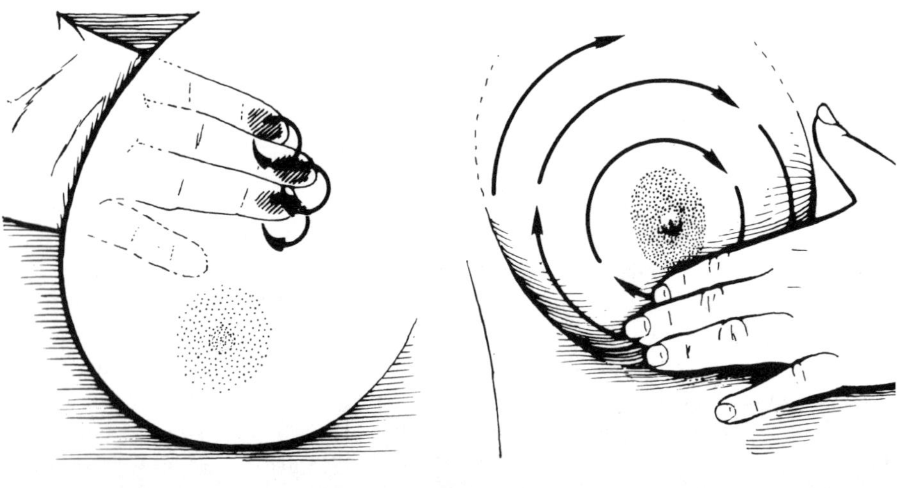

FIGURE 3. Diagram of breast self-examination. (From illustrations by David Factor in Beach RK: Routine breast exams: A chance to reassure, guide, and protect. Contemp Pediatr 4:73–74, 1987, with permission.)

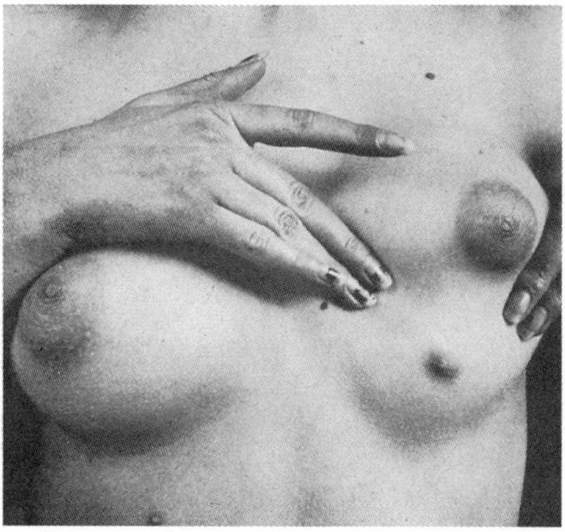

FIGURE 4. Polythelia.

Athelia (absence of nipples) and **amastia** (absence of breast tissue) are other congenital anomalies, but they are extremely rare. Amastia is associated with the rare Poland syndrome, which consists of aplasia of pectoralis muscles, rib deformities, webbed fingers, and radial nerve aplasia. Amastia sometimes is related to inadvertent surgical removal of the breast bud in infancy during chest wall surgery.

Breast atrophy may be seen in patients with severe weight loss or eating disorders. The weight loss causes a decrease in both the glandular and fatty elements of the breast. Hypoestrogenism is an additional mechanism, apart from weight loss, for breast atrophy in patients with eating disorders. Other conditions causing low estrogen secretion, high androgen production, or a combination of both also may cause breast atrophy. Scleroderma may cause unilateral or localized breast atrophy.

Juvenile hypertrophy is pathologic overgrowth of the breasts, which may be unilateral or bilateral (Fig. 5). This condition occurs at puberty with rapid, often painful, breast growth. Girls with this condition may present with severe physical sequelae of enlarged breasts. Sequelae include significant fugal intertrigo, tissue necrosis, and rupture of the skin. Mechanical consequences such as backache, postural kyphosis, and shoulder soreness from brassiere straps also may occur. However, the overriding concerns usually are cosmetic. At present, experience with medical management is limited, although some benefit using danazol (an antiestrogen) has been reported. Surgery is the mainstay in the management of this condition. Reduction mammoplasty is the procedure of choice, and often up to 500 gm of breast tissue requires excision. Adolescents with juvenile hypertrophy may suffer severe psychological consequences. Supportive counseling should always be offered pre- and postsurgery. Girls and their families need to understand the risks and benefits of surgery, including scars, infection, and potential difficulties with breast-feeding.

Tuberous breast deformity occurs when there is breast hypoplasia with protuberant and overdeveloped areola (Fig. 6). Because the base of the breast is underdeveloped and the nipple–areolar complex is overdeveloped, it has the appearance of a tuberous root, which explains the name. The glandular elements often are contained within the distended nipple–areolar complex. This

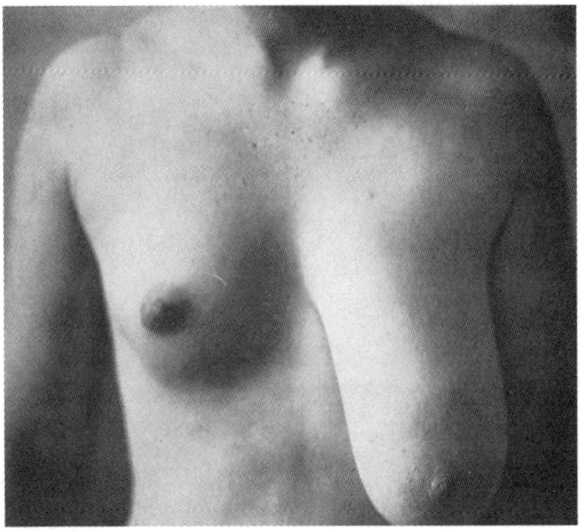

FIGURE 5. Juvenile hypertrophy (unilateral).

type of deformity may be seen in girls who have been taking exogenous hormones for treatment of premature ovarian failure, gonadal dysgenesis, or abnormalities of gonadotropin-releasing hormone secretion, but it also occurs in the absence of hormonal treatment. Tuberous breast deformity may be managed conservatively, and plastic surgery is reserved only for the most severe cases. Conservative management includes offering reassurance and counseling services to the adolescent.

Breast asymmetry is a normal variant. Frequently, in early puberty (SMR 2–4), one breast may be larger than the other, but catch-up growth usually occurs by SMR 5. Almost 25% remain asymmetrical until adulthood. The pubertal patient needs to be reassured about the likelihood of catch-up growth. However, surgical correction should be performed at SMR 5 (1–2 years after menarche) if marked asymmetry persists. The surgeon should be careful not to correct the asymmetry before SMR 5 because such correction may result in inadvertent removal of normal breast tissue. Surgery consists of either reducing the large breast or augmenting the small one, depending on the anatomy.

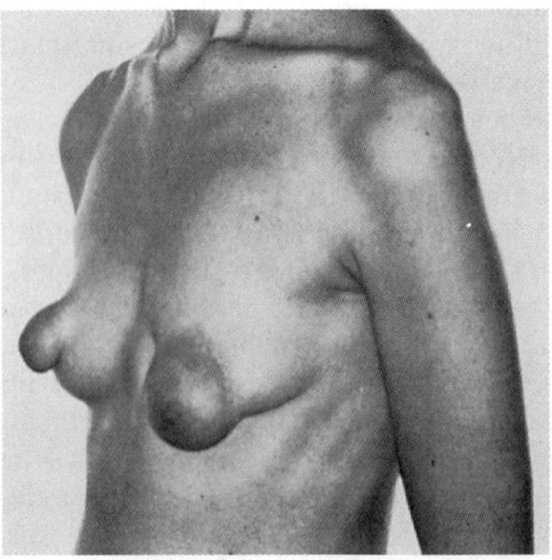

FIGURE 6. Tuberous breast.

BREAST INFECTIONS

Mastitis or infection of the breast tissue usually is associated with lactation. However, it also may occur in nonlactating adolescents. Infection most often develops beneath the areola and at the margin between the areola and the normal skin. Mastitis may occur secondary to trauma, during sports, during sexual activity, or after plucking of periareolar hair. The other predisposing factors are duct ectasia, metaplasia of duct epithelium, and macrocystic disease. The organisms that cause mastitis are *Staphylococcus aureus, Streptococcus pyogenes, Micrococcus* sp., *Escherichia coli,* and *Pseudomonas aeruginosa*. In the early stages of the infection, the patient presents with a warm and tender breast. Later, the presentation may include a tender, fluctuant breast mass with tender axillary lymph nodes. When superficial, the infection can be managed conservatively with hot compresses and oral antibiotics. A first-generation cephalosporin (e.g., cephalexin or cephradine) is the drug of choice. Recently, the use of macrolide antibiotics, in particular azithromycin, has been found to be effective. Breast abscesses may require incision and drainage.

NIPPLE DISCHARGE

Physiological nipple discharge is serous, unilateral, or bilateral. It occurs from multiple ducts and is nonspontaneous in nature. The cause of the discharge is excessive breast manipulation by either the patient or her sexual partner. The use of a poorly fitting brassiere also may result in a similar complaint. Stimulation of the breast results in two neurologic reflexes. The first reflex develops via the anterior pituitary that inhibits dopamine and stimulates prolactin. The second reflex works via the posterior pituitary by stimulating the release of oxytocin.

Pathological nipple discharge is classified by the color of the discharge. It could be bloody, serous, or milk-like (galactorrhea).

Bloody or serous discharges in adolescents are often the presentation of an intraductal papilloma. There is abnormal proliferation of the mammary epithelium, which projects into the duct lumen causing a blockage of the duct. Minimal local trauma causes rupture of the vascular stalk, resulting in a bloody discharge. In 50% of cases, a mass can be palpated under the involved duct. Surgical excision of the duct is the treatment of choice.

Dark brown discharge is seen with mammary duct ectasia. This is a clinical syndrome of nipple discharge, nipple inversion, breast mass, and/or nonpuerperal periareolar mastitis. There may be fibrosis of the underlying breast and skin dimpling. Hyperprolactinemia also has been associated with mammary duct ectasia. Patients have undiagnosed prolactinomas. The relationship between hyperprolactinemia and the inflammation is not exactly known. Some authors believe that the inflammation leads to a neurogenic hyperprolactinemia. In some patients with hyperprolactinemia (e.g., due to a prolactin-secreting adenoma), there is galactorrhea, which predisposes the patient to secondary infection. The treatment of choice is surgical excision of the duct and any associated mass.

TABLE 2. Causes of Hyperprolactinemia

1. **Physiologic states**
   a. Pregnancy
   b. Lactation
   c. Sleep
   d. Stress
   e. Nipple stimulation
2. **Drugs**
   a. Dopamine receptor agonist
      i. Phenothiazines
      ii. Butyrophenones
      iii. Metoclopramide
      iv. Risperidone
      v. Thioxanthines
   b. Dopamine-depleting agents
      i. Methyldopa
      ii. Reserpine
   c. Hormones
      i. Estrogens
      ii. Antiandrogens
      iii. Oral contraceptive pills
   d. Others
      i. Opiates
      ii. Verapamil
3. **Central nervous system disease**
   a. Pituitary tumors
      i. Prolactinomas
      ii. Growth hormone–secreting adenomas
      iii. Nonfunctioning chromophobe tumors with pituitary stalk compression
   b. Hypothalamic and pituitary stalk disease
      i. Granulomatous diseases, especially sarcoidosis
      ii. Craniopharyngiomas and other tumors
      iii. Cranial irradiation
      iv. Stalk section
      v. Metastatic carcinoma
4. **Miscellaneous**
   a. Primary hypothyroidism
   b. Chronic renal failure
   c. Cirrhosis
   d. Chest wall trauma (including surgery, herpes)

Serosanguinous discharge is seen in "jogger's nipple." Nipple injury results from prolonged contact with an irritating material like a brassiere or other rough-surfaced clothing or seam. A raw and bleeding nipple also may develop from other forms of exercise besides running. There may be persistent pain associated with cold-induced thermal injury, called "bicyclist nipple." During outdoor exercise, moisture from perspiration, evaporation, and wind chill all lower the nipple temperature, resulting in nipple soreness and sensitivity to touch and temperature change. "Jogger's nipple" can be prevented by use of a plastic bandage over a coating of petroleum jelly before exercise and use of a properly fitted sports brassiere. The use of wind-breaking material over the chest and avoidance of cold weather are beneficial in the prevention of nipple trauma in athletes. An abrasion can be treated conservatively by wound care and treatment of secondary infection, should it occur.

GALACTORRHEA

A milk-like discharge from the nipple is described as galactorrhea. In all patients with galactorrhea, pregnancy must be ruled out. The discharge is not necessarily white but can be water-like.

Pathophysiology

The final pathway causing galactorrhea is inappropriate secretion of prolactin. This hormone is under the control of a prolactin-releasing factor (PRF) and a prolactin-inhibiting factor (PIF), both secreted from the hypothalamus. The PRF has not been identified in humans, although it exists in fowl.

Thyrotropin-releasing hormone (TRH) from the hypothalamus is a potent stimulator of prolactin, and it is possible that it has a role similar to PRF in fowls. PIF is dopamine itself, a potent inhibitor of prolactin release. Dopamine is secreted by the basal hypothalamus into the portal system and thus to the anterior pituitary. Normally, prolactin is under chronic tonic inhibition because of the presence of PIF. If this mechanism is disturbed, the result is increased secretion of prolactin (hyperprolactinemia) and thereby secretion of milk from the breast (galactorrhea).

Local factors such as breast manipulation (sexual stimulation, physical activity) act in a similar manner as prolonged suckling, inhibiting release of PIF and resulting in galactorrhea. Other local factors associated with galactorrhea, such as trauma, thoracotomy scars, herpes zoster, and cervical spinal lesions, influence prolactin secretion by the afferent neural arc and thereby stimulate suckling.

Medications such as the phenothiazines and other drugs cause galactorrhea by hypothalamic suppression. They either deplete dopamine levels or block the dopamine receptors, thus decreasing PIF. Excessive estrogen, as in high-dose oral contraceptive pills, leads to secretion of prolactin via the hypothalamic suppression. However, the low-dose pills currently in use are less likely to cause galactorrhea.

Stress may inhibit hypothalamic PIF, leading to increased prolactin levels. Hypothalamic lesions, lesions of the pituitary stalk, or stalk compression may physically reduce production or delivery of PIF and allow excessive production of prolactin. Elevated levels of TRH in hypothyroidism may stimulate prolactin secretion.

Tumors of the anterior pituitary may result in increased levels of prolactin independent of PIF. Apart from secreting prolactin, the expanding tumor may compress surrounding structures, interfering with the secretion of other tropic hormones. This infrequent but serious disease has disabling endocrinologic, neurologic, and ophthalmic consequences. Tumors of the central nervous system (CNS), like craniopharyngioma, also may secrete prolactin. Secretion of prolactin from nonpituitary sources such as lung and renal tumors is possible, although rare.

Clinical Presentation

The adolescent girl with hyperprolactinemia may have varied presentations. She may come with a nipple discharge or menstrual dysfunction such as dysfunctional uterine bleeding, luteal phase defects, or amenorrhea. She may present with mild hirsuitism and signs of anovulation. Girls with pituitary tumors may present with headaches and/or visual field defects. Pituitary tumors associated with lactotroph (cells that secrete prolactin in the anterior pituitary) hyperplasia may present with classical signs of galactorrhea and amenorrhea.

Laboratory and Imaging Studies

Necessary laboratory investigations depend on the symptoms of the patient (Fig. 7). Adolescents who have menstrual irregularities should have a progesterone challenge test and measurement of levels of thyroid-stimulating hormone

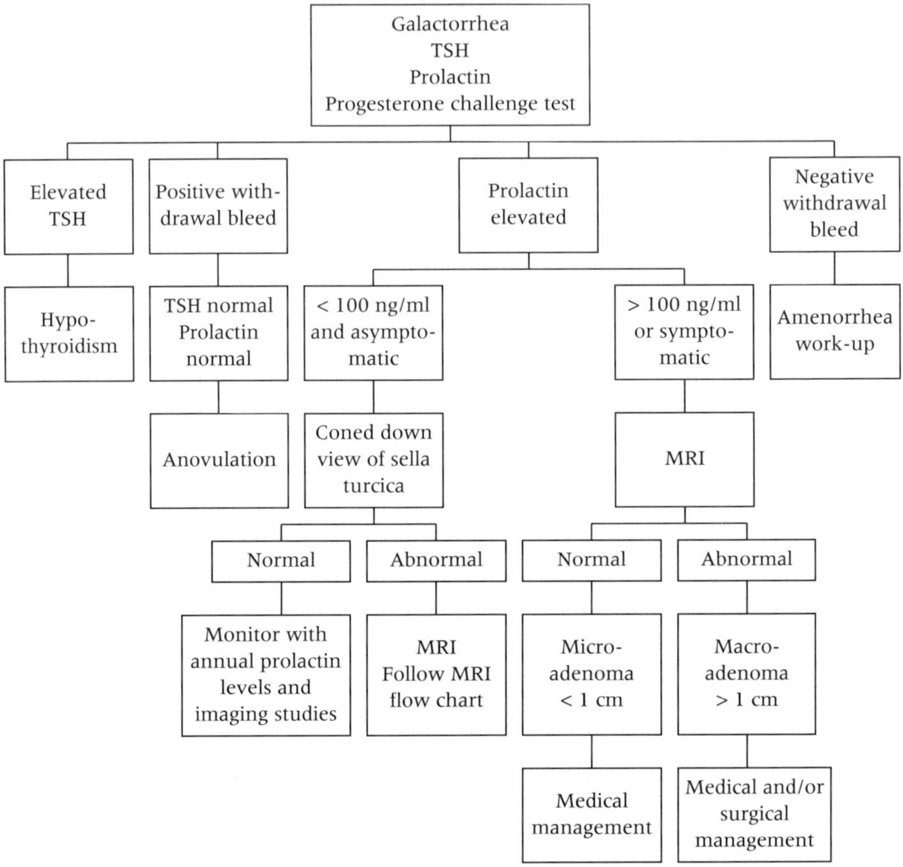

FIGURE 7. Evaluation of galactorrhea.

(TSH) and prolactin. The prolactin levels are most accurate if drawn in the morning after the patient has remained supine for 20–30 minutes, with no recent breast examination or stimulation. The adolescent should be relaxed and not acutely stressed so as to falsely elevate prolactin levels. Generally, serum prolactin levels > 100 ng/ml suggest tumor. Serum levels in this range are usually associated with abnormal imaging studies, CNS symptoms, or a history of primary malignancy.

Patients in whom a pituitary adenoma is suspected should undergo radiological imaging. The imaging procedure of choice is magnetic resonance imaging (MRI) of the hypothalamus and pituitary. The MRI is essential to differentiate between intrasellar lesions such as microadenomas and large "nonfunctioning" adenomas from suprasellar lesions such as craniopharyngiomas, germinomas, and meningiomas.

Management

Adolescents with galactorrhea with prolactin levels of less than 100 ng/ml and normal imaging studies should be offered medical management with bromocriptine or annual surveillance. Patients desiring pregnancy or in whom the galactorrhea is a cosmetic problem also should be offered bromocriptine. Bromocriptine, a dopamine agonist, is the only drug that has been approved by the FDA for use in the United States. It is the therapy of choice for patients with microadenomas. Therapy is started at a low dose of 0.625–1.25 mg once a day with a snack at bedtime and gradually increased to 2.5 mg twice a day. Patients may respond at lower doses. The most common side effects of the medication are nausea, vomiting, fatigue, nasal stuffiness, and postural hypotension. The drug is expensive but can abolish galactorrhea in all patients, including those with nonhyperprolactinemic galactorrhea. Size decreases most rapidly in the first 3 months of therapy. Treatment success is evaluated by assessing clinical manifestations, serum prolactin levels, and tumor size by MRI.

Adolescents with macroadenomas (adenoma > 1 cm) and higher levels of serum prolactin usually require surgery after pretreatment with bromocriptine. Transsphenoidal microsurgery is a safe procedure but is associated with up to an 80% recurrence rate.

BREAST MASSES

Anxiety and panic usually are the first responses in the adolescent and her parent once a breast mass is discovered (Fig. 8). Luckily, malignancy is extremely rare. Most palpable breast masses in adolescent girls are either fibroadenomas or benign cysts. Tumors of adjacent structures, particularly in thin girls, may be mistaken for a breast mass. These include tumors of the rib, chest wall, and dermal tissue.

Fibroadenoma

In surgical series, fibroadenomas account for 54–94% of histological diagnoses of breast masses and are the most common masses found in adolescents. On clinical examination, the fibroadenoma is encapsulated, rubbery, mobile, and nontender. It often is found in the upper outer quadrant of the breast and is unilateral in 75% of cases. There is no associated nipple discharge. On ultrasound, the mass has the classic features of a well circumscribed, homogenous, hypoechoic mass. Management depends on the size of the mass. If the fibroadenoma is ≤ 3 cm in diameter, they should be observed for 2–4 months. Excisional biopsy may be considered if the patient is symptomatic or if there is no regression in 6 months. However, if the mass is > 3 cm, rapidly enlarging, or has an unusual presentation, an excisional biopsy should be performed.

Breast Cysts

The nonpathologic, physiologic response to cyclic hormonal changes has been called a fibrocystic disease of the breast. Some authors now prefer to use the term "fibrocystic changes" because this common condition is not a disease process. The cause of the cystic changes is relative hyperestrogenism. The changes appear to be an inflammatory response in the stroma and alveolar tissues to the interaction of the hormones estrogen and progesterone. Histology

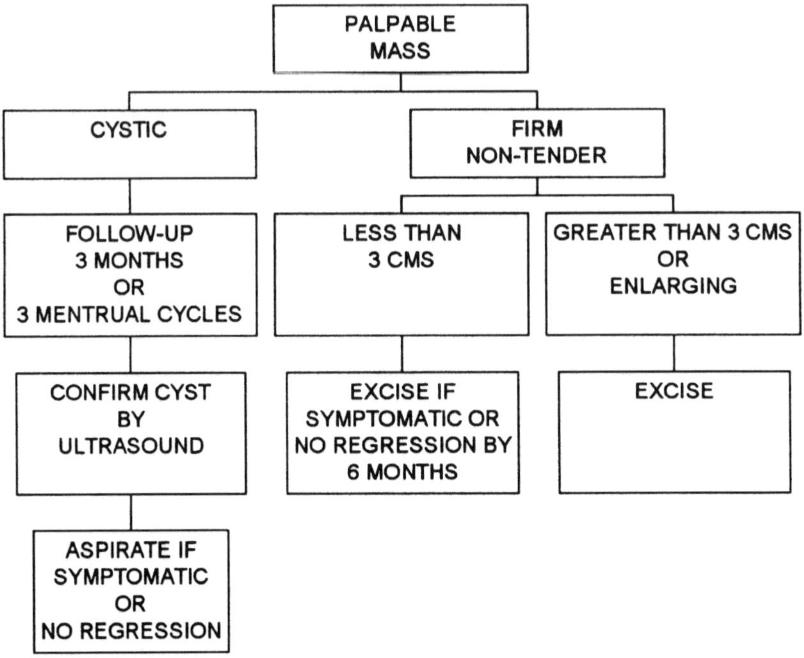

FIGURE 8. Evaluation of a breast mass.

shows both cystic and epithelial proliferative changes in the ductal tissue. The most common presentation of the condition in adolescents is breast pain or discomfort, particularly in the premenstrual phase of the menstrual cycle. The patient may also note swelling, tenderness, and nodularity of the breast. On palpation, the breasts are nodular without the presence of a discrete mass. These physical findings change with the menstrual cycle, resolving during the follicular phase and recurring during the luteal phase. Occasionally, a discrete mass can be palpated. Diagnosis of a cyst is made on ultrasound (showing a smooth, fluid-filled mass) and/or needle aspiration of cyst fluid.

The treatment depends on the severity of symptoms. In mild cases, a well-supported brassiere helps to prevent inflammation and stretching of supportive ligaments. Girls with moderate pain may require nonsteroidal antiinflammatory medication, whereas more severe cases may be treated with oral contraceptive pills.

Giant Juvenile Fibroadenoma

Giant juvenile fibroadenoma is a variant of fibroadenoma. It generally occurs at a younger age than classical fibroadenoma. Giant juvenile fibroadenoma can be single or multiple and is found in African-American girls. This mass is benign and rapidly enlarges to > 5 cm in diameter. It often distorts the breast parenchyma and may result in pressure necrosis of the skin. There is good recovery of breast architecture after surgical excision, and most patients do not require breast reconstruction.

Cystosarcoma Phyllodes

Cystosarcoma phyllodes is a rare primary tumor that usually is benign but may be of low-grade malignancy in adolescent girls. Histologic features such as stromal cellularity, nuclear atypia, mitotic activity, necrosis, and nature of tumor margins determine the malignant classification. The lesion is large (average of 6 cm) and circumscribed, and the overlying skin may be stretched because of the size of the tumor. It is the most common primary breast malignancy in adolescents, but is rare in patients younger than 20 years of age. Additional physical findings may include skin retraction, nipple discharge, and nipple retraction. The presence of lymphadenopathy should suggest lymphoma rather than a primary breast malignancy. The histology of the tumor does not correlate well with biological behavior; therefore, local excision is advised with close follow-up. Occasionally, metastases occur via the hematogenous route, in which case aggressive treatment with surgery, chemotherapy, radiation, and sometimes hormonal therapy is recommended.

Hematoma

Trauma to the breast can produce a hematoma. The possibility of physical and/or sexual abuse must always be considered in patients with a hematoma. Management consists of antiinflammatory medications and breast support with a sports brassiere or elastic wrap.

Fat Necrosis

Fat necrosis presents as a small, firm, immobile mass, usually associated with a previous history of trauma. It is rare in adolescents, and it does not enlarge but resolves slowly with time.

Malignancy

Breast malignancy is rare in adolescents. In two of the largest series by Ferguson et al. and Seltzer et al., no biopsy specimens from patients under 20 years old were positive for carcinoma of the breast. Only 0.2% of cases of carcinoma occur before the age of 25 years. Malignancies other than carcinomas are more likely in adolescent girls. Fewer than 1% of biopsies are positive in girls under 22 years old. Rhabdomyosarcoma, lymphoma, neuroblastoma, acute leukemia, liposarcoma, fibrosarcoma, Hodgkin's disease, and lymphoma have all been reported as presenting as breast masses in adolescents.

The clinical presentation depends on the type of malignancy. Constitutional symptoms such as anorexia, weight loss, and fatigue may be present as well as signs of anemia, axillary lymphadenopathy, hepatosplenomegaly, and masses elsewhere in the body. Any breast mass that is enlarging should be biopsied.

Our knowledge of adolescent breast carcinoma is limited because of the rarity in this population. No clear factors identifying the adolescent at risk have been found. However, risk factors in the adult population have been identified. These include radiation to the chest and family history of breast cancer.

Recently, in 1997, provisional recommendations for patients who have been identified with one of the breast cancer genes (BRCA-1 or BRCA-2) were published. They include monthly self-examination beginning at ages 18–21 years, annual or semiannual clinical breast examination at ages 25–35 years, and annual mammography screening beginning at ages 25–35 years.

BREAST IMAGING

Ultrasonography is the imaging procedure of choice in adolescent girls with breast masses. It is effective in distinguishing a solid from a cystic tumor. Under ultrasound guidance, cysts may be aspirated directly. The most common mass in adolescent girls, fibroadenoma, has characteristic features on ultrasound, which further enhance its utility in this age group.

Unlike for adult women, mammography is not recommended for diagnosis and screening in adolescent girls. The structural architecture of the adolescent breast differs significantly from that of the adult breast. The adolescent breast contains relatively larger amounts of fibroglandular tissue than fatty tissue, which hinders the detection of breast masses by mammography. The best use of mammography is in high-risk patients with large breasts that are clinically difficult to examine.

Computed tomography (CT) is useful to determine the tissue of origin of a mass palpated in the breast. Tumors arising from the chest wall and adjacent structures are likely to be fixed and independent of the breast, and CT is the diagnostic procedure of choice to differentiate them from breast masses.

CONCLUSION

Clinicians taking care of adolescent girls play a significant role in reassuring patients regarding the normalcy of breast development. The health care provider has a unique opportunity while examining the adolescent's breast to reassure her and teach her to respect her body and build a positive body image. The teaching of breast self-examination should serve only as a mechanism for developing good habits in later years and not as a rigid prescription that provokes anxiety and overconcern about malignancy.

SUGGESTED READING

1. Corpron CA, Black CT, Singletary SE, Andrassy RJ: Breast cancer in adolescent females. J Pediatr Surg 30:322–324, 1995.
2. Davis AJ, Kulig JW: Adolescent breast disorders. Adolesc Health Update 9:1–8, 1996.
3. Greydanus DE, Patel DR, Baxter TL: The breast and sports: Issues for the clinician. Adolesc Med 9:533–550, 1998.
4. Simmons PS: Diagnostic considerations in breast disorders of children and adolescents. Obstet Gynecol Clin North Am 19:91–102, 1992.
5. Neinstein LS: Breast disease in adolescents and young women. Ped Clin North Am 46:607–629, 1999.

CHAPTER 18

Common Dermatologic Problems

Peter G. Burk, M.D.

The epidemiology of skin diseases changes dramatically from childhood to adolescence. Common childhood skin diseases are still seen, but diseases associated with increased activity of sebaceous glands produce a high incidence of seborrheic dermatitis and acne. Fungal diseases such as tinea versicolor become much more common. All adolescents, but especially adolescent females, become increasingly concerned about their body image. Skin diseases may cause psychological distress in adolescents because of their visibility. Clinicians have to deal not only with the increased prevalence of skin diseases during adolescence but also with the distorted image of the "perfect" skin seen in advertisements in teen magazines.

ECZEMATOUS DISEASES

Atopic Dermatitis

Eczematous diseases are inflammatory processes involving the epidermis. Subacute eczema is characterized by the presence of erythema and scaling. With more acute eczematous dermatoses, bullous eruptions may occur. The most common eczematous disease is atopic dermatitis. This chronic pruritic eruption often is found in individuals with other atopic diseases such as hay fever and asthma or in families with a strong history of atopy. Atopic dermatitis is characterized by a chronic, itchy, inflammatory dermatitis that preferentially affects the neck and the antecubital and popliteal fossae. Many adolescents with atopic dermatitis also eventually develop eczematous dermatitis of the hands and feet. Atopic dermatitis is made worse by excessive dryness of the skin. Thus, it is usually worse in winter because of decreased humidity. In addition, excessive washing and bathing of the skin, which adolescents often do, tend to make atopic dermatitis worse. Some individuals also have flares during the summer during periods of heat and humidity.

Contact Dermatitis

Contact dermatitis is an inflammatory eczematous reaction of the skin to specific allergic contactants. Contact dermatitis is a cellular, type-4 immunologic reaction that is mediated in the skin by Langerhans cells in the epidermis. Langerhans cells process the allergic antigen and present it to sensitized T-lymphocytes, which release cytokines, producing inflammation. Allergic contact dermatitis is a self-limited process lasting 10 days to 2 weeks after an acute exposure. The most common type of contact dermatitis is poison ivy or rhus dermatitis. This reaction usually is seen during the summer and is characterized by the onset of linear inflammatory lesions, which become vesicular or bullous. It is intensely pruritic and, if present on the hands and face, may produce swelling and extreme discomfort. Other allergens such as nickel or rubber products produce a chronic eczema in the areas of direct contact. Identification and removal of the allergen from contact with the skin allow the process to be cleared. Many adolescent girls develop nickel-related contact dermatitis because of earrings, wristwatches, belt buckles, or snap fasteners on the hip. The distribution of the rash is a clue to the identity of the offending item of apparel.

Lichen simplex chronicus or localized neurodermatitis is a chronic localized type of eczema. The cause of this process is unknown, but when it begins, it produces a chronic cycle in which the individual scratches and itches continuously. Scratching produces a scaling and thickening of the skin in the area of the dermatitis with hyperpigmentation, called lichenification.

Management

Treatment of eczematous dermatitis depends on the severity of the disease. Severe generalized atopic dermatitis and localized severe allergic contact dermatitis may need to be treated with short courses of systemic steroids. Prednisone in doses of 40–60 mg for several days and then decreased over the next week to 10 days may be extremely helpful in severe generalized acute eczematous dermatitis. Localized acute eczematous dermatitis may be treated topically. If crusting and oozing are present, local compresses with antibacterial Burrow's solution (1:40 dilution) applied several times a day may reduce the exudation and allow the skin to heal. For subacute and chronic eczema, topical steroids are of great benefit. Medium- to high-potency topical steroids such as fluocinonide or clobetasol may clear the inflammation. It is important, however, not to use these higher-potency steroids on intertriginous areas or on the face because they may produce thinning and atrophy of the skin. For intertriginous and facial lesions, it is better to use 1–2.5% hydrocortisone cream or Westcort cream (0.2% hydrocortisone valerate). If the cutaneous lesions become secondarily infected, it is important to use oral antibiotics to treat the infection. Most skin infections arise from gram-positive bacteria and respond well to erythromycin and dicloxacillin. Antihistamines also are useful for control of the pruritus. Sedating antihistamines such as Benadryl and hydroxizine should be used only at night. Newer antihistamines such as Claritin or Zyrtec may be better for patients with chronic atopic dermatitis because they are nonsedating and act for 24 hours.

PAPULOSQUAMOUS DISEASES

Seborrheic Dermatitis

Inflammatory skin lesions with scaling papules and plaques characterize papulosquamous skin diseases. Seborrheic dermatitis is the most common papulosquamous disease. It is relatively uncommon in the preadolescent child, but at puberty, with the increase in sebaceous activity, it occurs more frequently. It is believed that seborrheic dermatitis represents an inflammatory reaction to products of bacteria and yeast reacting with sebum. Clinically, seborrheic dermatitis presents with erythema and scaling of the sides of the nose, eyebrows, and behind the ears. Scaling of the scalp is also quite common. The lesions in the scalp tend to have a diffuse erythema with fine scale (dandruff). More widespread seborrheic dermatitis can occur on the chest and in the axilla and inguinal folds. Seborrheic dermatitis may be made worse because of the common misperception that it represents dryness of the skin rather than inflammation. This perception may lead adolescents to stop washing their faces or shampooing their hair, which often makes seborrheic dermatitis worse.

Psoriasis

Psoriasis becomes more prevalent in adolescence. Psoriasis presents in two very different ways. It may have a slow onset of red, discrete, scaly plaques (0.5–3.0 cm) with a thick scale, which occur in the scalp, elbows, knees, and on the buttocks, especially in the gluteal fold. Alternatively, psoriasis may present as a generalized acute eruption with small, 0.5-cm, red scaly papules. This generalized form, called guttate psoriasis, can occur after streptococcal infections. Psoriasis is a genetic disease and is inherited in an autosomal dominant fashion. The age of onset of skin lesions and clinical course are quite variable, however. Psoriasis tends to be a chronic disease with exacerbations and remissions. Psoriasis that begins in childhood or early adolescence is often a more generalized and severe form than that occurring later in adolescence or adulthood.

Pityriasis Rosea

Pityriasis rosea is a distinctive clinical syndrome that develops acutely and then disappears spontaneously after 1–2 months. The initial lesion, which is called the herald patch, is a 2–3-cm, red scaly plaque with raised borders that often is confused with a dermatophyte infection of the skin. The second phase of pityriasis rosea is the onset of a generalized eruption with pink, slightly scaly, oval papules, which are 0.4–0.8 cm in diameter and distributed over the trunk and upper arms, extending onto the thighs and buttocks. This eruption, which occurs 1–2 weeks after the initial herald patch, may be quite pruritic. Clinically, it is important to differentiate pityriasis rosea from secondary syphilis. Secondary syphilis also may have a generalized papulosquamous eruption. Clinically, however, the rash of syphilis is somewhat different because the lesions are round and may extend to the palms and soles. It is useful to obtain a serologic test for syphilis to differentiate the two diseases.

Management

Treatment of papulosquamous diseases depends on the disease and the area of involvement. Seborrheic dermatitis is responsive to mild steroids such as hydrocortisone (1–2.5%) cream. This low-potency steroid is also safe to use on the face and ears for long periods of time, if necessary. Inflammation of the scalp may be treated with a medium-potency topical steroid such as fluocinonide solution 0.05%. It is also important to treat the scaling of the scalp by using antiseborrheic shampoos. Therapeutic shampoos such as T/Gel, selenium (Selsun Blue), or zinc parathion (Head and Shoulders) are also effective in reducing the scale and inflammation of the scalp. These shampoos also are useful in treating scalp psoriasis. Psoriasis is a more difficult disease to treat than seborrheic dermatitis. Usually it responds only to high-potency, class 1 topical steroids, such as Psorcon and clobetasol. These topical steroids have higher systemic absorption and can cause adrenal suppression. Chronic use may produce atrophy of the skin. There is a new topical vitamin D compound, Dovonex (0.005% ointment), which may be effective in controlling psoriasis and is safe to use for long periods of time. This compound may be used in conjunction with topical steroids. Generalized severe psoriasis may need to be treated with ultraviolet-B therapy, psoralens, and psoralen compounds with ultraviolet light (PUVA) therapy, or systemic antimetabolites such as methotrexate. Pityriasis rosea is relatively easy to treat under most circumstances. Topical steroids reduce the pruritus, but they do not clear the lesions. Pityriasis rosea is a self-limited disease and will disappear spontaneously after 4–8 weeks.

VASCULAR INFLAMMATORY DISEASES

Inflammatory pathologic processes involving blood vessels in the skin produce widely different clinical effects. Mild inflammation of the blood vessels with sudden local edema of the skin results in urticaria or hives. More intense inflammation produces erythematous maculopapular eruptions. Intense inflammation of the blood vessels with disruption of the vessels themselves produces a vasculitis with palpable purpura.

Urticaria

Acute urticaria is an extremely common syndrome in adolescents. It is characterized by the onset of transitory local edema of the skin producing wheals (hives). These lesions are extremely pruritic, and individual lesions fade within a period of hours. The pathophysiology of urticaria is believed to result from the degranulation of mast cells and the release of histamine and other vasoactive substances. Urticaria may result from an IgE-mediated allergic reaction to insect bites, foods, or drugs. In addition, there are non–IgE-mediated degranulating reactions. Some of these occur after ingestion of shellfish, aspirin-like substances, and opiates. In well over half the cases of acute urticaria, no specific causal exciting factor may be found.

Patients who present with erythematous eruptions consisting of macules and papules have morbilliform eruptions. These eruptions may occur with viral infections or as an allergic reaction to drugs. The drug eruptions can be somewhat more pruritic and more inflammatory than the morbilliform viral exanthems.

Purpura and Petechiae

Vasculitis with purpura is a cutaneous sign that must be taken seriously. Palpable purpuric lesions resulting from vascular inflammation and disruption of blood vessels characterize vasculitis. The lesions may be small, 0.1–0.2-cm petechial lesions or larger purpuric papules or pustules that are 0.5–1.0 cm in diameter. The lesions are seen more often on the lower extremities. Vascular purpura may be associated with drug eruptions, collagen vascular diseases, or an idiopathic process such as Henoch-Schoenlein purpura. It is important to look for evidence of vasculitis in the gastrointestinal tract or kidneys and to look for clinical evidence of arthritis. Purpuric pustules also may be a manifestation of bacterial septic processes. One such bacterial process is disseminated gonorrhea, which always must be considered in the differential diagnosis of purpuric lesion in adolescents.

Management

Treatment of urticaria depends on its severity. Mild, generalized urticaria is often controlled with oral antihistamines. H-1 blocker antihistamines, such as diphenhydramine (Benadryl), are given in doses of 25–50 mg, 4 times a day. However, these antihistamines are extremely sedating. Newer nonsedating antihistamines such as Claritin or Zyrtec also are effective in many patients with acute urticaria. Patients with severe urticaria or who also have angioedema should be treated with epinephrine (0.3 ml of 1:1000 dilution, subcutaneously). Also they may need a short course of oral prednisone (40–60 mg orally, once a day).

Morbilliform eruptions are treated with antihistamines and topical steroids as a palliative measure. Vasculitis may need to be treated with systemic steroids, but it is important to determine if an underlying systemic process is producing the vasculitis. If such a process is found, it should be treated specifically.

BACTERIAL SKIN INFECTIONS

Bacterial skin infections result from disruption of the integrity of the skin and consequent growth of pathogenic bacteria in the epidermis or in hair follicles. Bacterial skin infections are more common in individuals with chronic atopic dermatitis because they have disruption of their epidermal integrity. Skin infections also are more common during the summer months when greater heat and humidity provide a better environment for bacteria to grow.

Impetigo

The most common skin infection is impetigo. This infection is characterized clinically by the development of honey-colored crusts with superficial, erosive skin lesions, which may be quite widespread. Impetigo is a superficial bacterial infection involving the upper epidermis and the dermis. It starts with breaks in the skin, which allow serum and other proteins to be colonized by pathogenic bacteria. The most prevalent skin pathogens are *Streptococcus viridans* and *Staphylococcus aureus*. If not treated, impetigo may produce a deeper skin infection such as cellulitis. Certain strains of streptococcal organisms may produce kidney disease with acute glomerulonephritis as a postinfectious complication.

Folliculitis

Folliculitis is a localized process characterized by a bacterial infection of the hair follicles. Clinically, small pustules at the site of the hair follicles (pilosebaceous units) are seen. These pustules are more common on the legs, especially in young women who shave their legs. Shaving allows breaks in the skin and allows bacteria to be disseminated locally. Folliculitis, if present for a long time, may become a deeper process, in which case it forms a furuncle. These abscess-like lesions may need to be surgically drained.

Management

Therapy of bacterial infections of the skin involves several factors. First, it is important to reduce the bacterial population on the skin and to remove serum and oozing material. This is especially true in impetigo. Infected areas may be washed with antiseptic soap such as Hibiclens, which contains chlorhexadine. Compresses of Burrow's solution also may remove some of the crusted materials. Topical antibiotics such as topical Neosporin and Bacitracin are only mildly effective. Mupiricin 2% (Bactroban) ointment is a more effective topical agent. If the lesions are widespread, it may be necessary to give oral antibiotics. It is generally effective to use either erythromycin or dicloxacillin in doses of 250 mg, 4 times daily, for 10 days to treat superficial bacterial infections. This treatment is done in conjunction with the use of antiseptic wash and antibiotic ointment, which reduce the bacterial population on the skin and may prevent reinfection.

VIRAL SKIN INFECTIONS

Herpetic Infections

Viral skin infections include acute herpetic infections and slow, tumor-like infections with warts and molluscum. Herpes simplex involving the face and lip is an extremely common cutaneous infection. The majority of adults have antibodies to herpes simplex type I virus. Type I herpesvirus may cause an acute infection of the mouth with herpetic gingivitis. More commonly recurring herpes labialis occurs with localized vesicular lesions at the border of the lip. It also may be found elsewhere on the face. Herpes labialis is manifested as grouped pruritic and painful vesicles that last for approximately 7–10 days before resolving spontaneously. Herpes simplex may be triggered by a number of different factors. It is more common after exposure to ultraviolet light or

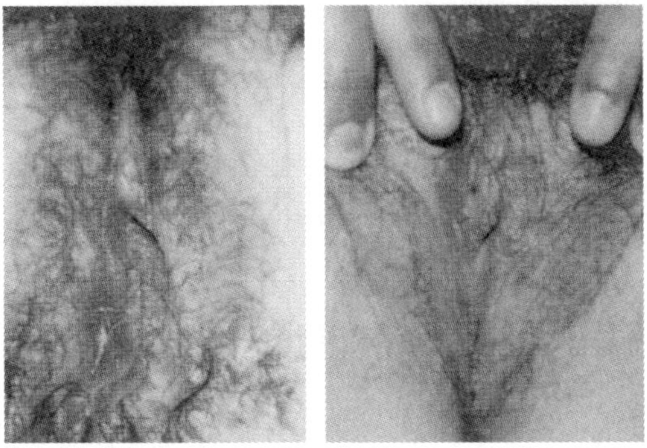

FIGURE 1. First episode of genital HSV infection with bilateral ulcerative lesions on vulva. (From McKendrick GDW, Sutherland S: An Introduction to Herpes Infections. London, Gower Medical for Wellcome Foundation Ltd., 1983, with permission.)

sunburn. It also may be set off by dental treatments involving trauma to the mouth or jaw. In addition, it may be triggered by other systemic viral infections, in which case it is called a "fever blister." Ten to twenty percent of adolescents and adults have recurrent herpes simplex infection of the lips.

Herpes progenitalis is caused by herpes virus type II, a virus closely related to herpes simplex type I. DNA from the two types of herpesviruses shares many viral antigens, but infection with one type of herpetic virus does not protect against infection with the other. Herpes progenitalis is extremely common in the sexually active population in the United States. As many as 25% of adolescents and adults become carriers of herpes progenitalis virus. Primary herpes type II infection in females may produce acute herpes vulvitis, an extremely painful condition with multiple vesicles over the vulvar and vaginal area (Fig. 1). Recurrent herpes progenitalis is a less severe process in both males and females. It is characterized by grouped vesicles, which may be preceded by several days by a painful or itching prodrome. These local infections last from 10 days to 2 weeks before spontaneously resolving. Herpes progenitalis also may occur on the buttocks and may be difficult to differentiate clinically from herpes zoster. Herpes progenitalis is infectious when blisters are present. Furthermore, it is believed that some individuals may secrete the virus even when no active lesions are visible. Herpes progenitalis may recur as often as monthly in some individuals.

Management

Treatment of herpes simplex and herpes progenitalis is now much more effective than it was in previous decades. The development of oral acyclovir has been a major advance. More recently, two new antiviral substances, famcyclovir and valacyclovir, which are much better absorbed than oral acyclovir, have been approved for the treatment of herpes progenitalis. The dosage of famcyclovir for herpes simplex and progenitalis is 250 mg, three times daily for 7 days, for new primary infections and 125 mg orally, three times daily, for recurrent infections. Valacyclovir is given in a dose of 500 mg, three times daily, for initial infections and 500 mg, twice daily for 7 days, for recurrent infections. These drugs should be used at the beginning of a recurrent episode at the first symptoms of burning or itching. Patients who have frequent recurrences of herpes progenitalis may be placed on daily suppressive therapy with famcyclovir or Valtrex. A small number of individuals, especially those who are immunosuppressed or have AIDS, have herpes simplex that is resistant to currently available antiviral medications. At this time, there are a few alternative agents to use for these patients.

Warts and Molluscum

Two types of slow-growing, viral skin infections produce papular eruptions of the skin. Papillomavirus is a DNA virus that infects the skin and produces warts or verrucae. Warts present as single or scattered verrucous keratotic papules, 0.2–0.8 cm in diameter, which may be on the glabrous skin, on the palms, or on the genitalia, depending on the strain of the papillomavirus. Papillomaviruses 1 and 3 produce common warts of the skin, palms, and soles. They are infectious processes and produce slow-growing epidermal papules, which are tumor-like and generally are not inflammatory. Certain types of warts, such as superficial plantar warts of the face, are extremely difficult to treat. Plantar warts on the soles of the feet may cause pain when walking. Genital warts are caused by different strains of papillomavirus (types 11 and 16 and others). Genital warts are soft, moist keratotic lesions that may be found in the genital or perirectal areas. Common skin warts are infectious and may be autoinnoculated as well as transferred from person to person, although the transfer rate is very low. Genital warts are extremely infectious.

Molluscum contagiosum is an infection of the skin with a different DNA virus than the papillomavirus. It produces a small, clear papule in the skin, which at first glance looks like a vesicle. Molluscum is an infectious process that can be transmitted from person to person. The individual may have anywhere from one to a large number of flesh-colored or semi-translucent, 0.2–0.4-cm papules over the skin. Molluscum also may involve the eye and produce a corneal keratitis. Generally speaking, molluscum infections are relatively self-limited, and most people who are infected eventually develop a clinical immunity to the virus.

Management

Verruca vulgaris and molluscum are superficial infectious processes, but because the lesions grow in a tumor-like way, they can be treated by various destructive measures, as are other types of benign growths. Warts respond to topical salicylic acid preparations, which act as keratolytics. These are available as over-the-counter products (Wart-off, Duofilm). If these preparations are applied to the warts on a daily basis and then removed with a rough surface such as an emery board, it is possible to debulk the wart. Small warts may be cleared by this treatment. This treatment is also preferred for plantar warts because it does not leave scars, which may be painful on a weight-bearing surface. Both warts and molluscum may be treated with destructive measures, including curettage, curettage with electrodesiccation, or cryotherapy with liquid nitrogen. It should be emphasized that individuals who are immunosuppressed have more difficulty in clearing their warts, and it may be quite difficult to cure warts or molluscum infection in individuals with a poor immune response.

FUNGAL SKIN INFECTIONS

Superficial fungal and yeast skin infections increase during adolescence. Some of these alterations are due to local changes in the skin that are mediated by alterations in sebaceous gland activity, which are triggered by increases in androgens during adolescence. The one fungal skin infection that decreases during adolescence is tinea capitis. This may be because the fungi involving the scalp are inhibited by free fatty acids formed by breakdown products of triglyceride fats in sebum.

Dermatophyte Infections

Dermatophyte infections are common in adolescents. They occur on the glabrous skin as annular erythematous lesions with a raised scaly border. They can be quite itchy. They gradually increase in size over a period of days to weeks and may involve many areas of the body. Those that occur on the arms, legs, and face (ringworm) are often secondary to exposure to animal sources, such as *Microsporum canis* from cats and dogs, or from being exposed to children with tinea capitis. Dermatophyte infections may also produce chronic, scaly red lesions on the feet, especially between the toes (athlete's foot). Dermatophyte infections of the inner crural area (jock itch) are very common in adolescent males but relatively uncommon in adolescent females. Young women may also develop a fungal folliculitis of the legs, which is spread by local infection of the hair follicles when shaving the legs.

Candida albicans

Candidiasis in intertriginous areas is more common during adolescence. It occurs in the inguinal folds and may be associated with a candidal vaginitis. It also may occur under the breast. Candidal infections may be diagnosed by the bright erythema of the lesion. They also may have burning symptoms as well as itching. There is often a certain amount of scale, and there may be surrounding satellite pustular lesions. Candidiasis is more common in individuals with diabetes and with immunodeficiency.

Tinea Versicolor

Tinea versicolor occurs almost exclusively after the onset of puberty. It is characterized clinically by discrete scaling papules with a fine scale, which may be hyperpigmented in winter or hypopigmented during the summer. Although it may cause mild itching, it usually is relatively asymptomatic and is more of a cosmetic problem. It occurs most commonly on the chest and back, but may extend to the neck and face and further down the trunk. Tinea versicolor is caused by the conversion of a normal skin organism, *Pityrosporum ovale*, from yeast to a fungal form. This conversion seems to occur because of a change in the sebaceous secretion of the skin on the chest and back secondary to sebaceous gland changes in adolescence. Tinea versicolor is a superficial infection and does not produce more deep-seated processes.

Management

Treatment of fungal skin infections depends on the type of fungus and the severity of infection. It is helpful that many of the new antifungal topical imidazoles are effective against dermatophytes, candidiasis, and also tinea versicolor. Topical clotrimazole (Lotrimin) or miconazole 2% cream (Micatin) may be applied twice daily for most superficial fungal infections. Second-generation topical antifungals such as spectazole or oxiconazole are somewhat more effective than clotrimazole. Individuals who have widespread dermatophyte infections or dermatophyte infections that involve the hair or nails may need to be treated with oral antifungals. Dermatophyte infections may be treated with oral griseofulvin, 10 mg/kg per day. They also may be treated with ketoconazole (200 mg, twice a day) or itraconazole (100 mg, twice a day). Candidiasis may be treated with the same topical antifungals and either ketoconazole or itraconazole orally for more widespread infections. Tinea versicolor is an extremely superficial infection that may be treated by washing with selenium sulfide shampoo (e.g., Selsun Blue), which is left on for 10–15 minutes daily. This treatment is followed by topical clotrimazole or other topical antifungals. Patients with severe tinea versicolor may be treated with oral antifungals, but this is usually not necessary.

DISEASES OF SEBACEOUS AND SWEAT GLANDS

Acne

Acne may occur 1–2 years before the onset of puberty in a mild form related to increased adrenal androgen secretion. At puberty, increased secretion of gonadal androgens causes a marked increase in the activity of sebaceous glands on the head, neck, chest, and back. Sebaceous glands have receptors for androgen hormones, and exposure to androgens increases the size and function of these glands. In genetically predisposed individuals this androgen-induced increase in sebaceous gland activity produces clinical acne. The exact pathophysiologic mechanism of acne is unknown, but the enlarged sebaceous glands allow high concentrations of *Propionibacterium acnes* to grow in the follicular openings. Rupture of the pilosebaceous follicles causes inflammatory pustules and cysts (Fig. 2). Other structures such as the apocrine sweat glands, which also have androgen receptors, increase in size at puberty as well. These structures may become inflamed and produce hidradenitis suppurativa.

Acne is extremely common during adolescence. It is characterized clinically by a range of lesions from small erythematous pustules, closed comedones, to blackheads, open comedones. Cystic acne is manifested by larger, deep cystic inflammatory lesions in the skin. These lesions occur primarily on the face, chest, and back. The onset of acne is variable from person to person. Adolescent males have more severe acne than adolescent females, although females may develop acne starting later in adolescence. There are distinct genetic factors in acne. Individuals in some families with severe acne are predisposed to develop the disorder in their early teens. Adolescent females who are obese and who have polycystic ovaries also have increased ovarian androgen secretion, which can produce both increased acne and hirsutism.

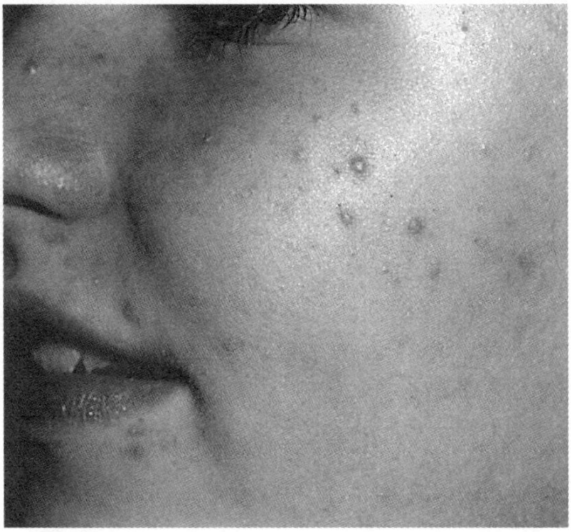

FIGURE 2. Mild inflammatory acne. (From Rabinovitz L: Acne vulgaris. Adolesc Med 8:77–86, 1997, with permission.)

Management

Treatment of acne depends on the severity of the disease. Superficial acne with pustules and papules usually does not produce scarring, but it may produce pigmentary changes in dark-skinned individuals. For this reason, it should be treated relatively aggressively in these patients. Superficial acne may be treated with a number of topical agents. Currently, the most effective agents include benzoyl peroxide in a 5–10% gel or as a wash form. Topical antibiotics also are effective. Topical erythromycin 2% and topical clindamycin 1% are available in solution gels, lotions, and plegette forms. The plegettes are useful for treating widespread lesions on the chest and back. More severe acne with widespread superficial pustules and cystic lesions should be treated with oral antibiotics in addition to topical treatment. Oral tetracycline is effective in many patients with acne. The most economical treatment is oral tetracycline given in a 500-mg, twice-daily dose. If this is not effective, oral doxycycline, 100 mg every day or twice a day, or minocycline, 100 mg every day or twice a day, is much more effective than tetracycline for controlling cystic acne. This distinction is important because cystic acne on the face and especially on the chest and back leads to permanent scarring. Antibiotic therapy must be continued as long as it is necessary for treatment. Most patients need to be treated for 6 months to 1 year.

In adolescent females oral contraceptives containing third-generation progestins recently have been shown to be effective in acne treatment for some patients. In individuals with severe cystic acne who are not responsive to topical agents and oral antibiotics, it may be necessary to consider using oral isotretinoin (Accutane). Isotretinoin works differently than other agents. It directly decreases the size of the sebaceous glands and sebaceous gland activity. It is very effective in severe cystic acne. Isotretinoin must be used in doses of 0.5–1.5 ml/kg for a period of 20 weeks. Isotretinoin is a known teratogen that causes severe birth defects in the fetus. It is absolutely imperative to start adolescent females on oral or injectable or implantable contraceptives before starting

Accutane therapy. They must be counseled regarding the necessity of considering an abortion if they become pregnant during the course of treatment with Accutane or up to 1 month afterward. Serum pregnancy tests, blood counts, liver enzymes, and triglycerides should be checked before therapy and at monthly intervals. The increased risk of birth defects continues for 1 month after stopping Accutane therapy. The majority of patients treated with Accutane respond well and have a long period of clearing or permanent remission of their acne. A smaller number require another course of treatment after another 6 months to 1 year.

Hidradenitis Suppurativa

Hidradenitis suppurativa is an inflammatory process of apocrine glands that occurs in genetically predisposed individuals, starting during puberty and occurring through adulthood. It is characterized clinically by chronic and recurrent inflammatory abscesses of anywhere from 1–2 cm in diameter, which occur in the axilla, buttocks, inner thighs, and under the breasts. It is worse in individuals who are overweight and also occurs more frequently in patients who have severe cystic acne. The abscesses in hidradenitis are often sterile, but may become infected with *Staphylococcus aureus* or other pathogens. Because these abscesses are painful, it is important to open and drain them to relieve the pressure. The lesion should be cultured, and, if infected, appropriate antibiotics should be given. Many individuals respond to long-term suppressive therapy with tetracycline, 500 mg 4 times a day, or doxycycline or minocycline, 100 mg twice a day. Local therapy may consist of using an antiseptic wash such as chlorhexidine to reduce the bacterial population. Some individuals also respond to topical erythromycin, which reduces the bacterial population in the area. Individuals who have persistent, serious cystic lesions that develop into abscesses may need to have local surgical excision of the involved areas.

DISEASES OF THE HAIR AND NAILS

Diseases of the hair and nails are not life-threatening but may cause cosmetic changes that are extremely distressing to the adolescent patient. One of the more common alterations in the hair is alopecia areata. Alopecia areata is characterized by the appearance of one or more round areas, anywhere from 1–5 cm in diameter, in which there is sudden total hair loss. There is no apparent clinical inflammation of the skin in these areas. There is no scarring or destruction of hair follicles. A more severe variant of alopecia areata is alopecia totalis, in which the hair is lost over the entire body, including the eyebrows and eyelashes. Alopecia areata is almost always a self-limited disease, and even without treatment the hair eventually regrows. The cause is unknown, but in many patients it seems to occur 1–2 months after a severe emotional stress or a severe illness. It also may be associated with thyroid disease, but this is not a causal association. Alopecia areata is treated with high-potency topical steroids such as clobetasol gel or local injections of Kenalog into the skin. Rogaine also may have some effect on helping the hair to regrow. It must be emphasized to the patient that it often takes several months to as long as a year for the hair to regrow.

Other sorts of diffuse hair loss include diffuse telogen hair loss, which can occur after severe illnesses or after pregnancy. In this disease, an increased number of hairs are lost per day over and above the 100–150 hairs normally shed daily. This increase may produce a total hair loss of as much as 25% of the hair on the scalp. It begins approximately 1–2 months and continues for up to 6 months after a severe illness or after pregnancy. The hair then begins to regrow to normal density.

Adolescent females in families with severe history of balding may develop the early onset of androgenic alopecia with male-pattern balding. This disorder is most often seen in young women with polycystic ovary syndrome who also have obesity, hirsutism, and acne.

Alterations of the nails are not common in adolescents, but diseases such as psoriasis may produce changes in the nails.

DISEASES OF PIGMENTATION

Alterations in pigmentation produce cosmetic changes that are extremely distressing to the adolescent patient, even though they do not represent severe illnesses. Both hyperpigmentation and hypopigmentation produce pigmentary alterations, which easily can be seen.

Vitiligo is a disease in which there is hypopigmentation or depigmentation of the skin occurring over exposed areas of the body. It starts with macular areas of depigmentation, which may be anywhere from one-half to several centimeters in diameter. These areas may occur over the face, hands, and elbows. They also may affect the genitalia. The cause of vitiligo is not known, but is believed to represent a possible autoimmune response to melanocytes. Vitiligo is a slowly progressive disease in most patients who develop a few areas of depigmentation that remain for long periods of time. A smaller number of patients may develop generalized vitiligo. It is important to use sunscreens to protect the areas of depigmentation, which are more sensitive to ultraviolet light. The areas of vitiligo may be treated with topical steroids over a period of time, which will cause repigmentation in some patients. Another available treatment is the use of psoralen compounds with ultraviolet light (UVA). This treatment, called PUVA therapy, may be successful in repigmenting patients. It is, however, an expensive and slow process with few patients developing total repigmentation.

Pigmentary problems also may be associated with inflammatory diseases of the skin. Eczema, as a chronic dermatitis, may produce either hyperpigmentation or hypopigmentation. The use of psoralen-containing perfumes may produce a hyperpigmented process called Berloque dermatitis after exposure to sunlight. Estrogen excess, especially during pregnancy but also from oral contraceptive pills, may produce hyperpigmentation of the cheeks, called melasma.

Hyperpigmentation may be treated with hydroquinone compounds. These are available as over-the-counter agents, but there are also prescription-strength compounds such as 3% hydroquinone solution (Melenex). Hydroquinone creams are used in conjunction with sunscreens to try to block additional hyperpigmentation from ultraviolet light. They may have some beneficial effect over a long period of time in hyperpigmentation of the face. Such creams have little effect on hyperpigmentation of the body or extremities.

PARASITIC INFECTIONS

The increased, close body contact in sexually active female adolescents may lead to exposure to agents of infestation. It should be emphasized that although scabies and pediculosis pubis can be spread by close body contact during sexual activity, they also may occur from close physical nonsexual activity or may spread within a family.

Scabies is a widespread infestation that occurs after exposure to a mite, *Sarcoptes scabiei*. The sarcoptes mite lives on humans. It is spread primarily by close physical contact and can live off humans only for up to 24 hours. Approximately 2 weeks after exposure to the scabies mite, individuals develop itching. Itching is a reaction to the bites and burrows of the mite in the skin. Scabies is characterized clinically by small pruritic papules and small burrows within the skin primarily in intertriginous areas. These occur around the abdomen and the breasts, in the inguinal area, and on the hands, especially in the finger webs and wrists. It is possible to do a scraping to identify a mineral oil specimen with the mites in the skin. Scabies is highly infectious. It spreads to other members of the family by close body contact or by sleeping in the same bed. Scabies is treated with Kwell lotion applied to the entire body from the neck down, overnight and repeated in 1 week. A newer treatment is with Elemite cream 5% applied to the body overnight. Clothes, bed linen, and towels need to be washed but do not necessarily need to be boiled. Anything that has not been worn or used in the 24 hours before treatment is noninfectious. After treatment the patients still may have itching that persists for a period of time. This itching may need to be treated with topical steroids and may represent an inflammatory reaction to the scabietic antigen left in the skin.

Pediculosis pubis or pubic lice is a common cutaneous problem in sexually active adolescents. The reaction is characterized by itching in the skin. On close examination of the skin, the clinician may see small white nits on the hair in the pubic area. There are also small violaceous purpuric areas where lice have bitten the skin. The lice themselves are small, 2–3 mm, and are light-colored and difficult to see. Pubic lice may be treated with Kwell shampoo for 10–15 minutes or Nix shampoo, which is an over-the-counter agent. If this is done and then repeated in 1 week later, most patients respond quickly.

SKIN DISEASES IN PREGNANCY

Many cutaneous lesions may occur during pregnancy. One of the most common and distressing to the patient is the development of striae or stretch marks. These are areas of atrophy that occur over the breasts, thighs, and abdomen. They may be violaceous initially and then become somewhat hyperpigmented. They still, however, retain their atrophic component. Striae are difficult to treat; however, they do improve spontaneously over a period of time. Some individuals are predisposed to develop striae. The development does not correspond to the amount of weight gain during pregnancy, but is probably an idiosyncratic reaction of certain individuals to the high levels of estrogen circulating during pregnancy. Emollients have little or no effect.

There may be some benefit from the use of topical Retin-A on the skin. This may be prescribed after childbirth.

Pruritic eruptive papules of pregnancy, which are given the acronym PUPP, are a common skin problem during pregnancy. PUPP is characterized by severe itching and small papular eruptions. It occurs especially in the second trimester of pregnancy and usually is not associated with any serious fetal problems. Affected individuals may be treated with low-potency topical steroids and Benadryl.

CUTANEOUS LESIONS OF AIDS

Sexually active adolescents may be exposed to the HIV virus and develop clinical AIDS. The practitioner taking care of these patients should look for cutaneous lesions that may be associated with AIDS.

Many skin diseases that occur as cutaneous manifestations of HIV infection are more severe clinical expressions of ordinary skin diseases. Seborrheic dermatitis that is extremely severe and does not respond well to therapy, tinea or candidal infections that are exaggerated, or severe molluscum warts should alert the clinician to the possibility that the patient may have HIV infection. In addition, herpes zoster occurs more frequently in HIV-infected individuals, and the development of herpes zoster in a sexually active adolescent should lead the practitioner to consider HIV testing.

Eosinophilic folliculitis is a characteristic cutaneous lesion of AIDS. This process, which is of unknown origin, occurs with a pruritic acneiform eruption over the face, chest, and back. Acneiform processes are usually not itchy, so this symptom should be a clinical tip-off. When the lesion is biopsied, a folliculitis with a mix of polymorphonuclear leukocytes and eosinophils is seen. This lesion is difficult to treat. If it is found, the patient certainly should have an HIV test because it is often associated with HIV disease.

CONCLUSION

Dermatologic problems frequently occur in adolescent girls and may cause considerable physical and psychological distress. Acne and eczematous lesions are most common but usually can be treated effectively with topical medication. Bacterial, viral, fungal, and parasitic infections also occur with some frequency, especially in sexually active girls. Many of these conditions can be diagnosed and treated by the primary care clinician, with referral to a dermatologist reserved for severe conditions and treatment failures.

SUGGESTED READING

1. Shapiro SC, Strasburger VC, Greydanus DE (eds): Adolescent Dermatology. Adolescent Medicine: State of the Art Reviews, Vol. 1, No. 2. Philadelphia, Hanley & Belfus, 1990.
2. Cohen BA: Pediatric Dermatology. Philadelphia, Mosby International, 1999.
3. Harper J, Oranje AP, Prose N (eds): Textbook of Pediatric Dermatology. Malden, MA, Blackwell Science, 1999.
4. Schachner LA, Hansen RC (eds): Pediatric Dermatology. New York, Churchill Livingstone, 1995.
5. Sahn EE: Dermatology Pearls. Philadelphia, Hanley & Belfus, 1999.

CHAPTER 19

Abdominal Pain

Sharon Rose Beier, M.D.
Susan M. Coupey, M.D.

Busy clinicians often are dismayed when faced with an adolescent girl complaining of abdominal pain. A thorough history and physical examination, including a gynecological examination (which may be her first), can take a lot of time, and still the diagnosis may be elusive. However, such diagnostic and therapeutic dilemmas also present an opportunity for the clinician to establish a trusting relationship with the adolescent patient and allow her to feel that her concerns are being heard even if a diagnosis is not immediately evident. How the young woman is approached may have a lasting impact on her future relationship with medical professionals and, perhaps, on her own future as well. This chapter discusses the evaluation, differential diagnosis, and management of both acute and chronic abdominal pain in adolescent girls. Although the differential diagnosis reaches well over a hundred possibilities, this chapter concentrates on the most common conditions seen in office practice.

PATHOPHYSIOLOGY

In order to interpret findings on history and physical examination correctly, a basic understanding of pathophysiologic mechanisms producing abdominal pain is helpful (Table 1). Visceral pain results when a hollow viscus such as the stomach or intestine, which normally is insensitive to touch, distends. The severity and acuity of pain depends on the rate and degree of distention of the viscus. Because abdominal viscera are innervated by multiple somatic nerves originating from both sides of the spinal cord, the pain, which may be dull and/or crampy, is usually midline, diffuse, and poorly localized.[1] An example of this type of pain is the initial vague periumbilical pain experienced when the appendix first becomes obstructed and begins to distend.

Somatic pain, on the other hand, is well localized. It results from inflammation of the parietal peritoneum, which is innervated along dermatomes. Peritoneal inflammation causes irritation of the overlying abdominal muscles, resulting in involuntary guarding and rebound tenderness.[1] An example of this type of pain is the localization to McBurney's point that occurs during the

TABLE 1. Mechanisms of Abdominal Pain

Trauma to abdominal muscles or nerves	Extraabdominal referred pain
Peritoneal inflammation or irritation	Neurogenic mechanisms
Hollow viscus or capsular distention	Metabolic changes
Increased or decreased bowel motility	Psychogenic mechanisms
Vascular insufficiency or infarct	

Adapted from Lavelle JM: A practical approach to non-traumatic, non-gynecologic abdominal pain in the adolescent patient. Adolesc Med 4:35–49, 1993.

course of acute appendicitis as the inflamed appendix begins to cause inflammation of the overlying parietal peritoneum.

Referred pain is pain that originates in one region but is experienced in another area of the body, usually the area of its embryologic origin. Examples of referred pain include backache seen with acute pancreatitis and right shoulder tip pain seen with acute cholecystitis.

DIFFERENTIAL DIAGNOSIS (Table 2)

During the course of eliciting the history and conducting a physical examination, the clinician should try to answer the following questions: Is the pain acute or chronic? If acute, is the condition emergent, possibly requiring surgical treatment, or can it be managed medically? If chronic, is the pain of organic or psychogenic etiology? Is the pain due to intraabdominal pathology, or is it extraabdominal referred pain or an abdominal manifestation of a systemic illness?

TABLE 2. Differential Diagnosis

Gastrointestinal
- Gastroenteritis
- Acid peptic disease (esophagitis, gastritis, duodenitis, ulcer)
- Appendicitis
- Intestinal obstruction or perforation
- Intraabdominal sepsis (abscess, peritonitis)
- Inflammatory bowel disease (abscess, megacolon)
- Mesenteric adenitis
- Constipation
- Lactose intolerance
- Cholecystitis or cholangitis
- Fulminant hepatitis
- Pancreatitis
- Hepatic, splenic, bladder rupture (trauma)

Gynecologic
- Pregnancy (ectopic, threatened or spontaneous abortion)
- Complications of therapeutic abortion (endometritis)
- Pelvic inflammatory disease
- Fitz-Hugh-Curtis syndrome

Gynecologic *(cont.)*
- Ovarian torsion
- Ruptured ovarian cyst
- Endometriosis
- Dysmenorrhea, mittleschmerz

Urinary tract
- Renal calculi
- Cystitis, polynephritis

Other
- Psychogenic
- Eating disorders (anorexia nervosa, bulimia nervosa)
- Pneumonia, pneumothorax, pulmonary embolism
- Diabetic ketoacidosis
- Malignancy
- Orthopedic (osteomyelitis, septic arthritis, aseptic necrosis, slipped capital-femoral epiphysis)
- Sickle cell disease (pain crisis, acute chest syndrome)
- Systemic lupus erythematosus

Girls with acute, severe, and potentially life-threatening abdominal pain are toxic-appearing and show signs of peritonitis, obstruction, and/or change in mental status.[2] They require a prompt surgical or gynecologic consultation and hospitalization for immediate stabilization, laboratory and imaging studies, and management.[3] Girls with acute but moderate pain may be in the early phase of an acute abdominal process, and hospitalization for close observation should be considered.[1] Those whose examination indicates a systemic medical illness as the cause for the abdominal pain (e.g., diabetes mellitus or systemic lupus erythematosis) should be treated appropriately for the underlying illness. Finally, girls with recurrent or chronic abdominal pain often have a normal physical examination, and they may require a complex outpatient medical, gynecologic, and psychosocial work-up to establish a diagnosis.

History

A detailed history is essential in diagnosing abdominal pain in adolescent girls (Table 3). At least some part of the history must be elicited from the girl herself, without her parents or others in the room, because the differential diagnosis includes conditions related to sexual behavior and other private and sensitive issues. It is important to consider both physical and emotional causes from the beginning, particularly when the pain is subacute or chronic. Careful evaluation for any history of physical, mental, and/or sexual abuse, domestic violence or traumatic events should be conducted. The patient needs to feel confident that her symptoms are taken seriously and that the

TABLE 3. Important Areas to Explore in the History

1. **Qualities of the pain** (preceding events; onset; frequency; duration; character; location; pattern; severity; what makes it better or worse; any associated symptoms such as nausea, vomiting, diarrhea, dysuria, urgency, frequency; any systemic symptoms such as fever, fatigue, lethargy, rash, arthralgias, bleeding, weight loss, or jaundice)
2. **Medical history** (trauma, previous abdominal surgery, chronic disease, allergies, medications or drugs, travel history, foreign visitors, drinking impure water, food-handling practices, family members or pets with abdominal symptoms)
3. **Stools** (frequency, shape, size, consistency, color)
4. **Diet** (appetite, restricted intake, vegetarian, fatty foods, fiber, amount of water, soda, caffeinated beverages, binging, self-induced vomiting, emetic use, laxative use)
5. **Menstrual history** (menarche, interval, regularity, duration of bleeding, amount of bleeding, associated pain, date of last menstrual period)
6. **Sexual history** (sexually active, age at first intercourse, number of partners, type of contraception used, history of previous pregnancies, history of sexually transmitted diseases, history of sexual abuse)
7. **Alcohol and substance use** (type of substances used, amount, frequency, route of administration, previous related health problems)
8. **Mental health** (sleep patterns; fatigue; lethargy; anhedonia; suicidal thoughts, plans or attempts; previous suicide attempts; history of psychological counseling or therapy, history of psychiatric hospitalizations or medications)
9. **Social history** (parents divorced, separated, or remarried; new family members; family illness or death; new rules or responsibilities; strict, demanding parents; lenient, uninvolved parents; get along with siblings and peers; school performance; recreation or sports activities; employment)

clinician will work in partnership with her to explore, understand, and treat the pain.

Many girls are embarrassed and uncomfortable discussing bodily functions. For example, when asked about constipation, a common cause of abdominal pain in teenage girls, many quickly deny it just to avoid having to talk about the subject. Questions should be phrased specifically and concretely, using words that the girl is likely to understand. Often a topic must be approached in two or three different ways to ensure an accurate understanding of the symptom. Abdominal pain may be the presenting complaint when a girl is concerned about a vaginal discharge, sexually transmitted disease, or pregnancy. It is always necessary to get a complete menstrual and sexual history while assuring the patient of confidentiality. Pregnancy and its complications must be kept high on the list of differential diagnoses, and a pregnancy test should probably be done on all girls with abdominal pain, even in the absence of a history of sexual activity or missed menstrual period.

Physical Examination (Table 4)

The physical examination should be gentle but thorough. Girls should be undressed and gowned, and careful attention should be paid to appropriate draping and chaperoning to address issues of modesty. Adolescent girls are often embarrassed, unsure, and insecure about their bodies. It helps the girl to relax if the clinician provides reassurance and explains each different step during the process of the examination. It is important for her to hear repeatedly what

TABLE 4. Important Features of the Physical Examination

1. **Vital signs** (help to assess acuity/severity, evaluate circulation and hydration status; elevated temperature suggests infection/peritonitis)
2. **Abdominal examination**
   a. **Observation** (distention, asymmetry, discoloration, scars, hernia)
   b. **Auscultation** (character of bowel sounds; may use stethoscope [so that the patients thinks you are listening] to press on abdomen to assess guarding and rebound tenderness)
   c. **Palpation** (instruct the patient to indicate the site of maximum pain, and start palpating from the point farthest away to localize tenderness. Look for the "closed-eye sign" [patients with nonspecific abdominal pain close their eyes during abdominal palpation, whereas those with organic pain keep a close watch on the doctor, hoping to avoid additional pain.[4]])
   d. **Other signs**
      i. Peritoneal irritation (psoas sign, obturator test, pain with sudden jarring movement [e.g., jumping or bumping the bed], referred pain to neck or shoulder, Murphy's sign)
      ii. Peritonitis (abdominal distention, abdominal muscle rigidity, rebound tenderness, guarding, decreased or absent bowel sounds, shock)
      iii. Intestinal obstruction (persistent vomiting, abdominal distention, decreased or absent bowel sounds)
3. **Pelvic examination** (look for external genital lesions, bleeding, abnormal discharge or odors; assess for friability of the cervix, indicating infection; assess for cervical motion tenderness by gently flicking your fingers at the lower part of the cervix; assess the size of the uterus for pregnancy; check for adnexal masses and tenderness.)
4. **Rectal examination** (palpate for a tender right lower quadrant mass, usually indicating appendicitis; check for rebound tenderness; palpate the cervix, uterus and adnexae if pelvic examination not done; check for impacted stool; perform guaiac test on stool.)

the clinician is doing, seeing, hearing, and feeling and to be reassured about what parts of the examination are normal and how any abnormal findings will be addressed. Because many girls are anxious and flinch when touched, it can be helpful to distract the patient by asking questions during palpation of the abdomen while closely observing her face to evaluate the severity of pain.

The location of the pain in the abdomen should help to narrow the differential diagnosis. If the pain is epigastric, consider esophagitis, gastrointestinal reflux, peptic ulcer disease, or pancreatitis. If there is right upper quadrant pain, think of hepatitis, Fitz-Hugh-Curtis syndrome, cholecystitis, or cholangitis. With bilateral acute lower quadrant pain, pelvic inflammatory disease is the most likely diagnosis. Unilateral lower quadrant pain may indicate appendicitis, ovarian torsion, ectopic pregnancy, or renal calculi. Diffuse lower abdominal pain may be associated with lactose intolerance, inflammatory bowel disease, or irritable bowel syndrome. With mild diffuse, periumbilical or left-sided pain, constipation, gastroenteritis, mesenteric adenitis, food poisoning, muscle strain, and psychogenic pain are considerations.[2]

ACUTE RIGHT UPPER QUADRANT PAIN

Clinical Case Vignette

A 19-year-old, previously healthy college student presented with a 5-day history of progressive, colicky abdominal pain with intermittent vomiting. She had no diarrhea, constipation, or fever. For the past few weeks, she had been on a restricted calorie diet to loose weight in preparation for her sister's wedding. No one in her family had similar symptoms. She was sexually active and had been taking oral contraceptives for the past 2 years but took no other medications. She had never been pregnant. She acknowledged smoking 1 pack of cigarettes per day but denied using alcohol or illicit drugs. On physical examination, she was moderately obese and had severe right upper quadrant and epigastric tenderness, with positive bowel sounds, no guarding, and no rebound tenderness. No abdominal masses were palpated, and the liver and spleen were not enlarged. Pelvic examination was unremarkable with no positive findings. Laboratory testing revealed a moderately elevated white blood cell count, moderately elevated liver function tests, as well as elevated amylase and lipase. Pregnancy test was negative. An ultrasound examination of the gallbladder revealed gallstones.

Acute Cholecystitis

Although cholelithiasis and acute cholecystitis are traditionally believed to be diseases of overweight, middle-aged women, in the past two decades these conditions have been seen with increasing frequency in adolescents.[5] The female-to-male incidence of cholelithiasis in teenagers is 20 to 1.[6] Reasons for the recent rise in the prevalence of gallbladder disease in young women include an increase in the prevalence of obesity in this age group and an increase in adolescent pregnancies. In addition, the typical adolescent fast-food diet, which is high in fat and low in fiber, promotes gallstone formation. The progestin-only contraceptive depot medroxyprogesterone acetate, which is known to accelerate gallstone formation in susceptible individuals, is increasingly used by adolescents and may be a factor in contributing to clinical illness.[7]

Most of the gallstones seen in adolescents (80%) are made of cholesterol. Stones form when the bile is supersaturated with cholesterol because of increased hepatic load from diets high in saturated fats and/or increased hepatic production that occurs in obesity. Gallbladder stasis related to the smooth muscle relaxant effect of high progesterone levels associated with pregnancy or long-acting contraceptives also promotes supersaturation of bile and cholesterol stone formation.

Diets that are high in fat and low in fiber promote gallstone formation even in normal-weight adolescents. Rapid weight loss and fasting as well as diets that are low in protein and calcium and high in carbohydrates, all of which are frequently consumed by adolescents, also promote gallstone formation. About 45% of female high school students in the United States report that they are currently trying to lose weight, and 49% report skipping meals in the past 7 days "to try to lose weight or to keep from gaining weight."[8] Given the high rates of obesity, poor diets, disordered eating, and pregnancy in American adolescent girls, it is not surprising that cholelithiasis is increasing in prevalence in this age group.

Pigment stones are common in adolescents with hemolytic anemias, including sickle cell disease, thalassemia major, and congenital spherocytosis. The prevalence of gallstones in 10–20-year-old youths with homozygous sickle cell disease is about 40%. Complications are frequent enough that all adolescents with sickle cell disease should be regularly screened for cholelithiasis by ultrasound.[9] Other conditions associated with gallstones in adolescents include spinal fusion, blunt abdominal trauma, ileal resection, cystic fibrosis, diabetes mellitus, Crohn's disease, and childhood cancers. Prolonged immobilization and total parenteral nutrition are additional risk factors for cholelithiasis.

Imaging studies are the key to making the diagnosis of cholelithiasis. After an overnight fast, an abdominal ultrasound usually shows the stones as echogenic forms within the gallbladder. A nuclear medicine technique, cholescintigraphy, is used to visualize the gallbladder and major bile ducts when acute cholecystitis is suspected. When acute pancreatitis, one of the most common complications of gallbladder disease, is suspected, an endoscopic retrograde cholangiopancreatography (ERCP) is performed. For adolescents with symptomatic gallstones, cholecystectomy is indicated. Laparoscopy, which is a much less invasive procedure than the traditional laparotomy, is the procedure of choice, when possible, for adolescents.

Fitz-Hugh-Curtis Syndrome

Fitz-Hugh-Curtis syndrome is a relatively common cause of acute right upper quadrant pain in adolescent girls, and the diagnosis is frequently missed. Fitz-Hugh-Curtis syndrome is defined as infection of Gilson's capsule of the liver and the surrounding peritoneum in association with sexually transmitted infections (STIs) of the lower genital tract.[10] It occurs more frequently in adolescents with STIs than in older women with STIs, and it is associated with both *Neisseria gonorrhoeae* and *Chlamydia trachomatis* infection. The pathophysiology is believed to involve tracking of organisms from the cervix and endometrial cavity through patent fallopian tubes and along the paracolic gutters to the liver capsule. Once the capsule of the liver is infected, the adolescent experiences severe right upper quadrant pain that is often pleuritic in nature. The pain may radiate to the shoulder. It may be associated with the lower abdominal pain of acute salpingitis or occur in the absence of any lower abdominal signs or symptoms.[11] When there are no associated symptoms of pelvic inflammatory disease (PID), clinicians may fail to consider the diagnosis of Fitz-Hugh-Curtis syndrome and may fail to do a careful sexual history and pelvic examination to test for STIs. The diagnosis can be made clinically with a positive sexual history and physical examination once laboratory and ultrasonographic findings have ruled out hepatitis, gallbladder disease, or pancreatitis. The only abnormal laboratory test with Fitz-Hugh-Curtis syndrome, besides a positive STI test, may be a mild-to-moderate elevation of the erythrocyte sedimentation rate (ESR). Liver function tests most commonly are normal because there is no infection of the liver parenchyma.

Once the diagnosis is made, the young woman should be treated immediately, without waiting for the STI test results from endocervical specimens. Antibiotic treatment for Fitz-Hugh-Curtis syndrome is the same as for PID, but because the infection of the liver capsule and peritoneum is superficial, it should respond rapidly with resolution of the upper right quadrant pain within 24–36 hours. The rapid response to appropriate therapy confirms the diagnosis even in the absence of positive STI test results. A late complication of Fitz-Hugh-Curtis syndrome is the development of "violin-string" adhesions from the liver capsule to the anterior abdominal wall.[12] These adhesions can cause chronic right upper quadrant pain. They are treated by lysis under laparoscopic visualization.

EPIGASTRIC PAIN

Clinical Case Vignette

A 17-year-old, high school girl complains of epigastric pain for the past 7 months. She describes the pain as sharp and stabbing, sometimes awakening her at night and often present in the morning. She denies weight loss, anorexia, vomiting or diarrhea, but reports that because she "feels full" soon after beginning to eat, she eats small amounts throughout the day. She is not on any special diet, eats relatively balanced meals, and is satisfied with her body image.

She tried antacids, with no relief. She took an over-the-counter histamine-2 receptor antagonist with good relief, but when she stopped the medication after 4 weeks, "the pain came right back." She has no chronic illness, has never been hospitalized, and has no allergies. Menarche was at age 12 years; she has 30-day cycles that last 4 days and is currently menstruating. She is sexually active with her first partner, her boyfriend of two years, and "almost always" uses condoms. She has never had an STI and had a normal pelvic examination 2 months ago.

She denies alcohol or illicit drug use and does not smoke. Her mother complains of a nervous stomach, and her father had surgery for colon cancer.

On physical examination, she was slender and appeared tired and mildly ill. Her height and weight were at the 60th percentile; she was tachycardic with a heart rate of 100 beats/minute and blood pressure of 80/60 mmHg. She had mild epigastric tenderness but an otherwise normal abdominal examination. Rectal examination revealed normal sphincter tone and no stool in the vault. Pelvic examination was not done. Laboratory testing revealed a mild microcytic anemia, negative urinalysis, negative pregnancy test, guaiac-positive stool, and positive serology for *Helicobacter pylori.* A barium study of the upper gastrointestinal tract with small bowel follow-through revealed no ulcers and a normal terminal ileum. Endoscopy of the upper gastrointestinal tract showed antral gastritis with no ulcers. Giemsa-stained biopsies were positive for *Helicobacter pylori,* which was confirmed by culture.

Acid Peptic Disease

Acid peptic disease may be associated with acute epigastric pain, especially if there is an ulcer. More often, however, this spectrum of conditions, including esophagitis, gastritis, and duodenitis as well as ulcers, presents as chronic recurrent epigastric pain.[13] Although peptic ulcers occur relatively infrequently during adolescence, there are important reasons to discuss acid peptic disease in this age group. Adolescent girls with the eating disorders anorexia nervosa and bulimia nervosa who induce vomiting for weight control often develop symptomatic esophagitis requiring assessment and treatment. Also, new findings associate *Helicobacter pylori* infection with antral gastritis and duodenal ulcers. Adolescents whose epigastric pain seems to improve with a course of acid suppression only to recur when the treatment is stopped, as occurred in the patient described in the case vignette, may be harboring *H. pylori* infection. All forms of acid peptic disease present with similar symptoms, including epigastric pain, particularly on awakening in the morning. Emesis relieves the pain in some individuals, and eating relieves it in others. Patients often experience early satiety and develop an eating pattern of "grazing" throughout the day while avoiding large meals. Half of the patients have stools positive for occult blood, and some may have anemia due to gastrointestinal blood loss.

H. pylori infection provokes a systemic immune response, and an enzyme-linked immunosorbent assay (ELISA) test measuring serologic IgG antibodies to the organism is available. This blood test, however, while it correlates very closely with infection, has a high rate of positivity in asymptomatic individuals, and its use for diagnosis is controversial. A negative serology does not rule out *H. pylori* infection; if suspected, endoscopy with biopsies for Giemsa staining, rapid urease testing, and culture of specimens from the gastric antrum and corpus should be done.[6] If the serology is positive, the patient is symptomatic, and if it is financially or geographically too difficult for her to have endoscopy, the patient should be treated; serology should show a significant decline or revert to negative within about 4 months of eradication of the organism. However, without endoscopy, other important disease processes may be missed.[6] Therapy for *H. pylori* infection includes an acid suppressor, antibiotics,

TABLE 5. Management of *Helicobactor pylori* Infection

1. Acid suppression for 4 weeks
   a. Histamine-2 blockers: **cimetidine**, 40–50 mg/kg/day divided every 6–8 hours, *or* **ranitidine**, 6–10 mg/kg/day divided every 8–12 hours
   b. Proton pump inhibitors: **omeprazole**, 0.5–2mg/kg/day divided every 12–24 hours

AND

2. Antibiotics for 2 weeks
   1. **Amoxicillin**, 1 gm twice daily, *or* **clarithromycin**, 500 mg twice daily, *and* **metronidazole**, 500 mg twice daily

AND

3. Enhance mucosal protection for 2 weeks
   a. **Pepto Bismol**, 2 tablets twice daily

and a mucosal protection enhancer (Table 5). With treatment, the patient should become clinically symptom-free within 2 weeks, and the *H. pylori* serology should be negative after 4 months. If the patient has persistent or recurrent symptoms, endoscopy is indicated.

LOWER QUADRANT PAIN

Clinical Case Vignette

A 14-year-old girl is brought to the emergency department by her mother with the chief complaint of "stomachache" for the past 2 weeks. The mother's biggest concern is that her daughter is eating and drinking very little and has had some fever and vomiting. Initially, the mother thought it was the "stomach flu," but now she thinks that it has lasted too long. The adolescent describes the pain as dull and crampy and states that it hurts all the time and is slowly getting worse. She points vaguely to her lower abdomen but is unable to indicate an area of maximal pain. When questioned alone without her mother, the patient said that her last menstrual period was between 2 and 3 weeks ago and was much heavier than usual with bad cramps. After being assured of confidentiality, the girl acknowledged that she has a 17-year-old boyfriend with whom she started to have sex 2 months ago. They do not use condoms. Her mother doesn't know about the boyfriend: "She would kill me if she knew." The adolescent has noticed some yellow vaginal discharge, claims that she has to urinate "all the time," but denies dysuria.

On physical examination the girl appeared to be in some distress but not toxic. She had a low-grade fever and tachycardia with a heart rate of 98 beats/minute; blood pressure and respiratory rate were normal. She had a soft abdomen with voluntary guarding and diffuse bilateral lower abdominal tenderness. There was no upper quadrant tenderness, no hepatosplenomegally, and bowel sounds were normal. Pelvic examination (her first) was remarkable for yellow, mucopurulent discharge from the cervical os, a friable cervix, marked cervical motion tenderness, and some bilateral adnexal fullness and tenderness. A sample from the endocervix was sent to the laboratory to test for *Chlamydia trachomatis* and *Neisseria gonorrhoeae*. Wet mount of the discharge revealed many polymorphonuclear leukocytes. Urine pregnancy test was negative, and urinalysis showed a few white cells and scattered epithelial cells; the specific gravity was 1.025. Complete blood count revealed a normal white blood cell count and no anemia. Erythrocyte sedimentation rate was elevated at 45 mm/hr.

The patient was diagnosed with pelvic inflammatory disease and admitted to the hospital.

Pelvic Inflammatory Disease

Pelvic inflammatory disease (PID) describes a group of inflammatory disorders of the upper genital tract in women, including any combination of endometritis, salpingitis, tuboovarian abscess, or pelvic peritonitis. Adolescent girls are at particular risk of developing PID. While PID is most often initiated by a sexually transmitted pathogen, such as *Neisseria gonorrhoeae* and/or *Chlamydia trachomatis*, cultures indicate that most established cases have a polymicrobial cause. Organisms that may be part of the vaginal flora, such as *Gardnerella vaginalis*, *Haemophilis influenzae*, *Streptococcus agalactiae*, anaerobes, and enteric gram-negative rods, can be involved as can the sexually transmitted organisms, *Ureaplasma urealyticum* and *Mycoplasma hominis*.[14] PID associated with *Chlamydia trachomatis* usually is subacute without fever or elevation of the white blood cell count, whereas that associated with *Neisseria gonorrhoeae* can be quite fulminant.[15]

Typically, PID presents with bilateral lower quadrant abdominal pain that is continuous and worsens with movement and sexual intercourse (Table 6). Other symptoms may include fever and chills, abnormal vaginal discharge and/or bleeding, nausea, vomiting, and anorexia. Right upper quadrant pain, indicative of perihepatitis or Fitz-Hugh-Curtis syndrome, may be present. Signs include lower abdominal tenderness, cervical motion tenderness, and adnexal tenderness. PID has a wide range of presentations and can be difficult to diagnose. However, it is a clinical rather than a laboratory diagnosis; samples for culture and testing are obtained from the endocervix, a site remote

TABLE 6. Diagnostic Criteria for Pelvic Inflammatory Disease

Minimum criteria: empiric treatment for PID should be started if all three of the following are present, in the absence of any other causes of abdominal pain such as pregnancy or appendicitis

- Lower abdominal tenderness
- Adnexal tenderness (unilateral or bilateral)
- Cervical motion tenderness

Additional criteria: to increase the specificity of the diagnosis because incorrect diagnosis and treatment may cause unnecessary morbidity.

- Oral temperature > 38.3° C (100.9° F)
- Abnormal cervical or vaginal discharge
- Elevated erythrocyte sedimentation rate or C-reactive protein
- Laboratory documentation of cervical infection with *Neisseria gonorrhoeae* or *Chlamydia trachomatis*

Elaborate criteria:

- Histopathologic evidence of endometritis on endometrial biopsy
- Tuboovarian abscess on sonography
- Laparoscopic abnormalities consistent with PID

From Sexually Transmitted Diseases, Treatment Guidelines. Albany, NY, New York State Department of Health, Bureau of Sexually Transmitted Disease Control, 1994, pp 106–112.

from the upper genital tract where the infection resides, and even if cultures are negative, the diagnosis should be made when signs and symptoms are suggestive. Diagnosis of chlamydia or gonorrhea infection is important in the treatment of sexual partners and for public health reasons.

Most adolescent girls aged 16 years or younger do better if they are hospitalized for the treatment of PID. Because of confidentiality issues and lack of parental monitoring, many young adolescent girls are unable to follow or tolerate an outpatient oral regimen of treatment. Long-term sequelae such as chronic pelvic pain, infertility, and increased risk of subsequent ectopic pregnancy are serious and warrant aggressive management. Other indications for hospitalization include pregnancy, a severely ill patient, signs of peritonitis, uncertain diagnosis including possible surgical emergencies, adnexal mass, inability to tolerate oral antibiotics, failure to respond to outpatient treatment, inability to return for follow-up within 72 hours, and HIV infection.[14,16] Treatment is outlined in Table 7.

All adolescents treated as outpatients should be reevaluated within 72 hours after beginning antibiotic treatment. At this visit the clinician should verify that the prescriptions have been filled and that the patient is taking the antibiotics as prescribed. A bimanual pelvic examination should indicate improvement in the signs of cervical motion tenderness and adnexal tenderness. Failure to improve

TABLE 7. Management of PID

Inpatient Management

Parenteral Regimen A

Cefoxitin, 2 gm IV every 6 hours *or* **cefotetan**, 2 gm IV every 12 hours

plus

doxycycline, 100 mg orally every 12 hours

Parenteral Regimen B

Clindamycin, 900 mg IV every 8 hours

plus

gentamicin, loading dose IV or IM (2 mg/kg of body weight), followed by a maintenance dose (1.5 mg/kg) every 8 hours

Both parenteral regimens should be given for at least 48 hours or for 24 hours after clinical improvement occurs. Therapy should be continued with oral doxycycline, 100 mg 2 times a day, or clindamycin, 450 mg 4 times a day for a total of 14 days of therapy.

Outpatient Management

Regimen A

Ofloxacin, 400 mg orally 2 times a day for 14 days

plus

metronidazole, 500 mg orally 2 times a day for 14 days

Regimen B

Ceftriaxone, 240 mg IM once

or

cefoxitan 2 gm IM *plus* **probenecid**, 1 gm orally in a single dose concurrently once

plus

doxycycline, 100 mg orally 2 times a day for 14 days

From Centers for Disease Control and Prevention: 1998 guidelines for treatment of sexually transmitted diseases. MMWR 47(RR-1):1–118, 1998.

clinically by the 72-hour visit is a strong indication to admit the adolescent to hospital. It must be stressed to the adolescent girl that her sexual partner must be treated regardless of whether or not he has symptoms. It is helpful to give a written note to the patient to give to her partner(s) specifying her diagnosis and indicating that treatment is necessary.

Ovarian Cysts

Abdominal ultrasound examinations are often a part of the investigation for abdominal pain in adolescent girls. Many of the patients have small ovarian cysts or multicystic ovaries. Isolated follicular cysts and polycystic ovary syndrome are common at this age. Intact ovarian cysts that are ≤ 5 cm in diameter do not cause abdominal pain. Serial ultrasonography usually shows resolution of such cysts without therapy.[17] Adolescent girls experience acute abdominal pain, however, if an ovarian cyst ruptures. In such cases, the ultrasound shows fluid in the cul-de-sac but no cyst. These girls often have an abnormal menstrual history and may have uterine bleeding 2 days after the cyst ruptures due to estrogen withdrawal. Hemorrhage into an ovarian cyst also is a cause of acute lower quadrant abdominal pain. This complication is suggested by a homogeneous increased echogenicity of the cyst fluid on sonography. Large, complex ovarian cysts such as teratomas and dermoid cysts are not often associated with acute abdominal pain; they are more likely to produce a chronic, heavy, dragging sensation in the lower abdomen.

Like testicular torsion, ovarian torsion is uncommon, but it causes severe lower abdominal pain and is a surgical emergency. Unless the diagnosis is quickly suspected and surgery is performed early, the gonadal vascular supply will be irreversibly compromised, and the ovary will have to be removed. Acute lower abdominal pain can be caused by an ovarian cyst acting as a lead point for torsion of the cyst itself or the whole ovary.[18] The young woman usually feels an abrupt onset of severe, crampy, unilateral, lower abdominal pain, with exquisite adnexal tenderness and often with vomiting, similar to the symptoms of ectopic pregnancy, appendicitis, PID, or renal colic. The symptoms of torsion may be intermittent as the ovary twists and untwists. A large adnexal mass, which may be solid, cystic, or complex, with or without fluid in the cul-de-sac, may be seen on ultrasound. Immediate surgical exploration is necessary with an ultrasound finding of an enlarged solid ovarian mass with peripheral cysts 8–12 mm in size. Color doppler can confirm the the absence of ovarian blood flow in cases of ovarian torsion, improving diagnostic accuracy.

Inflammatory Bowel Disease

Inflammatory bowel disease includes Crohn's disease (granulomatous colitis), a transmural inflammation that can occur in any region of the gastrointestinal tract, and ulcerative colitis, a mucosal inflammation limited to the large bowel. The peak age of onset for both diseases is during adolescence. Presenting symptoms include abdominal pain, diarrhea with mucus and/or blood, rectal bleeding, weight loss, and intermittent fevers. More subtle clinical manifestations include anemia that is unresponsive to iron therapy, delayed puberty, amenorrhea, recurring oral apthous ulcers, reduced growth velocity, atypical anorexia with early satiety, diet-responsive diarrhea, protein-losing enteropathy, postprandial pain, recurring episcleritis/uveitis, chronic active hepatitis, perianal fissures, rectal tags, fistula, abscess, and large-joint synovitis/arthritis.[6]

Complications and acute, severe presentations of inflammatory bowel disease are beyond the scope of this chapter. When the diagnosis is considered, patients should be referred to a gastroenterologist for further diagnostic work-up and management, but the primary care physician should continue to follow the patient to address the biopsychosocial issues that are important for adolescents. Such issues include delayed physical and sexual development and difficulty achieving a degree of independence from parents who may be overprotective. Also, it is difficult for an adolescent girl to feel comfortable in social interactions with peers when she constantly has to seek the nearest bathroom.[6] Adolescents with inflammatory bowel disease have a high frequency of depression and need support, which may include peer groups, individual counseling, and family counseling.

CHRONIC ABDOMINAL PAIN

Clinical Case Vignette

A 15-year-old girl was seen with a chief complaint of persistent abdominal pain for more than a year. She described the pain as constant, most often around the umbilicus but sometimes on the right or left side. The pain is usually dull but is sometimes sharp and burning. She occasionally takes Tylenol, but it does not help. The pain is not related to eating, defecating, or menses. Although embarrassed when asked about bowel movements, she denied constipation or diarrhea, as well as fever, nausea, and vomiting. She eats three meals and two snacks a day, with lots of fried foods, loves to eat ice cream, drinks several cokes every day, and hardly ever eats fruits and vegetables. She never drinks water. She does not exercise regularly. Before leaving the room, the patient's mother expressed concern that her daughter had lost some weight, which the daughter denied. When questioned about body image, the girl acknowledged that she thought she was "ugly" but that her body size was okay. She denied binging or purging, but did say that once or twice a month, when she is completely stressed out, she throws up and then falls asleep and feels much better. She has no chronic illnesses and no allergies. Menarche was at age 11 years. Her periods are fairly regular, but she has skipped 1 or 2 months in the last year. She broke up with her last boyfriend 4 months ago and has had two other boyfriends. She was sexually active with all three boyfriends. She has never been pregnant and never had any STIs. She denied smoking, drinking, or drug use. Her social life used to consist of "hanging out" with girlfriends at the mall, but she says that her mother is making her stay home now because she has been doing poorly in school. She has no idea what she wants to be in the future. She finds it difficult to concentrate and often just sits and watches television. She says that her mother, a waitress, who was born in another country, does not understand her and is constantly criticizing her. She has no brothers or sisters and never knew her father; her stepfather left a couple of years ago. She refused to answer any further questions about her stepfather; she shrugged her shoulders and looked at her hands. She denied depression, abuse, or suicidal thoughts or attempts.

On physical examination, the patient was a pretty, slender girl in no distress, but she appeared ill at ease. She rarely made eye contact and her posture was poor. Vital signs were normal. The entire examination, including abdominal and pelvic examination, was completely normal. Complete blood count, erythrocyte sedimentation rate, electrolytes, and liver function tests were normal. Pregnancy test was negative. Gonorrhea and chlamydia tests were negative. Her urinalysis showed a specific gravity of 1.020. Stool guaiac was negative. *Helicobacter pylori* serology was negative. Abdominal ultrasound was normal. Abdominal x-ray showed a small amount of stool in the descending colon.

The patient was asked to keep a food diary and to note any change in pain symptoms or stool patterns as well as how she was feeling each day. Because of her poor self-image, she was referred to a social worker experienced in counseling adolescents and their families. At her follow-up visit, she brought a meticulously kept diary. In the section in which she wrote about her feelings, she repeatedly wrote "sad, tired, or angry." After her fourth visit with the social worker, she revealed that her stepfather had molested her for years and told her he would harm her mother if she ever told anyone. With the help of the social worker, she told her mother, and they began family therapy. Over the following year, her abdominal pain gradually receded. Her family life, social life, and school grades gradually improved.

Psychosomatic Pain

Psychosomatic disorders are frequently the underlying cause of chronic abdominal pain in adolescent girls. In a study at a midwestern high school, students with frequent abdominal pain symptoms and/or headaches were more likely to report greater emotional risks, including sadness, loneliness, tension, and sleep disturbances, and also greater behavioral risks, including sexual activity, drug use, and minor delinquency, than those without somatic symptoms.[19] Therefore, it is of utmost importance when investigating chronic abdominal pain in adolescent girls to take a comprehensive social history exploring her home, school, and peer relationships, as well as her participation in risky behaviors. As with the patient described in the case vignette, it may take several visits before the adolescent trusts the clinician enough to reveal abuse or other traumatic life events. A few laboratory tests, such as a complete blood count, erythrocyte sedimentation rate, and urinalysis, are used to decrease the suspicion of significant renal disease or inflammatory bowel disease. Abdominal ultrasonography usually is not helpful with this type of chronic pain when the physical examination is normal.[20]

Psychosomatic symptoms are organic expressions of psychological stress. Abdominal pain and headache are the most common symptoms associated with psychological stress in adolescent girls. There are often primary physiologic alterations such as altered bowel function or increased gastric acid production associated with psychosomatic pain. Clues to diagnosing psychosomatic abdominal pain include a history of chronic pain with little objective evidence of impairment. The pain is vague, diffuse, and difficult to describe or pinpoint. It may be associated with recent illness. The patient may seem disconnected with and curiously unconcerned about the severe symptoms she is reporting. There may be someone else in the family with similar symptoms who becomes an unconscious role model for the girl. There should be positive evidence for acute or chronic psychosocial stressors, which may include severe illness or death of a loved one, family dysfunction with or without abuse, sexual abuse, dysfunctional peer relationships, family moves, or school changes. The physical examination is normal, and there is no evidence of growth failure, delayed puberty, or weight loss. Laboratory and radiologic studies are within normal limits.

The best approach to the diagnosis and treatment of psychosomatic abdominal pain is to pursue both physical and psychosocial causes right from the beginning. If organic disease is pursued vigorously initially with many tests and imaging studies, it reinforces the patient's preoccupation with physical symptoms, closing the door to dealing with the psychological possibilities and failing to educate the adolescent and her family about the reality of the mind–body relationship. When the clinician exhausts all physical diagnostic possibilities and then attempts to refer the patient to a mental health professional, the family may feel as if they were referred to a therapist because the clinician did not know what was wrong. Instead of following up with the therapist, they may seek another medical opinion (doctor shopping). At the outset, the clinician should explain to the girl and her family that sometimes traumatic or painful events that the patient has not dealt with may make themselves felt physically and repeatedly until they are resolved. Some people get headaches, some develop chest pain or breathing problems, and some get stomach pains. It also helps to explain to the patient and her family that, in any case, she has had this pain for quite a while, and it may take a long time to resolve it. Seeing a therapist, having someone to talk with as she goes through the work-up, will help her to deal with the pain and the process better. Even when there are positive findings for treatable causes, such as lactose intolerance, *H. pylori*, or chronic constipation, the abdominal pain is unlikely to fully resolve unless the psychologic stressors are treated as well. Besides a referral for supportive therapy, teaching the patient relaxation techniques, having her keep a journal, and prescribing daily physical exercise are some of the ways that may help her to deal with stress.

Lactose Intolerance

An important cause of recurrent chronic abdominal pain in adolescents is lactose intolerance. In a recent study of 137 children and adolescents with recurrent abdominal pain, 24% were found to have lactose intolerance.[21] No clinical parameter differentiated these patients from those with pain but without lactose intolerance; therefore, a formal evaluation for lactose malabsorption is recommended for adolescents presenting with recurrent abdominal pain.

Adolescents with lactose intolerance typically present with gastrointestinal symptoms of crampy pain, diarrhea, bloating, boborygmi, and flatus.[22] Approximately 90% of Asian and 80% of African-American adolescents have some degree of lactose intolerance. Hispanic and native American adolescents also have high rates of lactose intolerance. Only about 15% of Caucasian adolescents of Northern European ancestry are lactose-intolerant. The history is usually unreliable when trying to elicit a relationship between symptoms and the ingestion of lactose-containing foods. The symptoms may vary in frequency and are nonspecific. There is usually a lag time of more than an hour between ingestion of lactose-containing food and the onset of the abdominal pain, so adolescents do not perceive the cause and effect relationship between the food and the pain.

As children age, a maturational reduction in lactase activity in the brush boarder of the small intestine may result in lactose intolerance. Lactase is the enzyme that hydrolyses lactose into glucose and galactose, the monosaccharides that are readily absorbed in the small intestine. When a lactase-deficient individual eats a large amount of lactose in dairy foods such as milk, ice cream, and cheese, the unhydrolysed, thus unabsorbed, lactose passes into the colon where it is fermented by anaerobic colonic bacteria. This fermentation process produces volatile fatty acids and free carbon dioxide and hydrogen gasses, which then can cause symptoms. A noninvasive hydrogen breath test demonstrates lactase deficiency by taking breath samples at fixed intervals after the ingestion of a lactose load. The samples are measured for hydrogen concentration; if there is a significant rise at 90 or 120 minutes, lactose malabsorption is likely.

Diagnosis is made by breath hydrogen testing, followed by a 2-week trial of a lactose-free diet. If the adolescent's abdominal pain improves during this time, a diagnosis of lactose intolerance can be made. Because this is an essential time for female adolescents to be eating dairy products to get the calcium that they need to build up their bones, it is important to restore dairy products to their diets. Foods containing lactose can be gradually reintroduced into the diet as tolerated. Yogurt is usually well tolerated by lactase-deficient adolescents, because lactase is released from the yogurt culture organisms (mainly lactobacilli), thus autodigesting the lactose.[23] In addition, most stores carry lactase-treated milk, and lactase drops and tablets can be taken before eating dairy foods.

Constipation

Constipation is common in adolescent girls with chronic recurrent abdominal pain. Largely because of dietary patterns that are low in fiber and high in fat, inadequate water intake, consumption of caffeinated beverages leading to mild dehydration, and a lack of daily exercise, constipation is endemic among adolescent girls. In the United States, 89% of girls, aged 12–18 years, do not consume the American Health Foundation's recommended amount of fiber in their diets.[24] Dietary fiber has been shown to increase the bulk and water content of the stool and to reduce gastrointestinal transit times, thus increasing the ease and frequency of defecation. A national survey by the U.S. Department of Agriculture indicates that a significant amount of teenage girls' daily fiber intake is from grains, mostly ready-to-eat cereals, and is consumed at breakfast.[24] The data indicated that 21% of girls skip breakfast and 52% eat noncereal breakfasts, thus partly explaining their inadequate fiber intake.

In addition to deficient intake of fiber by girls on adequate caloric diets, girls who are dieting to lose weight consume even less fiber, and are at greater risk for developing symptomatic constipation. Almost all girls with anorexia nervosa and many with bulimia nervosa are constipated. Diffuse chronic abdominal pain may be the initial symptom that brings girls with eating disorders in for medical care. Many adolescent girls, whether they have a clinical eating disorder or not, occasionally use laxatives. They may then develop a vicious cycle of constipation and increasing laxative use.

A bowel habit history is usually unreliable when trying to diagnose constipation in adolescent girls. It is an embarrassing subject, and most girls minimize or completely deny symptoms. The pain associated with constipation is usually vague and periumbilical. It is often worse after meals and may occur several times a day, lasting from a few minutes to a few hours. On abdominal examination, a sausage-shaped mass made up of hard stool often can be palpated in the descending colon, indicating constipation even in the absence of a positive history.

The treatment of constipation in an adolescent girl is as problematic as is the diagnosis. It is inadequate to tell her to increase the fiber in her diet by eating cereal for breakfast ("I don't have time for breakfast"), drinking prune juice ("I hate prunes!"), or eating more fruits and vegetables ("I only like cucumbers"). Treatment with an initial purging with a laxative and then 1 month of the stool softener, docusate sodium (Colace), 100 mg 3 times daily, demonstrates to the adolescent how much better she feels when having regular bowel movements. At the same time, changes should be made slowly in her diet, adding some cereal in the morning the first week (even if it means bringing some to school as a snack), then adding a new fruit and vegetable each week. Ask her to explore the produce section of the supermarket with her friends or family to discover new fruits and vegetables to try. She also should be encouraged to increase her water intake by one glass each week until she is drinking 6-8 glasses per day. At the same time, she should attempt to decrease her caffeine intake. Ask her to walk each day, increasing the amount each week until she is able to walk briskly at least a half hour per day. These changes should produce regular bowel habits, but emphasize as well that these healthy lifestyle changes also will give her more energy, boost her spirits, and make her skin glow.

CONCLUSION

Acute and chronic abdominal pain, which often indicate serious anatomic, physiologic, infectious, or psychologic diseases, are common complaints in adolescent girls. The pain may be related to sexual behaviors, abnormal eating behaviors, or serious peer or family relationship dysfunctions. Because of the possibility that the underlying cause of the abdominal pain may be related to behavioral dysfunction, it is of the utmost importance that the medical interview be conducted in private and that confidentiality be clearly acknowledged. In the diagnosis of abdominal pain in the adolescent girl, appropriate physical examination, laboratory testing, and imaging studies are all important, but the medical history is usually key. It may be necessary to enlist the help of a social worker, nutritionist, psychologist or psychiatrist or to have the girl return a number of times until she feels comfortable enough to reveal her true concerns. In this age group, effective treatment of abdominal pain of many causes requires attention to both physiologic and psychosocial issues.

REFERENCES

1. Lavelle JM: A practical approach to nontraumatic, nongynecologic abdominal pain in the adolescent patient. Adolesc Med 4:35–49, 1993.
2. Berman S: Acute abdominal pain. In Berman S: Pediatric Decision Making, 3rd ed. St. Louis, Mosby, 1996.
3. Neblett WW, Pietsch JB, Holcomb GW, et al: Acute abdominal conditions in children and adolescents. Surg Clin North Am 68:415, 1988.
4. Gray DW, Dixon JM, Collin J: The closed-eye sign: An aid to diagnosing nonspecific abdominal pain. BMJ 297:837, 1988.
5. Evans JS: Adolescent gallbladder disease. Adolesc Med 6:417–436, 1995.
6. Lake AM: Chronic abdominal pain in childhood: Diagnosis and management. Am Fam Physician 59:1823–1830, 1999.
7. Meyer WJ, Wiener I, Emory LE, et al: Cholelithiasis associated with medroxyprogesterone acetate therapy in men. Res Commun Chem Pathol Pharmacol 75:69–84, 1992.
8. Centers for Disease Control and Prevention: Body weight perceptions and selected weight management goals and practices of high school students—United States, 1990. MMWR 40:741–750, 1991.
9. Radel E: Advances in the treatment of adolescents with sickle hemoglobinopathies. Adolesc Med 5:271–292, 1994.
10. Wald ER: Pelvic inflammatory disease in adolescents. Adv Pediatr Infect Dis 9:171, 1994.
11. Katzman DK, Friedman IM, McDonald CA, Litt IF: *Chlamydia trachomatis* Fitz-Hugh-Curtis syndrome without salpingitis in female adolescents. Am J Dis Child 142:996–998, 1988.
12. Reichert JA, Valle RF: Fitz-Hugh-Curtis syndrome. JAMA 236:266–268, 1976.
13. Drumm B, Rhoads JM, Stringer DA, et al: Peptic ulcer disease in children: Etiology, clinical findings, and clinical course. Pediatrics 82:410–441, 1988.
14. Centers for Disease Control and Prevention: 1998 guidelines for treatment of sexually transmitted diseases. MMWR 47(RR-1):1–118, 1998.
15. Neinstein LS, Himebaugh KS: Pelvic inflammatory disease. In Neinstein LS: Adolescent Health Care, A Practical Guide, 3rd ed. Baltimore, Williams & Wilkins, 1996, pp 909–923.
16. Sexually Transmitted Diseases, Treatment Guidelines, 1994. Albany, NY, New York State Department of Health, Bureau of Sexually Transmitted Disease Control, 1994, pp 106–112.
17. Warner BW, Kuhn JC, Barr LL: Conservative management of large ovarian cysts in children: The value of serial pelvic ultrasonography. Surgery 112:749–755, 1992.
18. Meyer JS, Harmon CM, Harty MP, et al: Ovarian torsion: Clinical and imaging presentation in children. J Pediatr Surg 30:1433–1436, 1995.
19. Beiter M, Ingersoll G, Ganser J, Orr DP: Relationships of somatic symptoms to behavioral and emotional risk in young adolescents. J Pediatr 118:473–478, 1991.
20. Shanon A, Martin DJ, Feldman W: Ultrasonographic studies in the management of recurrent abdominal pain. Pediatrics 86:35–38, 1990.
21. Webster RB, DiPalma JA, Gremse DA: Lactose maldigestion and recurrent abdominal pain in children. Digest Dis Sci 40:1506–1510, 1995.
22. Hyams JS: Chronic abdominal pain. Adolesc Med 6:305–315, 1995.
23. Kolars JC, Levitt MD, Aouji M, Savaiano DA: Yogurt—An autodigesting source of lactose. N Engl J Med 310:1–3, 1984.
24. Saldanha LG: Fiber in the diet of U.S. children: Results of national surveys. Pediatrics 96:994–997, 1995.
25. Silen W: Cope's Early Diagnosis of the Acute Abdomen, 18th ed. London, Oxford University Press, 1991.

CHAPTER 20

Menstrual Dysfunction

Alvin F. Goldfarb, M.D.

Understanding and managing menstrual dysfunction in the adolescent require knowledge of the normal developmental maturation of the neuroendocrine system that controls reproduction. Clinicians also must be able to recognize and evaluate the many congenital, endocrine, nutritional, and psychosocial conditions that can present as menstrual dysfunction in the adolescent girl. These tasks are best accomplished with an adequate understanding of reproductive endocrinology coupled with an approach to the adolescent and her family that respects her emerging autonomy and the sensitive nature of problems related to menstruation. This chapter discusses neuroendocrine regulation of reproduction, disorders causing delayed puberty, evaluation and management of secondary amenorrhea and oligomenorrhea as well as of dysfunctional uterine bleeding and dysmenorrhea.

MATURATION OF THE HYPOTHALAMIC–PITUITARY–OVARIAN AXIS

The neonate is born with a structurally complete reproductive endocrine mechanism, which remains quiescent, however, until the peripubertal period.[1] The precise nature of the intrinsic inhibitory restraint to gonadotropin-releasing hormone (GnRH) secretion by the hypothalamus that inhibits pubertal development during childhood has not been completely clarified. At puberty, various neurotransmitters interact to influence the secretion of GnRH and hence the synthesis and release of gonadotropins. An increase in pituitary gland secretion of the gonadotropins follicle-stimulating hormone (FSH) and luteinizing hormone (LH) heralds the onset of puberty. The administration of a gonadotropin-releasing hormone agonist (GnRHa) elicits several different patterns of gonadotropin release, depending on the stage of development of the individual. Prepubertal children show a minimal but significant rise in LH after GnRHa administration. However, a marked increase in LH response to GnRHa is seen in pubertal girls and boys.[2] The increase in pituitary LH reserve and sensitivity to GnRHa is a hallmark of puberty. In contrast, FSH shows sex-specific change in response to GnRHa (females release significantly more FSH than males) but no maturational alteration.

Enhanced secretion of LH during sleep is another maturational change first seen in the peripubertal and pubertal periods.[2] The demonstration of sleep-associated enhanced LH secretion in agonadal patients during puberty indicates that this process is not dependent on gonadal function but represents a maturational change in the central nervous system (CNS). Pulsatile GnRH secretion at the hypothalamic level activates the pituitary to increase LH and FSH release. The increased secretion of gonadotropins stimulates the ovaries to begin follicular development and estrogen production, which, in turn, stimulates the growth of the breasts and uterus in pubertal girls. The development of the positive feedback mechanism, whereby an increasing circulating level of estradiol triggers an LH surge and ovulation, is a late maturational phase of gonadotropin secretion. Maturation of the positive feedback mechanism may not occur until several years after puberty is initiated. In prepubertal or early pubertal girls no rise in LH can be induced even though estradiol levels are similar to those found in fully mature ovulating young women.

In addition to the maturational timetable of reproductive endocrine control in the CNS, nutrition and disease also serve as modifiers of normal sexual maturation in girls. Menarche occurs in 95% of all girls when they reach approximately 47 kg in weight with 13% body fat.[3] The average age at menarche is 12.8 years for white girls and 12.2 years for African American girls.[4] Mean ages for various pubertal milestones are listed in Table 1. Diagnosis of problems of sexual maturation should use the Tanner classification (see chapter 1).

DELAYED SEXUAL MATURATION AND PRIMARY AMENORRHEA

Evaluation

Girls with no signs of sexual maturation by their thirteenth birthday need to be evaluated. Breast development (thelarche) begins at a mean age of approximately 9 years for African American girls and 10 years for white girls in the United States; thus no breast development by the thirteenth birthday is well

TABLE 1. Mean Ages of Pubertal Changes in Girls in the United States

Age (yr)	Characteristic
8–10	Breast budding Beginning of height spurt Growth of bony pelvis Female contour fat deposition
10–11	Appearance of pubic hair (may precede breast budding in 10%)
11–12	Appearance of vaginal secretions Growth of internal and external genitalia Increase in vaginal glycogen content and lowering of pH
12–13	Pigmentation of areolae and growth of breasts Increase in amount of pubic hair Menarche Acne (in 75–90%)
14–15	Arrest of skeletal growth

beyond the range of normal.[4] The evaluation process begins with an adequate history and physical examination. A good antenatal and postnatal history is essential. Children with chronic diseases such as sickle cell anemia, cystic fibrosis, or renal disease may have delayed sexual maturation. On physical examination, simple findings such as height, weight, signs of estrogen effect, and texture of the skin and hair can be used as clues in the diagnosis and evaluation of pubertal delay. Careful examination for breast budding, early pubic hair growth, and Tanner staging should be done.

The most helpful laboratory test to begin the evaluation is a serum FSH level. If the level is elevated (hypergonadotropic hypogonadism), the problem is in the ovary and the diagnosis is primary ovarian failure. In cases of ovarian failure, a karyotype should be done to look for XO or XY gonadal dysgenesis. Very low or absent levels of FSH (hypogonadotropic hypogonadism) indicate that the problem is central and the hypothalamic–pituitary axis should be further evaluated. The most common cause of hypogonadotropic hypogonadism is constitutional delay of puberty. However, this is a diagnosis of exclusion. Attempts to use GnRHa testing to differentiate constitutional delay from other forms of hypogonadotropic hypogonadism have not been successful if the child does not show any early signs of puberty.[5] A history of systemic disease and malnutrition suggests reversible hypogonadism due to hypothalamic suppression. A history of increased intracranial pressure, abnormal vision, or neurological symptoms demands imaging studies of the sella turcica to diagnose tumors of the pituitary or hypothalamus. Deficiency of pituitary hormones (thyroid-stimulating hormone, adrenocorticotropic hormone, growth hormone) suggests the possibility of idiopathic hypopituitarism. Table 2 shows causes of delayed puberty in girls.

Girls with constitutional delay of puberty often have a family history of a similar type of late development in a parent or relative and will have delayed bone age. Often, these children are smaller than average throughout childhood, suggesting that all body tissues may be slow in maturing. This theory agrees with the idea that a certain level of general physical maturity must be attained before the hypothalamic–pituitary mechanism is activated. Once these girls enter puberty, however, they go through the normal stages at rate similar to that of girls with on-time puberty.

If menarche has not occurred within 4–5 years after the onset of breast development, delayed or arrested pubertal development with primary amenorrhea

TABLE 2. Causes of Delayed Puberty in Girls

	Site of Defect	Gonadotropin Levels	FSH/LH Response	Estrogen Levels
Constitutional delay	Delayed maturation	Low	Prepubertal	Low
Reversible hypogonadism	Hypothalamus or pituitary	Low	Prepubertal or absent	Low
Permanent hypogonadism	Hypothalamus or pituitary	Low	Prepubertal or absent	Low
Hyperandrogenism	Adrenal or ovary	Low	Prepubertal	Low
Ovarian failure	Ovary	High	Accentuated	Low

may be diagnosed. Short stature and very low weight can give important clues to the diagnosis of malnutrition. Prolonged delayed puberty may be noticed in combination with malnutrition such as that found with anorexia nervosa or with systemic disease such as inflammatory bowel disease or hypothyroidism.[6] Delayed puberty in athletic children should not be attributed to the exercise before excluding other conditions. Nevertheless, intense athletic training in childhood, particularly gymnastic and ballet training, is associated with delayed puberty.[7] Severe psychological stress related to abuse or family dysfunction has been associated with delayed puberty and primary amenorrhea. Functional ovarian hyperandrogenism, adrenal hyperplasia, and androgen-producing tumors are associated with delayed menarche. These conditions present with physical signs of virilization such as acne, hirsutism, or obesity, and laboratory tests confirm increased androgen levels.

Primary amenorrhea with complete, normal, on-time pubertal development is not true delayed puberty but must be considered in the differential diagnosis of absent menarche. Girls with primary amenorrhea usually have a congenital genital anomaly with obstruction to menstrual flow. Imperforate hymen can be diagnosed easily on physical examination by observing a bulging hymen. In the Mayer-Rokitansky-Küster-Hauser syndrome (müllerian agenesis), there is congenital atresia of the vagina and/or the uterus.[8] Genital examination readily demonstrates the presence of a small dimple where the vaginal opening should be. This syndrome often is associated with renal agenesis and other urinary tract anomalies. An algorithm for the evaluation of delayed sexual maturation and primary amenorrhea is depicted in Figure 1.

Management

Patients with irreversible ovarian, pituitary, or hypothalamic failure should be treated with hormone replacement therapy (HRT). Treatment should begin between the ages of 13 and 15 years and be continued throughout life.[9] Therapy started earlier than age 13 may cause premature closure of the epiphyses, ultimately resulting in short stature. HRT is essential for development of secondary sexual characteristics, prevention of osteoporosis, and the maintenance of good health, particularly cardiovascular health.

A suggested HRT regimen is to begin with conjugated estrogen tablets (Premarin), 0.3 mg orally for 6 months. Starting hormonal therapy with this very low dose minimizes side effects and excessive breast stimulation. After 6 months the dose is doubled to 0.625 mg orally daily and continued for an additional 6 months. After 1 year of continuous estrogen administration, a progestin, medroxyprogesterone acetate, is introduced in a cyclic fashion using 10 mg orally daily from the first to the tenth of each calendar month. The dose of conjugated estrogens may be increased to 0.9 mg, then 1.25 mg orally daily. The adolescent should begin having regular menstrual cycles in the second year of therapy. Once regular cycles are established and secondary sexual characteristics have developed, some girls prefer the convenience of low-dose combination oral contraceptives for replacement therapy.

Girls in whom an eating disorder or severe psychological stress is suspected should be referred to a psychotherapist experienced in working with adolescents

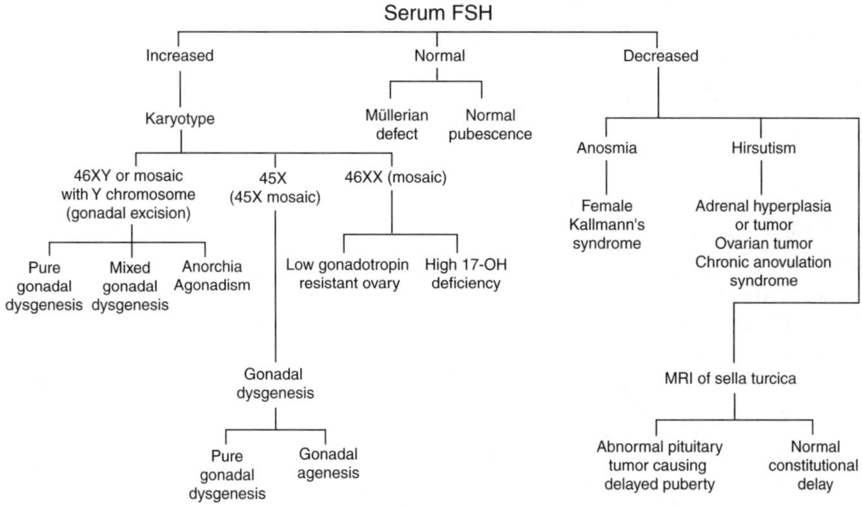

FIGURE 1. Evaluation of delayed sexual maturation.

for diagnostic evaluation and management. Patients with suspected congenital anomalies should be referred to a pediatric and adolescent gynecologist for further work-up and possible surgical correction. In girls for whom gonadal removal is indicated because of the presence of Y chromosomal material, but who have a uterus, it is suggested that the uterus not be removed. With modern methods of assisted reproductive technology, there is always a possibility that they may become gestational mothers using a donor ovum that can be fertilized by their husbands' sperm.

SECONDARY AMENORRHEA AND OLIGOMENORRHEA

Secondary amenorrhea is defined as no menstrual periods for 6 months or more in an adolescent who had been menstruating regularly. Oligomenorrhea is defined as irregular, infrequent periods for a period of 1 year or longer. Most of the conditions that present as primary amenorrhea also can present as secondary amenorrhea or oligomenorrhea.

Evaluation

A complete history and physical examination is essential for accurate diagnosis of these menstrual dysfunctions. In most instances information should be gathered from the adolescent herself, without parent(s) present. Because pregnancy is a common cause of secondary amenorrhea in the adolescent age group, a detailed sexual history should be elicited and a pregnancy test performed at the initial office visit. Additional important areas to pursue in the history include weight changes, body image, athletic activity, and stressors such as death in the family or moving into a new environment. Important signs to note on physical examination include excessive thinness, obesity, hirsutism, acne, or galactorrhea.

After a negative pregnancy test, it is helpful diagnostically to give the patient a progesterone challenge test (PCT) using medroxyprogesterone acetate, 10 mg orally daily for 10 days. If the adolescent has a withdrawal bleed 2 or 3 days after stopping the progestin, there is adequate gonadotropin stimulation of the ovaries, which causes them to secrete enough estrogen to cause proliferation of the endometrium. In such cases, the endometrium is exposed to unopposed estrogen, and the adolescent is at risk for dysfunctional uterine bleeding and, if the condition persists, endometrial carcinoma. If, on the other hand, the patient fails to bleed, there is inadequate gonadotropin secretion to stimulate ovarian estrogen production and endometrial growth (hypothalamic suppression or failure), or there is ovarian failure. For patients who fail to bleed with the PCT, serum levels of FSH and LH should be performed. Individuals with severe weight loss, intense exercise regimens, eating disorders, or poor nutrition, and who have low body fat, usually are unresponsive to the PCT. Such patients have low gonadotropins, particularly LH, and the diagnosis of hypothalamic amenorrhea can be made.[10] If there is no obvious explanation for the hypothalamic suppression, investigations to rule out a CNS tumor should be considered.

Premature Ovarian Failure

Ovarian failure is associated with high gonadotropins, particularly FSH. The young woman may give a history of hot flashes and/or other vasomotor symptoms. Mosaic varieties of gonadal dysgenesis, autoimmune disease, radiation, chemotherapy, or rarely, a systemic febrile illness can result in ovarian failure with secondary amenorrhea. Autoimmune disorders associated with premature ovarian failure include thyroiditis, myasthenia gravis, hypoadrenalism, hypoparathyroidism, and mucocutaneous candidiasis.[11]

Exercise-related Amenorrhea

Exercise-induced amenorrhea is found most often in high-intensity runners and ballet dancers. It is more common in athletic girls who also have disordered eating and are very thin.[12] Amenorrheic athletes who are hypoestrogenic are at risk for osteopenia and stress fractures. They may have the so-called female athletic triad of amenorrhea, disordered eating, and osteopenia. Nutritional counseling as well as multivitamin and calcium supplementation should be recommended to such patients. A reduction in the intensity of training, if possible, also is helpful. However, HRT to reduce the risk of fracture should be considered if the amenorrhea is longstanding.

Anorexia Nervosa

Amenorrhea associated with anorexia nervosa is due to impaired gonadotropin secretion.[13] FSH and LH levels are very low and measure in the prepubertal range, cortisol levels are elevated, prolactin levels are normal, thyroid stimulating hormone (TSH) and thyroxine (T_4) levels are normal, but triiodothyronine (T_3) levels are low. The adolescent with anorexia nervosa may have constipation, cold intolerance, bradycardia, hypotension, and dry skin. This condition should be diagnosed quickly by taking a confidential, careful dietary, body image, and psychosocial history, and the adolescent should be referred to a psychotherapist for further evaluation. HRT is sometimes used to protect the bones in girls with anorexia nervosa who fail to regain their menses after a year or more of treatment.

Thyroid Disorders

Adolescents who experience a withdrawal bleed with the PCT should have thyroid function studies performed. Hypothyroidism is a subtle disease that is associated with menstrual dysfunction, and the diagnosis may be missed if the relevant laboratory studies are not performed.

Hyperprolactinemia

Hyperprolactinemia disrupts pituitary gonadotropin secretion. Menstrual dysfunction ranges from cycles with a short inadequate luteal phase to amenorrhea. Galactorrhea may or may not be present. Patients with amenorrhea and galactorrhea may have an abnormal sella turcica due to either a tumor or the so-called empty sella syndrome. Visual field testing and radiologic imaging by computed tomography scan or magnetic resonance imaging are a necessary part of the evaluation. Prolactin-secreting pituitary adenomas are classified as microadenomas if they are under 10 mm in diameter and macroadenomas if they are over 10 in diameter. Other conditions sometimes associated with hyperprolactinemia include hypothyroidism and polycystic ovary syndrome. Treatment of hyperprolactinemia depends on the patient's needs. Most adolescents are treated to reverse the galactorrhea and restore the menses. If a macroadenoma is present, medical treatment may be indicated to shrink the tumor before surgery. The mainstay of medical treatment is the dopamine receptor agonist, bromocriptine mesylate, in an initial dose of 1.25 mg at bedtime, gradually increasing to 5–7.5 mg daily. Pergolide mesylate, a much more potent dopamine receptor agonist approved for use in Parkinson's disease, is now an acceptable method of treatment for hyperprolactinemia with fewer side effects than bromocriptine. When oral administration causes nausea, vaginal application may be suggested as an alternative.

Hyperandrogenic Amenorrhea

Functional ovarian hyperandrogenism or polycystic ovary syndrome (PCOS) is among the most common endocrinopathies in women, affecting an estimated 10% of all women after puberty. Nevertheless, it is often overlooked by physicians, especially in adolescents, and even when recognized, it often is not treated. Adolescent girls with the condition may not manifest the classic signs and symptoms described in adult women of obesity, hirsutism, enlarged polycystic ovaries, and infertility. More importantly, however, they often have the changes in insulin and lipid metabolism that can have implications for future health. Since the original studies of Stein and Leventhal, it has been recognized that symptoms of PCOS commonly begin at menarche. Recent studies by Apter have suggested that adolescents with PCOS, as compared with controls, exhibit augmented LH pulsatility with earlier reversal of the normal pubertal pattern of sleep-related pulsatility.[14] The disorder is believed to have an autosomal-dominant inheritance with premature male pattern baldness as the male phenotype. Late-onset 21-hydroxylase deficiency (nonclassic congenital adrenal hyperplasia) is a less common cause of hyperandrogenic amenorrhea in adolescents. This condition also is associated with secondary amenorrhea and polycystic ovaries, but unlike adolescents with PCOS, adolescents with 21-hydroxylase deficiency usually have moderate-to-severe acne and hirsutism and more often have other signs of virilization such as clitoromegaly. Androgen-secreting tumors usually are characterized by rapid onset of virilizing signs.

Pathophysiology

Apart from hyperandrogenism, a major characteristic of hyperandrogenic amenorrhea is chronic anovulation. A popular hypothesis for the development of chronic anovulation starts with the presence of excessive amounts of androgen that undergo conversion to estrogen in skin and adipose tissue.[15] This acyclic estrogenic milieu induces inappropriate LH secretion, which stimulates the theca cells in the ovarian stroma, producing an abundance of ovarian androgens. The altered intraovarian environment leads to the arrest of follicular maturation and ultimately atresia. These atretic follicles do not have the ability to aromatize androgen to estradiol. Thus, under persistent LH stimulation the ovary secretes inordinately high amounts of androstenedione and testosterone, worsening the hyperandrogenism. Yen was the first to postulate that the adrenal gland is an important contributor to the perimenarcheal onset of PCOS.[15] Obesity and emotional stress at puberty are associated with increased adrenal activity. An exaggerated adrenarche with excess adrenal androgen secretion may result in increased peripheral conversion to estrogen, thus beginning the pathophysiologic cycle described earlier. The androgenic basis for the inappropriate estrogen production eventually undergoes a shift from adrenal to ovary.

Insulin resistance with hyperinsulinemia commonly is associated with PCOS.[16] It is suspected that insulin resistance is secondary to either the obesity or hyperandrogenism associated with this condition. The latter may be the more important factor because women with PCOS who are not obese also demonstrate insulin resistance. The clinical association of hyperandrogenism, insulin resistance, and acanthosis nigricans has been termed the HAIR-AN syndrome. Women with PCOS have a high risk of developing type 2 diabetes mellitus as they age. Other metabolic changes found with PCOS include higher mean serum levels of low-density lipoprotein (LDL) cholesterol than in weight-matched controls. The preponderance of evidence points to an increase in cardiovascular risk factors for women with PCOS, particularly with onset in adolescence.

Evaluation

In evaluation of hyperandrogenic amenorrhea, total testosterone and dehydroepiandrosterone sulfate (DHEAS) determinations are screening tests to rule

TABLE 3. Differential Diagnosis of Hyperandrogenism

1. Idiopathic hirsutism	5. Congenital adrenal hyperplasia
2. Polycystic ovary syndrome	6. Masculinizing tumors of the adrenal or ovary
3. Cushing's syndrome	7. Hypothyroidism
4. Obesity	

out a neoplastic source of androgen secretion. Total testosterone > 200 ng/dl or DHEAS > 700 μg/dl are suggestive of an adrenal or ovarian tumor and require further evaluation.[17] Other useful laboratory tests include thyroid function tests, free testosterone, which is a sensitive marker of ovarian hyperandrogenism, and LH, which is elevated in PCOS with an LH to FSH ratio greater than 3 to 1. 17α-hydroxyprogesterone levels are elevated in congenital adrenal hyperplasia; early morning levels > 1000 ng/dl establish the diagnosis and levels > 400 ng/dl are suggestive.[17] In addition, because DHEAS is an exclusive marker of adrenal androgen production, a significant elevation raises suspicion of a primary adrenal disorder. A dexamethasone suppression test and an ACTH stimulation test should be performed to further evaluate adrenal gland function. Occasionally, the use of sonography or other imaging studies to evaluate the size of the ovaries and adrenal glands may be in order. The differential diagnosis of hyperandrogenic amenorrhea is presented in Table 3.

Management

In the adolescent who is not interested in becoming pregnant, drugs that decrease the secretion of androgens and block the action of androgens at the target organ level are used in managing hyperandrogenic amenorrhea.[16] This drug treatment improves acne and hirsutism and restores regular menstrual cycles. Low-dose combination oral contraceptive pills (OCPs) are the mainstay of treatment for PCOS. OCPs suppress ovarian androgen production and increase the levels of sex hormone–binding globulin circulating in the blood, thus lowering free testosterone levels. Spironolactone, which blocks the conversion of testosterone to 5-hydroxytestosterone, the active androgen at the cellular level, may be used in conjunction with OCPs. Cyproterone acetate, an antiandrogen that is not approved for use in the United States, is effective and has been used extensively in other countries. Congenital adrenal hyperplasia is treated with hydrocortisone or prednisone to suppress the adrenal gland. The response to medical therapy of androgen disorders may be disappointing to both the physician and the patient. Anatomic changes of hyperandrogenism such as deepening of the voice and clitoromegaly are not reversible. Insulin resistance associated with PCOS is not amenable to hormonal therapy. Therefore, management of hyperinsulinemia should be considered separately from the hyperandrogenic disorder. Obesity and dyslipidemia are best handled by a team approach with a nutritionist who is sensitive to the emotional needs of the adolescent. Weight reduction alone can reverse the abnormal endocrine dynamics seen in patients with PCOS. If type 2 diabetes mellitus develops, treatment with the oral antihyperglycemic drug, metformin, may be indicated. The treatment of hyperandrogenism is summarized in Table 4.

TABLE 4. Treatment of Hyperandrogenism

1. Oral contraceptives
2. Antiandrogens: cyproterone acetate, spironolactone
3. Dexamethasone, prednisone, hydrocortisone
4. GnRH agonists
5. Cosmetic hair removal: shaving, waxing, tweezing, electrolysis

EXCESSIVE UTERINE BLEEDING

Irregular heavy menstrual bleeding in adolescent girls most commonly is a symptom of anovulation, systemic disease, or pregnancy. Causes are listed in Table 5. Unlike in the perimenopausal woman, organic disease of the uterus rarely is the cause of excess uterine bleeding in the adolescent. Dysfunctional uterine bleeding (DUB), which is defined as irregular, painless menstrual bleeding that is prolonged, excessive, and unpatterned, is associated most often with anovulation.

Although many menstrual cycles in the first few years after menarche are anovulatory, most perimenarcheal adolescents have regular menses and do not bleed excessively. In a World Health Organization (WHO) study of early adolescents, 19% of the girls achieved regular cycles within the first 3 cycles after menarche, and by the end of 2 years, 67% had achieved regular menstrual cycles.[18] Median cycle length was 31 days, slightly longer than the 28-day cycles experienced by adult women. The study documented that fewer than 0.5% of bleeding episodes within the first 2 years after menarche lasted longer than 10 days, while the mean duration of bleeding was 4–5 days.[18] Recent data demonstrate that the frequency of ovulation during adolescence depends upon the age at menarche; the earlier menarche occurs, the sooner regular ovulation is established. Apter et al. found that the length of time after menarche until 50% of the cycles were ovulatory was 1 year when age at menarche was younger than 12 years but increased to 3 years and 4.5 years when the ages at menarche were between 12 and 12.9 years and equal to or older than 13 years, respectively.[19] Furthermore, Apter's data demonstrate that it may take up to 7 years after menarche before 90% or more of the cycles are ovulatory, yet by this time the large majority of young women have regular cycles.

Physiology of Ovulatory and Anovulatory Cycles

An orderly sequence of hormonal and endometrial events is responsible for the regular and limited bleeding that is associated with ovulatory cycles.

TABLE 5. Causes of Abnormal Uterine Bleeding

Pelvic Causes	Extrapelvic Causes
Pregnancy	Coagulation defects
Malignancy	Endocrinopathies
Infection	Systemic diseases
Vaginal lesions	Medications
Cervical lesions	
Uterine pathology	
Ovarian factors	

Repetitive patterns of gonadotropin release result in ovarian follicular development and estrogen secretion during the follicular phase of the cycle. A midcycle LH surge triggers ovulation. Subsequent gonadotropin release in the luteal phase of the cycle is responsible for the secretion of progesterone as well as estrogen from the corpus luteum, followed by withdrawal of both hormones. Estrogen stimulates the production of both estrogen and progesterone receptors on endometrial cells. So long as estrogen is secreted in an unopposed (i.e., without concomitant progesterone) continuous manner, the endometrium continues to grow (proliferative phase). The effects of progesterone on the endometrium during the luteal phase of the cycle are to halt growth and stabilize the tissue (secretory phase). Progesterone decreases the quantity of both estrogen and progesterone receptors in the endometrium. With fewer estrogen receptors, stimulation of growth is halted. The binding of progesterone to its own receptors results in predecidualization of the endometrial stroma and is a stabilizing influence. Once the corpus luteum begins its demise and estrogen and progesterone secretion decrease, an orderly sequence of hormonal (prostaglandin-mediated) and vascular events occurs universally throughout the endometrium, leading to a complete sloughing and well-controlled bleeding.

Pathologic anovulation associated with PCOS and other disorders often produces irregular and prolonged episodes of heavy bleeding.[20] In the absence of organic pelvic causes, most DUB in the adolescent age group is secondary to anovulation, and in most cases of anovulation the possibility of PCOS must be considered. In these patients, progesterone either is never produced or is produced only during the infrequent ovulatory cycle. Numerous follicles are continuously being stimulated to grow by an abnormal secretion of gonadotropins. Increased androgen secretion from the ovarian theca cells (also resulting from abnormal gonadotropin secretion) causes premature follicular atresia. The continuous unopposed secretion of estrogen from multiple follicles results in overgrowth of the endometrium, which becomes significantly thicker than it does in ovulatory cycles. The thickened endometrium is unstable and sloughs irregularly, causing abnormal bleeding. In addition, bleeding occurs if the abnormal gonadotropin pattern is interrupted and estrogen levels decrease. In either case, shedding of the unstable and excessively thickened endometrium is neither a universal nor an orderly event. Hence, the resultant bleeding is prolonged and uncontrolled.

Causes of Excessive Uterine Bleeding

In the adolescent, systemic causes of excessive uterine bleeding include coagulation defects such as von Willebrand's disease (factor VIII deficiency), platelet abnormalities, idiopathic thrombocytopenic purpura, and leukemia. Ten percent of all adolescent girls who develop any of these coagulopathies have excessive uterine bleeding as their presenting symptom. Endocrine disorders that can be associated with irregular heavy menstrual bleeding include hypothyroidism, hyperthyroidism, Addison's disease, and Cushing's disease. These endocrinopathies may present as anovulation, irregular menstrual bleeding, or secondary amenorrhea due to premature ovarian failure. Certain infectious diseases that affect the liver are sometimes associated with excessive uterine bleeding, most commonly infectious mononucleosis. Adolescent girls with other conditions causing hepatic damage, including autoimmune hepatitis, cirrhosis, or toxins such as alcohol, also may have excessive menstrual bleeding. The liver damage results in impaired conjugation and detoxification of ovarian steroids.

Threatened abortion, ectopic pregnancy, normal pregnancy, or trophoblastic disease can result in excessive and irregular uterine bleeding, usually accompanied by painful cramps but not always. Pregnancy must be ruled out in any adolescent girl presenting with a menstrual irregularity. As a rule, malignancy of any of the pelvic organs is rare in adolescents. However, spotting and staining may be associated with human papillomavirus infection of the cervix (see chapter 22) or cervical polyps. Endometrial polyps and uterine myomas (fibroids) are rare in the adolescent age group as are ovarian tumors. Functional ovarian cysts are not associated with excessive bleeding. In addition, abnormal bleeding in the adolescent may be a sign of sexually transmitted endometrial infection or cervicitis. Finally, trauma, infections, or foreign bodies in the vagina may present with irregular bleeding.

Evaluation

The assessment of abnormal uterine bleeding must begin by obtaining important facts that relate to the onset of the problem, including the nature, amount, and timing of the bleeding; whether or not there is associated pain; any event that preceded the onset of the symptoms; the presence of known systemic or psychosocial pathology; the possibility of pregnancy; relevant past medical and family history; and a determination of whether or not the bleeding constitutes an emergency. The physical examination is directed initially toward assessing hemodynamic stability by noting any pallor, tachycardia, or orthostatic hypotension. Subsequently, identification of signs of systemic disorders (e.g., cachexia, jaundice), bleeding disorders (e.g., petechiae, purpura), and endocrinopathies should be a priority. Hyperandrogenism is identified by the presence of excessive hair and signs of masculinization; thyroid disorders may be signaled by a goiter; galactorrhea may be demonstrated with hyperprolactinemia. Genital inspection is directed toward confirmation of the source of bleeding and identification of any masses, trauma, or foreign objects. Any girl who is sexually experienced should have a full speculum and bimanual pelvic examination with testing for sexually transmitted infections and assessment of uterine size and adnexal masses or tenderness.

Determination of the amount of blood loss and degree of urgency in management is best made with an immediate complete blood count (CBC) with a differential and platelet count. Coagulation studies should be obtained on all patients with evidence of severe anemia and very heavy or prolonged bleeding and all patients who require hospitalization. It is imperative to obtain not only a prothrombin time (PT) and partial thromboplastin time (PTT) but also a total platelet count, bleeding time, and clotting time. Patients with von Willebrand's disease may have normal PT and PTT studies and can be identified only by a prolonged bleeding time. In addition, all patients should have thyroid function studies done because hypothyroidism may have a subtle presentation with no overt signs or symptoms. Consideration for further hormonal evaluation should

TABLE 6. Laboratory Evaluation of Abnormal Uterine Bleeding

Pregnancy test	Bleeding time
CBC, platelet count	Thyroid function studies
Prothrombin time (PT), partial thromboplastin time (PTT)	Pelvic ultrasound
	Others as indicated

be made at the initial blood sampling, depending on signs and symptoms. Most clinicians do a pregnancy test on all adolescents, regardless of a positive history of sexual activity. Table 6 lists the laboratory evaluation of abnormal bleeding.

Management

In the adolescent age group, management of excessive uterine bleeding is almost exclusively medical and surgical intervention rarely is indicated. Regimens of progestin with or without estrogen are the best initial hormonal approach for these patients.[21] For most adolescents with DUB, especially those who have bled excessively and for prolonged periods of time, a regimen using a combination oral contraceptive pill is most appropriate.[20,22] Lo/Ovral® has been a favorite because it contains the potent progestin, norgestrel. However, any low-dose combination OCP may be used. Therapy should begin with 4 tablets daily until bleeding has stopped completely, tapering to 1 tablet per day over 21 days. After 3 weeks, a withdrawal bleed may be allowed, and OCPs are continued for 3–6 months to control the menstrual bleeding while anemia is corrected and iron stores are replenished. Concomitant antiemetics to treat the nausea associated with high doses of estrogen may be necessary when the patient is taking more than one OCP per day. If the bleeding has been of short duration and it appears that enough endometrium remains to allow progestin-induced stabilization, the adolescent may be treated with progestin alone. Medroxyprogesterone acetate (Provera®), 10 mg, or norethindrone acetate (Aygestin®), 5 mg, may be given in tapering doses beginning with 1 tablet, 4 times daily for 4 days; then 1 tablet, 3 times a day for 3 days; and finally 1 tablet, 2 times a day for 2 weeks. This entire course of therapy extends treatment over 3 weeks and tapers slowly enough to avoid breakthrough bleeding.

If hormonal therapy does not control the bleeding within a reasonable length of time, dilatation and curettage (D&C) and hysteroscopy are indicated. D&C allows a complete emptying of the uterine cavity and more efficient uterine contractility. In addition, it enables diagnosis of the rare uterine neoplasm or other unusual pathology. For adolescents who are comfortable with pelvic examinations, an endometrial biopsy with emptying of the uterine cavity can be done in the gynecologist's office using a Novak curette and a 10-ml syringe or a Vibra aspirator, which may be easier to pass through the cervix. However, this type of office procedure is rarely required and even more rarely tolerated by adolescent girls.

DYSMENORRHEA

Pain with menses or dysmenorrhea is the most common menstrual dysfunction in adolescents. Nearly two-thirds of 12–17-year-old girls report some degree of crampy abdominal pain recurring with most menstrual periods, and a significant number of girls miss school on a monthly basis because of this menstrual disorder.[23] The clinician should screen for dysmenorrhea by history because many adolescents will not report it unless specifically asked. Primary dysmenorrhea is the most common type. It is not associated with pelvic pathology but may be accompanied by diarrhea, vomiting, headache, and generalized malaise in its moderate or severe forms. Secondary dysmenorrhea results from obstruction to menstrual flow or other pelvic pathology.

Primary Dysmenorrhea

The pathophysiology of primary dysmenorrhea is related to excessive secretion of prostaglandin $F_{2\alpha}$ and vasopressin by the endometrium. These hormones stimulate uterine contractions and increase resting myometrial tone, resulting in myometrial ischemia and pain. Primary dysmenorrhea occurs only with ovulatory cycles. The prevalence increases each year after menarche as regular ovulation becomes established, from 31% in the first year to 72% in the 5th year (Fig. 2).[23] Girls with primary dysmenorrhea will often have a history of other family members with menstrual pain. In addition, they may have loose bowel movements at the time of menses because prostaglandins also cause diarrhea. Nausea and/or vomiting are nonspecific symptoms that may occur with any moderate-to-severe pain and are not helpful in differentiating primary from secondary dysmenorrhea. A full pelvic examination may not be indicated in a virginal girl with mild and typical symptoms of primary dysmenorrhea, but examination of pelvic structures should be conducted for moderate or severe symptoms. Management of primary dysmenorrhea focuses on decreasing endometrial prostaglandin secretion with nonsteroidal antiinflammatory drugs (NSAIDs). This class of drugs inhibits the action of the enzyme prostaglandin synthetase. Oral administration of naproxen sodium (Anaprox DS), 550 mg every 12 hours; ibuprofen (Motrin), 400 mg every 6 hours; or mefenamic acid (Ponstel), 500 mg

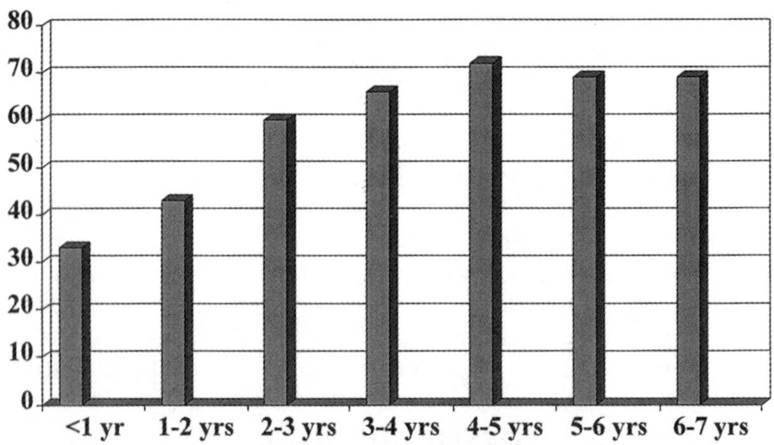

FIGURE 2. Prevalence of dysmenorrhea by gynecologic age (%). (Adapted from data supplied in Klein JR, Litt IF: Epidemiology of adolescent dysmenorrhea. Pediatrics 68:661–664, 1981, with permission.)

initially, followed by 250 mg every 6 hours for the first 2 or 3 days of the menses, usually is effective. Both ibuprofen and naproxen sodium are available in lower-dose, over-the-counter formulations. Because it only requires twice daily dosing and has a rapid onset of action, naproxen sodium may promote better compliance in adolescents. Oral contraceptive pills and depot medroxyprogesterone acetate contraceptive injection (DMPA) also are highly effective as treatments for primary dysmenorrhea because they produce endometrial hypoplasia with resultant reduction in prostaglandin synthesis and secretion.

Secondary Dysmenorrhea

Secondary dysmenorrhea should be considered when severe pain begins at menarche, suggesting outflow tract obstruction. Congenital anomalies such as bicornuate uterus with one obstructed horn will present as a pelvic mass and moderate to severe dysmenorrhea. Surgical intervention usually is required. Acute problems such as pelvic infection or complications of pregnancy may present as an isolated painful period. In such cases, a detailed sexual history and pelvic examination should be done with testing for sexually transmitted infections. Endometriosis should be suspected in girls who present with increasing chronic pelvic pain that may be both cyclic and acyclic and that fails to respond to NSAID or OCP therapy.[24] Laparoscopy with biopsy is necessary to make the diagnosis. Atypical lesions including opaque nodules, flame lesions, and clear vesicles are commonly seen in adolescents, whereas adult women are more likely to have typical blue-black endometriotic lesions. Management generally consists of a combination of surgical excision, cautery, or laser vaporization of the lesions and medical treatment with continuous OCP therapy or GnRH agonists such as leuprolide or nafarelin.[25] Because of the "menopausal" side effects of GnRHa treatment, particularly bone mineral loss, the length of treatment should be limited to no more than 6 months, and consideration should be given to estrogen "add-back" therapy.

CONCLUSION

Menstrual dysfunction in adolescent girls can be a diagnostic dilemma for the clinician and a distressing problem for the patient and her parents. In early adolescence, menstrual problems are likely to result from congenital anomalies of the reproductive organs, chromosomal abnormalities, or immaturity of the hypothalamic–pituitary–ovarian axis. In later adolescence, menstrual dysfunction more often occurs as a result of behavioral or psychosocial disorders and endocrinopathies, particularly anovulation associated with PCOS. A thorough history eliciting both physiologic and psychosocial data, including sexual behavior and eating and exercise habits, should be conducted in private. The history in combination with a careful physical examination, including genital inspection and pelvic examination, if indicated, and appropriate laboratory investigations reveal the diagnosis in the majority of cases. Apart from appropriate medications to manage menstrual dysfunction, many adolescent girls also require psychological counseling, nutritional advice, and meaningful information concerning their reproductive health.

REFERENCES

1. Winter JSD, Faiman C, Reyes FL: The gonadotropins of the fetus and neonate: Their ontogeny, function and regulation. In Flamigni D, Givens JR (eds): The Gonadotropins: Basic Science and Clinical Aspects in Females. New York, Academic Press, 1982, pp 157–165.
2. Kaplan SA, Grumbach MG: Physiology of puberty. In Flamigni D, Givens JR (eds): The Gonadotropins: Basic Science and Clinical Aspects in Females. New York, Academic Press, 1982, pp 167–176.
3. Frisch RE, Revelle R: The height and weight of girls and boys at the time of initiation of the adolescent growth spurt in height and weight, and the relationship to menarche. Human Biol 43:140–159, 1971.
4. Herman-Giddens ME, Slora EJ, Wasserman RC, et al: Secondary sexual characteristics and menses in young girls seen in office practice: A study from the pediatric research in office settings network. Pediatrics 99:505–512, 1997.
5. Migeon CJ: Delayed puberty in girls. In Flamigni C, Givens JR (eds): The Gonadotropins: Basic Science and Clinical Aspects in Females. New York, Academic Press, 1982, pp 3302–3325.
6. Coupey SM: Anorexia nervosa. In Friedman SB, Fisher M, Schonberg SK, Alderman EM (eds): Comprehensive Adolescent Health Care, 2nd ed. St. Louis, Mosby, 1998, pp 247–262.
7. Frisch RE, Wyshak G, Vincent L: Delayed menarche and amenorrhea in ballet dancers. N Engl J Med 303:17–19, 1980.
8. Bergh PA, Breen JL, Gregori CA: Congenital absence of the vagina—Mayer-Rokitansky-Küster-Hauser syndrome. Adolesc Pediatr Gynecol 2:73–85, 1989.
9. Layman LC: An update on the treatment of hypogonadism, part 1: Hypergonadotropic hypogonadism. Adolesc Pediatr Gynecol 7:83–193, 1994.
10. Berga SL, Mortola JF, Girton B, et al: Neuroendocrine aberrations in women with functional hypothalamic amenorrhea. J Clin Endocrinol Metab 68:301–308, 1989.
11. Betterle C, Rossi A, Dalla Pria S, et al: Premature ovarian failure: Autoimmunity and natural history. Clin Endocrinol 39:35, 1993.
12. Bullen B, Skrinar G, Breitins I, et al: Induction of menstrual disorders by strenuous exercise in untrained women. N Engl J Med 312:1349–1353, 1985.
13. Golden NH, Shenker IR: Amenorrhea in anorexia nervosa: Etiology and implications. Adolesc Med 3:503–517, 1992.
14. Apter D, Butzow T, Laughlin GA, Yen SSC: Accelerated 24-hour luteinizing hormone pulsatile activity in adolescent girls with ovarian hyperandrogenism: Relevance to the developmental phase of polycystic ovarian syndrome. J Clin Endocrinol Metab 79:119, 1994.
15. Yen SSC: Chronic anovulation due to CNS-hypothalamic pituitary dysfunction. In Yen SSC, Jaffe RB (eds): Endocrine Disorders in Reproductive Endocrinology. Philadelphia, W.B. Saunders, 1991.
16. Franks S: Polycystic ovary syndrome. N Engl J Med 333:853, 1995.
17. Ibanez L, Neusse P, Zampoli M, et al: Source localization of androgen excess in adolescent girls. J Clin Endocrinol Metab 79:178, 1994.
18. World Health Organization Task Force on Adolescent Reproductive Health: World Health Organization multicenter study on menstrual and ovulatory patterns in adolescent girls. J Adolesc Health 7:236–244, 1986.
19. Apter D, Vihko R: Early menarche, a risk factor for breast cancer, indicates early onset of ovulatory cycles. J Clin Endocrinol Metab 57:82–86, 1983.
20. Bayer SR, DeCherney AM: Clinical manifestations and treatment of dysfunctional uterine bleeding. JAMA 269:1823, 1993.
21. Goldfarb AF: Dysfunctional uterine bleeding. In Goldfarb AF (ed): Clinical Problems in Pediatric and Adolescent Gynecology. New York, Chapman and Hall, 1996, pp 61–68.
22. Iglesias EA, Coupey SM: Menstrual cycle abnormalities: Diagnosis and management. Adolesc Med 10:255–273, 1999.
23. Klein JR, Litt IF: Epidemiology of adolescent dysmenorrhea. Pediatrics 68:661–664, 1981.
24. Laufer MR, Goietein L, Bush M, et al: Prevalence of endometriosis in adolescent girls with chronic pelvic pain not responding to conventional therapy. J Pediatr Adolesc Gynecol 10:199–202, 1997.
25. Economy KE, Laufer MR: Pelvic pain. Adolesc Med 10:291–304, 1999.

CHAPTER 21

Disorders of the Vulva, Vagina, and Cervix

David Muram, M.D.

Physicians who care for adolescent girls are often faced with a variety of genital complaints, including vaginal discharge, vulvar pruritus, and lesions of the vulva that present in various combinations and cause distressing symptoms. Because it is difficult to separate disorders of the vulva from those of the vagina, they are discussed together in this chapter.

DIAGNOSTIC TECHNIQUES

The diagnosis of most external genital disorders can be made by history and physical examination, supplemented by simple office tests such as wet mounts, appropriate cultures, and biopsies. The physical examination may be aided by a magnifying device such as a colposcope.

Wet smear or wet mount is useful to evaluate vaginal discharge. The examiner places a drop from a mixture of saline and vaginal secretions on a glass slide and examines the preparation under the microscope using both low- and high-power magnifications. The discharge is evaluated for color, character, odor, and pH. Mixing of vaginal secretions with a 10% solution of potassium hydroxide (KOH) facilitates the identification of *Candida* sp. Liberation of a distinct fishy odor immediately after the addition of KOH is one of the diagnostic features of bacterial vaginosis. This odor is attributable to volatile amines in the vaginal fluid, presumably resulting from anaerobic bacterial metabolism. Specific tests are required to isolate specific pathogens, such as *Chlamydia trachomatis* or *Neisseria gonorrhoeae*.

When the patient does not respond to therapy, it may be necessary to discontinue all treatments, because the appearance of the genital lesions may have been altered by previous treatment regimens. The adolescent should be reevaluated several days later. An incorrect initial diagnosis also may be the cause of treatment failure, and a histologic examination may be required. Using local anesthetic, a full-thickness vulvar biopsy can be obtained with a Keyes dermal punch. Cervical biopsy instruments may be used to obtain vaginal or cervical samples.

VULVAR AND VAGINAL INFLAMMATION

Lactobacilli help to control the vaginal microflora and maintain its steady state. Lactic acid, produced during lactobacillus metabolism as well as by vaginal epithelial cells, provides a low vaginal pH in which lactobacilli continue to thrive. Changes in pH or glycogen status within the vaginal environment adversely affect lactobacilli, thereby permitting other organisms to predominate. Antibiotics, douches, alkaline secretions during menses, alkaline soaps, and poorly controlled diabetes mellitus are among the more common causes of changes in vaginal microflora.

Once the normal vaginal flora are replaced by a pathogen, the vaginal mucosa becomes irritated and inflamed. The inflammation process results in an increase in production of vaginal secretions and a change in odor or color of the discharge. Symptoms of pruritus and vulvar irritation are common, including burning, dyspareunia, vulvar dysuria, or ill-defined discomfort of the genitalia. Pelvic pain, abnormal uterine bleeding, and other signs of pelvic inflammatory disease may be evident if an ascending infection is present. Table 1 outlines the differential diagnosis of vaginal discharge.

Physiologic Discharge

Vaginal secretions may increase in early adolescence, causing a physiologic discharge (leukorrhea). It is clear or yellow-white in appearance, mucoid in texture, and nonirritating. Dried secretions may cause vulvar pruritus and stain the patient's underwear. Evaluation of the discharge by microscopy shows normal flora with the absence of leukocytes or pathogenic bacteria. The pH of the secretions is less than 4.5, and there is no foul odor. Good perineal hygiene should be encouraged, and the patient should be reassured that this is not a disease.

Cervical Ectopy

Ectopy represents the extension of the columnar epithelium of the endocervix onto the visible ectocervix. Ectopy is normally found during adolescence and gradually recedes as squamous metaplasia replaces the ectopic columnar epithelium. Oral contraceptive use is associated with the persistence or reappearance of ectopy. The cervical os may contain clear or slightly cloudy mucus. Ectopy may make the cervix more susceptible to infections with *N. gonorrhoeae, C. trachomatis,* or HIV by exposing a larger area of susceptible columnar epithelium. If cervicitis supervenes, the area of ectopy may become

TABLE 1. Common Causes of Vaginal Discharge

Physiologic	Inflammatory	Sexually Transmitted Infections
Hormonal changes	Foreign body	Gonorrhea
Cervical ectopy	Bacterial	Chlamydial infection
	Nonspecific vulvovaginitis	Salpingo-oophoritis
	Bacterial vaginosis	(pelvic inflammatory disease)
	Candidal infection	Condylomata acuminata
	Trichomonal infection	

edematous and fragile, with bleeding induced by gentle swabbing. Because cervical ectopy is normally present in young adolescent girls, they are more likely to develop sexually transmitted infections, if sexually active, than older adolescents and adult women.

Vaginal Adenosis

Vaginal adenosis is the presence of glandular epithelium resembling that of the endocervix and associated with transverse cervical and vaginal ridges. Such changes are encountered in about two-thirds of females exposed in utero to maternally administered diethylstilbestrol (DES) and related synthetic compounds. The risk of clear-cell carcinoma is estimated at 0.14–1.4 per 1000. Clear cell carcinoma has not been described in prepubescent girls or in those younger than 14 years of age. Thus, the American College of Obstetrians and Gynecologists recommends that a thorough gynecologic evaluation, including colposcopy, be performed on all DES-exposed females at menarche or by age 14, whichever comes first. Vaginal adenosis is often asymptomatic and requires no therapy. Treatment of clear-cell adenocarcinoma involves radical surgical excision because the lesion is invasive.

Nonspecific Vulvovaginitis

Adolescents may develop nonspecific vaginitis, often caused by *Escherichia coli*, beta hemolytic streptococci, or coagulase-positive staphylococci. Obese adolescents are more susceptible to these infections, usually because of poor perineal hygiene. The symptoms and signs of nonspecific vulvovaginitis are similar to those of other vaginal infections. Therapy, however, is directed toward the symptoms and the prevention of recurrences. A change to cotton underwear, use of loose-fitting clothing, removal of irritants, and improved perineal hygiene are often sufficient to alleviate the condition.

Foreign Bodies

Foreign bodies in the vagina induce an intense inflammatory reaction and result in a blood-stained, foul-smelling discharge. Usually the adolescent does not recall inserting the foreign object or will not admit to it. The most commonly found foreign bodies are tampons that were inserted during the last menstrual cycle. Upon insertion of the speculum, the tampon appears in the vagina as an amorphous gray mass, which can be easily removed with ring forceps.

Urethritis and the Urethral Syndrome

Dysuria occurs quite frequently in adolescents with urinary tract infections (UTIs), but this symptom often is attributed to vulvovaginitis, which in many settings is more common than UTI. Dysuria in the absence of pyuria is not associated with uropathogens or sexually transmitted pathogens, whereas pyuria is seen in patients infected with a sexually transmitted infection (STI): *C. trachomatis, N. gonorrhoeae*, and occasionally herpes simplex virus (HSV). The dysuria associated with vulvar disease or vulvovaginitis is often described as "external," because it is caused by painful contact of urine with the inflamed labia or introitus.

Among girls with acute dysuria and frequency, the first step in diagnosis is to exclude the possibility of a UTI. The next step is to differentiate cystitis from urethritis or vaginal infection. STI etiology is suggested by young age, more than one current sexual partner or a new partner within the past month, or coexisting mucopurulent cervicitis. Thus a pelvic exam should be done on all sexually active girls with dysuria. Bacterial cystitis is suggested by acute onset, hematuria, or suprapubic bladder tenderness. Urine cultures positive for a conventional urinary pathogen (e.g., *E. coli*) in a concentration of $> 10^2$/ml indicate probable bacterial UTI, whereas sterile pyuria suggests acute urethral syndrome due to *C. trachomatis* or *N. gonorrhoeae*, and appropriate cultures from the cervix and urethra are indicated. Treatment with doxycycline, 100 mg twice daily for 7 days, alleviates dysuria in women with sterile pyuria but not in women with UTI or without pyuria.

Bacterial Vaginosis

Bacterial vaginosis accounts for 40–50% of cases of vulvovaginitis. It occurs when the normal flora are replaced by *Gardnerella vaginalis, Mycoplasma hominis, Bacteroides* species, or *Mobiluncus* species. Some women are more susceptible because they lack the H_2O_2-producing strains of lactobacilli that usually inhibit the growth of the etiologic pathogens.

While many women remain asymptomatic, the common presenting symptom is an abnormal vaginal discharge. The discharge is typically thin, homogenous, and gray with a foul, "fishy" odor. The discharge usually is noted at the introitus and adherent to the vaginal walls. The mucosal surface often appears normal without signs of acute inflammation. The vaginal pH is greater than 4.5, and on mixture of the fluid with a 10% KOH solution a "fishy" odor may be noticed ("whiff" test). The positive whiff test is caused by the release of amines produced by the microorganisms. Microscopic evaluation of a saline wet mount shows stippled vaginal epithelial cells ("clue cells"). Clue cells are vaginal epithelial cells coated with coccobacillary organisms. They have a granular appearance and indistinct borders. Few, if any, leukocytes are noted. Routine cultures are not helpful, and the diagnosis of bacterial vaginosis is confirmed on the basis of clinical features and wet-mount observations. The demonstration of many clue cells by wet-mount microscopy and the documentation of characteristically altered vaginal flora by Gram stain are the most sensitive, specific, and objective criteria for the diagnosis of bacterial vaginosis in adolescents with characteristics symptoms and/or signs.

The treatment of bacterial vaginosis consists of a 7-day course of metronidazole, 500 mg, administered orally twice a day. A single 2-gram dose improves patient compliance, but the failure rate is higher. Clindamycin, either orally or intravaginally, is an alternative regimen. It is unclear whether an asymptomatic patient should be treated, although in light of the potential for an ascending infection, it may well be necessary to treat asymptomatic women. Sexual partners are not treated, unless infections recur.

Candidal Vulvovaginitis

Candidal vulvovaginitis is fairly common in adolescents, accounting for about 25% of vulvovaginitis among women. Risk factors include pregnancy, combination oral contraceptives, diabetes mellitus, use of broad-spectrum antibiotics, immunosuppressive states, luteal phase of the menstrual cycle, and increased body moisture associated with tight or restrictive clothing. *Candida albicans* accounts for 80–95% of all yeast isolated from the vagina. Other candidal species (e.g., *C. tropicalis* and *C. glabrata*) are becoming more prevalent as the causative agent in vulvovaginitis, particularly in patients who fail initial therapy.

The presenting complaint in candidal vulvovaginitis is usually severe vulvar pruritus. Secondary vulvar dysuria and dyspareunia also may be present. There may be a small amount of white or yellow, curd-like discharge without an odor. Examination reveals diffuse erythema and hyperemia of the vulva. Inflammation may extend to the perianal region or toward the inner thighs. Excoriations, desquamated areas, white plaques, and satellite lesions may be identified.

The diagnosis is made by the observation of fungal hyphae and buds on a wet-mount preparation. Leukocytes and epithelial cells are usually present. The pH is less than 4.5. Culture can be used if the diagnosis is in doubt.

Predisposing factors should be assessed and, if possible, corrected. Traditional therapy consists of any of the imidazoles given intravaginally. There is little difference in efficacy among miconazole, clotrimazole, tioconazole, butoconazole, and terconazole vaginal formulations. Cutaneous candidiasis of macerated areas responds to measures that reduce moisture and chafing plus a topically applied antifungal agent in a nonocclusive base. Systemic treatment of candidal vulvovaginitis with ketoconazole or fluconazole is more convenient than topical treatment, but the potential for adverse effects is higher. In adolescent females, the shorter-course therapy promotes patient compliance. Treatment of the male partner is not recommended. In patients with frequent recurrences, prophylactic postmenstrual therapy with intravaginal clotrimazole (500 mg each month) or suppressive therapy with low-dose oral ketoconazole (100 mg daily for 6 months) may be beneficial.

Trichomonal Infection

Trichomonas vaginalis, a motile protozoan, accounts for 15–20% of cases of vulvovaginitis. The organism often is transmitted through sexual contact. The presenting complaints are usually vaginal discharge, dysuria, and vulvar pruritus. The discharge ranges from scant to profuse, usually is malodorous, and may be yellow, green, or gray. The trichomonads produce carbon dioxide, which causes the discharge to appear frothy. On examination, vulvar and vaginal erythema are common. Punctate hemorrhages of the vagina and cervix ("strawberry cervix") are visibly noted in about 20% of cases. Such cervical involvement may result in postcoital bleeding, which may alter the color of the discharge.

The diagnosis is made by the microscopic examination of the wet-mount preparation, when motile, flagellated, tear-shaped organisms are seen. Vaginal pH in patients with trichomoniasis is generally greater than 5.0. Cultures are highly sensitive but rarely required to confirm the diagnosis.

Treatment consists of a combination of local vulvar care and antibiotic therapy. Metronidazole (Flagyl) remains the drug of choice. A one-time dose of 2 gm has a comparable cure rate to a 7-day treatment (90%). Vaginal treatment with 0.75% metronidazole gel is not highly effective for vaginal trichomoniasis. Metronidazole is not recommended during the first trimester of pregnancy. Alcohol must be avoided for 24 hours after its use because of occasional disulfiram-like effects. Sexual partners should be treated simultaneously with the single-dose regimen. Other nitroimidazoles, such as tinidazole and ornidazole, have longer half-lives than metronidazole but have not been shown to give better results in trichomoniasis. Metronidazole-resistant strains may require treatment with a higher dose for a longer period. The habitual use of condoms and postcoital douching with an acid preparation solution may be used in selected patients as preventive therapy.

SEXUALLY TRANSMITTED INFECTIONS

Sexually transmitted infections (STIs) take on significant importance because of the high rates of infections during adolescence and because many STIs have the greatest impact on future health. Many teenagers infected with an STI are asymptomatic, do not recognize symptoms when present, or fail to associate the symptoms with a disease. Sexually active adolescents have a particularly high rate of upper genital tract infections (pelvic inflammatory disease [PID]) but appear to have less PID-associated tubal damage and infertility than older women. With repeated infections, however, the infertility rate increases approximately 3-fold for each infection.

Chlamydial Infections

Chlamydia sp. is the most prevalent sexually transmitted infection in the United States. Among adolescents, chlamydial infections are diagnosed more commonly than gonorrhea. The causative organism is *Chlamydia trachomatis*, an obligate intracellular parasite. As many as 75% of women with uncomplicated chlamydial infection have no symptoms or signs of infection. The organism infects the endocervix most commonly, but most infections fail to demonstrate sufficient inflammation to cause clinical signs. When present, the most common clinical signs are a yellow or green mucopurulent endocervical discharge and hypertrophic ectropion (an area of cervical ectopy that is edematous, congested, and bleeds easily upon manipulation).

The urethra is also a common site for *C. trachomatis* infection. Infected women present with symptoms of dysuria and frequency, but urine cultures for other common urinary tract pathogens are negative. *Chlamydia* sp. can be isolated in as many as 65% of such patients. *C. trachomatis* may ascend from the endocervix into the upper genital tract, leading to asymptomatic and symptomatic PID.

In most circumstances, the diagnosis is based solely on clinical grounds and the presence of reported risk factors. Risk indicators include: young age, nonwhite race, single marital status, use of oral contraceptives, suspicion of PID, and male sex partners with urethritis. Screening should be expanded to include sexually active young women with a new sex partner within the past 2 months and more than 2 partners in the preceding 2 months.

Chlamydial culture remains the gold standard for clinical purposes, but it is expensive and technically difficult. The yield of chlamydial cultures is adversely affected by specimen collection techniques, sites of sampling, the numbers of sites sampled, and specimen transport and storage conditions. Antigen detection methods, such as direct fluorescent antibody staining and enzyme-linked immunosorbent assays, have offered appealing alternatives to the use of bacteriologic cultures. These tests are less expensive, more rapid, and can be used in any physician's office. The highest sensitivity and specificity are found in patients from high-prevalence settings (e.g., STD clinics). The use of nonculture tests in low-risk populations may not be appropriate when the prevalence of *C. trachomatis* is less than 10%. In recent years, nucleic acid probes have gained popularity and are now used to detect chlamydia in urethral and cervical specimens.

Doxycycline, 100 mg orally twice daily for 7 days, is currently the drug of choice because of improved patient compliance and an excellent pharmacokinetic profile. No clinically significant evidence of resistance has been noted. Alternatively, single-dose oral azithromycin (1 gm orally) is recommended. Although associated with better compliance than a 7-day regimen, single-dose azithromycin is more expensive. Therapy of chlamydial infection during pregnancy consists of erythromycin base or equivalent, 500 mg orally 4 times daily for 7 days, or single-dose azythromycin.

Gonorrhea

Gonorrhea is an infection of the mucous membrane of the urethra and genital tract caused by *N. gonorrhoeae,* a gram-negative diplococcus. The incubation period for *N. gonorrhoeae* is roughly 1 week, with symptoms generally appearing 2–7 days after exposure. Acute uncomplicated gonorrhea in females often causes dysuria, increased vaginal discharge, abnormal menstrual bleeding due to endometritis, and anorectal discomfort. Compression of the urethra through the anterior vaginal wall against the symphysis pubis may express urethral exudate, which can be examined by Gram stain and culture. The inflammation may extend to the vestibular glands, Skene's glands, and Bartholin's glands. Acute inflammation of Bartholin's gland is usually unilateral. The acutely infected duct is surrounded by a red halo and exudes pus at the posterior third of the labium majus. Occlusion of the duct results in formation of a Bartholin's abscess. Rectal infection, assumed to occur by local spread of infected cervical secretions, is relatively common in patients with urogenital infections and often asymptomatic, although it may present as irritation or tenesmus.

Infection extends to the fallopian tubes in at least 15% of women with gonorrhea. This extension tends to occur soon after acquisition of infection or during menstruation and results in acute endometritis with abnormal menstrual bleeding and midline low abdominal pain and tenderness, followed by acute salpingitis (see PID).

A presumptive diagnosis of gonorrhea may be made when the typical, gram-negative intracellular diplococci are seen on a Gram-stained smear of urethral or endocervical exudate. Selective media (i.e., Thayer-Martin medium) are most useful for recovering the organism. After inoculation, the medium should be placed in a chamber with 70% humidity and an atmosphere containing 3–10% carbon dioxide to permit growth of the gonococci. In recent years, nucleic acid probes have gained popularity and are now used to detect gonococci in urethral and cervical specimens.

Because of the widespread and steadily increasing resistance to penicillin, the 1993 STD Treatment Guidelines from the Centers for Disease Control and Prevention (CDC) recommend the use of penicillinase-resistant regimens (e.g., ceftriaxone, 125 mg intramuscularly, combined with doxycycline, 100 mg orally 2 times/day for 7 days). For patients who cannot take ceftriaxone, the preferred alternative is single-dose spectinomycin, 2 gm intramuscularly. Patients who receive therapies that are not effective against penicillin-resistant *N. gonorrhoeae* must have a test-of-cure performed. Treatment of asymptomatic carriers and sexual partners is cost-effective in communities with high prevalence of asymptomatic infections. Concurrent treatment with doxycycline or azythromycin for coexistent chlamydia is recommended.

Disseminated Gonococcal Infection

Disseminated gonococcal infections (DGI) occur in 0.5–3% of patients with untreated urogenital gonorrhea. Patients typically present either with symptoms and signs of gonococcemia or with purulent arthritis affecting one or two joints. Typical clinical manifestations, in addition to malaise and fever, include skin lesions, arthralgia, and tenosynovitis. The typical skin lesion of DGI consists of a necrotic pustule on an erythematous base. The arthritis is a migrating polyarthritis involving the wrist, metacarpal, ankle, and knee. The onset of symptoms follows the menstrual period in approximately 50% of patients. Other common manifestations of DGI include mild myopericarditis and toxic hepatitis. Endocarditis and meningitis are infrequent but severe complications.

The definitive diagnosis of DGI is based on the isolation of gonococci from the blood, skin lesions, synovial fluid, or cerebrospinal fluid. In some patients, the diagnosis is based on the typical clinical manifestations and the concurrent isolation of *N. gonorrhoeae* from the lower genital tract or rectum or, at times, from a sexual partner. The recommended treatment of patients with systemic infections (DGI, meningitis, endocarditis) is high-dose, intravenous ceftriaxone or an equivalent beta lactamase–resistant antibiotic.

Pelvic Inflammatory Disease

PID usually refers to infection ascending from the endocervix to the endometrium and/or fallopian tubes. Intrauterine infection may be primary (spontaneously occurring and usually sexually transmitted) or secondary (following invasive intrauterine surgical procedures or parturition). In adolescent girls, PID is almost always a consequence of an STI. Recognized risk factors for the development of PID are summarized in Table 2. The most common aerobic

TABLE 2. Risk Factors Associated with the Development of Pelvic Inflammatory Disease

Demographic and Social Indicators	Sexually Transmitted Infections	Uterine Instrumentation	Other
Young age Low socioeconomic status Single marital status	Inactivation of mucosal immune mechanisms, e.g., secretory IgA by *Neisseria gonorrhoeae* proteases	Insertion of an intrauterine contraceptive device Dilatation and curettage Termination of pregnancy Hysterosalpingography	Douching Menstruation

organisms include *E. coli, Haemophilus influenzae*, group B streptoccoci, and *G. vaginalis*. The most frequently recovered anaerobic bacteria include *Bacteroides, Peptostreptococcus*, and *Peptococcus* species. *N. gonorrhoeae* and *C. trachomatis* may be recovered from up to 80% of patients with acute PID.

The clinical presentation of PID varies from no symptoms to severe peritonitis. Abdominal pain (less than 10 days' duration) is the most common symptom encountered in patients with PID. Other historical indicators of variable significance include recent onset of menses, increased dysmenorrhea with the last period, irregular menses (menorrhagia), recent onset of pelvic dyspareunia, and symptoms of proctitis. Gastrointestinal symptoms, such as nausea and vomiting, diarrhea, and anorexia, also may occur. Up to 15% of patients with PID present with perihepatitis (Fitz-Hugh-Curtis syndrome) as part of the clinical picture.

The clinical diagnosis of PID is imprecise. Clinical signs that have the strongest degree of correlation with laparoscopically proven PID include abnormal vaginal discharge, temperature above 38°C, and a palpable adnexal mass. The abdominal pain usually is described as dull or aching. In some cases, pain is lacking or atypical. Abnormal uterine bleeding precedes or coincides with the onset of pain in about 40% of women with PID, symptoms of urethritis occur in 20%, and symptoms of proctitis occasionally are seen in women with gonococcal or chlamydial infection.

Speculum examination shows evidence of mucopurulent cervicitis in most women with gonococcal or chlamydial PID. Cervical motion tenderness is produced by stretching of the adnexal attachments on the side toward which the cervix is pushed. Bimanual examination reveals a uterine fundal tenderness due to endometritis and abnormal adnexal tenderness due to salpingitis, which usually, but not necessarily, is bilateral. Adnexal swelling is palpable in about one-half of women with acute salpingitis, but evaluation of the adnexae in a patient with marked tenderness is not reliable, even by an experienced examiner. An initial temperature > 38°C is found in only about one-third of patients with acute salpingitis, and fever is not required for the diagnosis.

Laboratory findings include elevation of the erythrocyte sedimentation rate (ESR) in 75% and elevation of the peripheral white blood cell count in up to 60% of patients with acute salpingitis. Microscopic examination of a saline wet-mount preparation of vaginal fluid shows predominance of polymorphonuclear leukocytes.

The diagnosis of acute PID is based primarily on the history of abdominal pain, the presence of tenderness to motion of the cervix and adnexae on bi-

TABLE 3. Criteria Useful for Diagnosing Pelvic Inflammatory Disease

Routine	Elaborate
Oral temperature > 38.3°C	Histopathologic evidence on endometrial biopsy
Abnormal cervical or vaginal discharge	Tuboovarian abscess on sonography
Elevated erythrocyte sedimentation rate and/or C-reactive protein	Laparoscopy
Culture or nonculture evidence of cervical infection with *Neisseria gonorrhoeae* or *Chlamydia trachomatis*	

manual examination, and signs of a lower genital tract infection. PID is present in 60% of patients presenting with these symptoms and signs. Table 3 lists additional criteria useful for the diagnosis of PID. The lack of substantial clinical signs mandates a high index of suspicion for clinicians evaluating adolescent girls and young women at risk for PID.

Early diagnosis and initiation of therapy are essential to minimize tubal scarring. Appropriate treatment must not be withheld from patients who have an equivocal diagnosis. Because delay in therapy may lead to progression of tubal scarring, it is better to err on the side of overdiagnosis and overtreatment. On the other hand, it is essential to differentiate between salpingitis and other pelvic pathology, particularly surgical emergencies such as appendicitis and ectopic pregnancy. An appropriate plan of management requires a thorough assessment of the severity of infection. All patients should have cervical cultures for *N. gonorrhoeae* and cultures or nonculture tests for *C. trachomatis*. Hospitalization should be used liberally (Table 4), especially for adolescents, although no objective evidence indicates that parenteral antimicrobial therapy results in better long-term outcomes. As bacteriologic data suggest a mixed infection in many patients, administration of broad-spectrum antibiotics is required, along with adequate support with intravenous fluids and analgesia. Many different treatment regimens have been evaluated and have proved to be highly effective in achieving clinical cure. Although no single regimen has been shown to be clearly superior, two basic regimens have been recommended by the CDC to provide broad-spectrum coverage for the pathogens most likely to be encountered (see Table 7, chapter 19). Patients managed on an outpatient basis require close follow-up (within 72 hours) to monitor response to therapy. Those not responding favorably should be hospitalized. The return visit also should be used to emphasize the need to avoid sexual intercourse and to refer sex partners for evaluation and treatment.

TABLE 4. Indications for Hospitalization of Patients with Pelvic Inflammatory Disease

Uncertain diagnosis
Exclusion of surgical emergency (e.g., appendicitis, ectopic pregnancy)
Suspicion of pelvic abscess
Pregnancy
Adolescent patients (unpredictable compliance)
Severe illness (precludes outpatient treatment)
Inability to tolerate outpatient regimen
Failure to respond to outpatient treatment
Inability to arrange clinical follow-up within 72 hr of starting antibiotics

Ulcerative Lesions of the Genitalia

The differential diagnosis of genital ulcers usually includes genital herpes, syphilis, and chancroid. Genital herpes is the most common cause of genital ulcers in the industrialized western countries, and syphilis is the second most common form of genital ulcer in almost all areas of the world. Lymphogranuloma venereum (LGV) and granuloma inguinale are rare in North America and Europe.

In a few cases, clinical findings include the typical herpetic vesicles and guide initial therapy, pending the results of further studies. Nevertheless, most genital ulcerations cannot be diagnosed confidently on clinical grounds. It is necessary to exclude syphilis by appropriate serologic studies in all cases. All lesions except those highly characteristic of infection with HSV should be subjected to dark-field examination or a direct immunofluorescence test for *Treponema pallidum*. An attempt should be made to isolate *Haemophilus ducreyi* if the genital ulcer is painful and inguinal lymphadenopathy is prominent. Enlarged, fluctuant lymph nodes should be aspirated for culture and Gram stain to detect *H. ducreyi* and pyogenic bacteria.

Ideally, treatment for genital ulceration should be withheld until the diagnosis is secure. However, immediate symptomatic treatment for acute genital ulcerations is sometimes necessary. Initial treatment in such cases generally includes 2.4 million units of benzathine penicillin G for possible primary syphilis. Prompt systemic therapy with acyclovir is indicated for patients with initial episodes of genital or anorectal herpes. When genital ulcers persist, a biopsy is indicated to exclude carcinoma and other nonvenereal dermatoses. All genital ulcers enhance the efficacy of sexual transmission and acquisition of HIV. Moreover, genital ulcers are most prevalent in inner-city populations with low socioeconomic status and high rates of prostitution and illicit drug use—independent risk factors for HIV infection. Therefore, a test for HIV infection should be considered for any adolescent girl with genital ulcerative lesions.

Genital Herpes Simplex

Herpes simplex virus (HSV) is a member of the herpesvirus family, which includes Epstein-Barr, cytomegalovirus, and varicella-zoster viruses. HSV has a predilection for cutaneous and mucous membrane sensory ganglia and persists in this neural tissue in a dormant state. The risk of recurrence after the first episode of genital herpes is more than 80% with HSV-2 infection and approximates 50% with HSV-1. Primary infection is associated with significant vulvar pain, dysuria, and, at times, urinary retention. Tender inguinal lymphadenopathy is typically present. Systemic symptoms are common, and patients may complain of fever, headaches, malaise, and myalgia. Severe complications (e.g., meningitis) may be encountered. Early in the course of the disease, the infected area shows vesicular lesions with associated inflammation and edema. With time, the vesicles break, forming ulcerative lesions with an erythematous base, often covered with a purulent exudate. The ulcers may coalesce and form a larger ulcer with a covering crust. Complete healing of the lesions usually occurs within 2 weeks, although it may take as long as 4–6 weeks.

Recurrent episodes are typically less painful with minimal systemic signs, a smaller mean number of lesions, and shorter mean duration of viral shedding.

Viral culture of the lesions is the most sensitive and specific method of diagnosis of mucocutaneous HSV. Vesicles and pustular lesions have the highest viral isolation rates; up to 90% produce positive cultures. Cytologic examination of lesional fluid is much less sensitive and provides less definitive information about viral types. Serologic testing is not useful for the diagnosis of HSV because commercially available tests do not differentiate reliably between type-specific and type-common antigens. With the exception of documentation of seroconversion in primary genital herpes infection or screening for evidence of past HSV infection, serologic testing should not be performed.

Antiviral therapy with oral or parenteral acyclovir is currently recommended in primary genital herpes infections. Acyclovir has been shown to accelerate healing of genital lesions, decrease the duration of viral shedding, and limit local and systemic symptoms. Treatment should be initiated as soon as the diagnosis is suspected, because benefits usually outweigh risks while waiting for culture results and the toxicity of acyclovir is quite low, especially with oral therapy. The recommended therapy for the first episode of genital herpes is oral acyclovir, 200 mg 5 times daily for 10 days.

Local adjunctive measures of the vulvovaginal lesions are important. Sitz baths with tepid water and Burrow's solution are soothing to the inflamed perineum. Pat drying or blow drying with a hair dryer on a low setting is followed by topical lidocaine gel or ointment. Patients can be encouraged to void in the sitz bath or tub to limit urine contamination of the lesions. Occasionally catheterization is needed if urinary retention is present or appears likely.

With recurrent genital HSV, initiation of oral therapy at the first sign of prodrome or lesions is only moderately effective in reducing the number of symptomatic days. Episodic therapy should be reserved for patients with infrequent but severe or prolonged recurrences. Patients with frequent recurrences generally benefit from prolonged suppressive therapy, regardless of severity.

Syphilis

Syphilis is caused by *T. pallidum*, which enters the body through invisible breaks in the skin or through intact mucous membranes lining the mouth, rectum, or genital tract. Approximately one-third of people exposed to a sex partner with syphilis will acquire the disease. The clinical features of untreated syphilis are divided into a series of clinical stages that are used as indicators of the length of infection and as a guide for therapy.

Primary Syphilis

Approximately 3 weeks after inoculation, the patient develops a macule or papule at the site of entry, usually around the genitalia. The ulcer is a painless, usually solitary lesion with raised, well-defined borders and a clean, indurated base. The chancre contains large numbers of spirochetes and is highly contagious. It is usually associated with nontender regional adenopathy, which may be unilateral or bilateral. Even without treatment, the chancre slowly heals in several weeks; the spirochetes, however, spread throughout the body.

Secondary Syphilis

Between 4 and 10 weeks after the appearance of the chancre, secondary syphilis occurs. The most prominent feature is a painless, nonpruritic, maculopapular rash that typically affects the limbs, including the palms and soles, and trunk. Systemic complaints consist of low-grade fever, myalgia, arthralgia, and adenopathy. Lesions referred to as mucous patches may form in the mouth and around the vagina and anus. Other highly contagious anogenital lesions are called condyloma lata, which can be described as broad-based, flat, beefy lesions of a pearly gray color. These lesions eventually resolve, and the disease enters its latent phase.

Latent Syphilis

During the latency period, serologic tests for syphilis are reactive, but there are no clinical signs of the disease. Latent syphilis of less than 1 year's duration is considered early latent, whereas latent syphilis of more than 1 year's duration is late latent. Differentiation of these two phases is designed to reflect differences in infectivity and to serve as a guide for therapy. Most adolescent girls diagnosed with latent syphilis on positive serologic testing will be in the early latent phase.

Tertiary Syphilis

Gummata, the chronic inflammatory lesions of tertiary syphilis, affect primarily the skin, subcutaneous tissues, and bone. This stage is virtually never seen in the adolescent age group. Central nervous system (CNS) involvement occurs at all stages of syphilis. Asymptomatic CNS disease, confirmed by cerebrospinal fluid cell and serologic abnormalities, may be present in some people.

The diagnosis of syphilis is based on the characteristic clinical features in conjunction with the appropriate serologic tests. During the primary and secondary states, *T. pallidum* can be observed on darkfield examination of chancres, condylomata lata, and mucous patches. Reactive nonspecific serologic tests, the rapid plasma reagin (RPR) or Venereal Disease Research Laboratory (VDRL), must be confirmed with specific antibody tests to *T. pallidum*. The commonly used specific tests include the fluorescent treponemal antibody–absorbed test (FTA–ABS), the microhemagglutination–*T. pallidum* test (MHA–TP), or the hemagglutination treponemal test for syphilis (HATTS). Patients with suspected central nervous system involvement may require an evaluation of the cerebrospinal fluid.

Penicillin remains the cornerstone of therapy for syphilis. The drug has remained effective because of the persistent sensitivity of *T. pallidum* to penicillin. The benzathine formulation readily achieves the sustained, moderately low serum levels required to eradicate the spirochete, which has a long division time. Treatment regimens are based on the stage of the disease at diagnosis. Benzathine penicillin, 2.4 million units intramuscularly in 2 separate injections, is the recommended treatment for patients with primary, secondary, and early latent disease. For patients who are allergic to penicillin, doxycycline, 100 mg orally twice daily for 14 days, is recommended. Patients with late latent syphilis, syphilis of unknown duration, or tertiary syphilis other than neurosyphilis should receive a longer course of therapy. Benzathine penicillin, 7.2 million units, administered in doses of 2.4 million units at weekly intervals for 3 weeks, is recommended. Patients who are allergic to penicillin should be treated with doxycycline for 4 weeks. Patients with neurosyphilis should be given aqueous crystalline penicillin G, 12–24 million units/day intravenously (2–4 million units intravenously every 4 hours) for 10–14 days, or procaine penicillin G, 2.4 million units/day intramuscularly, given with probenecid, 500 mg orally 4 times daily for the same period.

Pregnant patients with syphilis should be treated with penicillin at the dose appropriate for the stage of disease. Because tetracyclines are contraindicated in pregnancy and because of unacceptably high failure rates to prevent congenital syphilis when alternative drugs (erythromycin) are used, pregnant women who are allergic to penicillin should undergo skin testing and desensitization in order to receive penicillin.

Patients should be cautioned about Jarisch-Herxheimer reactions after treatment for early syphilis. These self-limited manifestations, which include myalgias, chills, headache, and postural hypotension, can be controlled with hydration and aspirin. Pregnant patients may experience preterm labor or fetal distress and should be treated in consultation with an obstetrician.

To assess response to treatment, follow-up serologic testing should be performed at 3, 6, and 12 months after treatment. At least a four-fold (two dilution) decline in titer is generally regarded as an appropriate response. Sexual partners of patients with early syphilis should be assumed to have incubating syphilis and should be treated as patients with early disease. All infected persons and their sexual contacts should be encouraged to undergo HIV counseling and testing.

Human Papillomavirus (HPV) Infections

Human papillomavirus (HPV) infections are discussed in detail in chapter 22. Briefly, genital warts are usually multifocal, and frequently involve large areas of the genital tract. The most common sites in females are the posterior fourchette, adjacent labia and perineum, and vaginal introitus, vagina, and cervix. Condyloma acuminatum is the most widely recognized manifestation of anogenital HPV infection. Inspection with the unaided eye may discern the typical cauliflower-like projections and, occasionally, the flat papular lesions. Application of 5% acetic acid for 5 minutes may augment the identification of flat lesions that are not readily apparent. Cytology and histology may be used in selected cases to confirm the diagnosis.

VULVAR DYSTROPHY

Vulvar pruritus may be caused by any of several vulvar or perineal dermatologic disorders. These conditions are often not limited to the vulva but affect other body areas as well. Lichen sclerosus of the vulva is a hypotrophic dystrophy. Although it is seen mainly in postmenopausal women, it occasionally affects children and adolescents. The symptoms consist of vulvar irritation, dysuria, and pruritus. Examination of the vulva shows flat, ivory-colored papules that may coalesce into plaques and in extreme cases may involve the entire vulvar skin. The lesions do not extend laterally beyond the middle of the labia majora, nor do they encroach into the vagina. The clitoris, posterior fourchette, and anorectal area are frequently affected. Affected areas are predominantly white, but some have pronounced vascular markings. The lesions tend to bruise easily, forming bloody blisters that are susceptible to secondary infections. In most patients the diagnosis can be established on the basis of clinical features. Pathologic confirmation is necessary in atypical cases. Histologically, the skin shows flattening of the rete pegs, hyalinization of the subdermal tissues, and keratinization. In young women hypotrophic lichen sclerosus has no malignant potential. Treatment consists of improved local hygiene, reduction of trauma, and short-term use of hydrocortisone creams to alleviate the pruritus. Treatment may be repeated when exacerbations occur.

GENITAL TRAUMA

Because the perineum and vulva are extremely vascular and the subcutaneous tissues are loosely arranged, an injury may cause rupture of blood vessels underneath the perineal skin. Blood accumulates under the skin and forms a hematoma, producing a rounded, tense, and tender swelling, the size of which depends on the amount of bleeding. A contusion of the vulva usually does not require treatment. A small vulvar hematoma can be controlled by pressure. A large hematoma or one that continues to increase in size should be incised, with removal of clotted blood removed and ligation of bleeding points. If the source of the bleeding cannot be found, the cavity should be packed with gauze and a pressure dressing applied. The pack is removed in 24 hours. Prophylactic broad-spectrum antibiotics may be advisable. The vulva should be kept clean and dry. When the urethra is obstructed by the hematoma, it is necessary to insert a suprapubic catheter. Pelvic radiographs may be necessary in some patients to rule out a fracture of the pelvis. Postcoital tears of the vagina are occasionally seen in adolescents. They represent surgical emergencies, and suturing under general anesthesia is required to stop the often massive bleeding.

NEOPLASMS OF THE VULVA AND VAGINA

Although uncommon, genital tumors must be considered whenever an adolescent is found to have a chronic genital ulcer, a nontraumatic swelling of the external genitalia, tissue protruding from the vagina, foul-smelling bloody discharge, abdominal pain or enlargement, virilization, or premature sexual maturation. Despite their rarity, virtually every type of genital neoplasm reported in adults also has been found in young girls, and about one-half of these tumors are malignant.

Most benign tumors of the vagina in children are unilocular cystic remnants of the mesonephric duct. Other benign neoplasms include teratomas, hemangiomas, simple cysts of the hymen, retention cysts of the paraurethral ducts, benign granulomas of the perineum, and condylomata acuminata. Small, asymptomatic cysts of the mesonephric (Gartner's) duct do not require surgery. Large cysts may interfere with urination or vaginal drainage and must be treated surgically. The cyst is opened, most of the accessible cyst wall is removed, and the edges are marsupilized to prevent reaccumulation of fluid.

Obstruction of a paraurethral duct may form a relatively large cyst, distorting the urethral orifice. Marsupialization or excision is the recommended treatment. Teratomas usually present as cystic masses arising from the midline of the perineum. Although a teratoma in this area may be benign, local recurrence may be a problem. Therefore, a generous margin of healthy tissue should be excised about the periphery. Capillary hemangiomas usually disappear as the child grows older and require no therapy. In contrast, cavernous hemangiomas are composed of vessels of considerable size, and injury to them may cause serious hemorrhage. For this reason, cavernous hemangiomas are best treated surgically.

Embryonal carcinoma of the vagina (botryoid sarcoma) is seen commonly in girls < 3 years old. In older girls, the neoplasm often affects the upper vagina or cervix. It arises in the submucosal tissues and spreads rapidly beneath an intact vaginal epithelium. The diagnosis is confirmed by histologic examination of a biopsy specimen.

Combination chemotherapy regimens—often vincristine, actinomycin-D, and cyclophosphamide—have been used in recent years with success. After the course of chemotherapy, the tumor is reexamined and biopsied. If viable tumor is present, limited surgical excision is indicated. Otherwise, additional courses of chemotherapy and radiotherapy are used for further reduction of tumor mass. Such therapy is continued until no viable tumor remains or local excision is feasible.

CONCLUSION

Vulvar and vaginal pathology is frequently encountered in adolescent girls and young women. A thorough menstrual, sexual, and gynecologic history as well as a genital and, if necessary, pelvic examination often establish the diagnosis. Simple office tests such as wet mount, cultures, and tests for STIs may be all that is necessary for confirmation. More extensive surgical diagnosis and treatment should be managed by an expert in pediatric and adolescent gynecology.

SUGGESTED READING

1. ACOG Technical Bulletin: Vaginitis. Committee on Technical Bulletins of the American College of Obstetricians and Gynecologists. Int J Gynaecol Obstet 54:293–302, 1996.
2. Batteiger BE, Jones RB: Chlamydia infections. Infect Dis Clin North Am 1:55–81, 1987.
3. Bump RC, Sachs LA, Bueshing WJ: Sexually transmitted infectious agents in sexually active and virginal asymptomatic adolescent girls. Pediatrics 77:488, 1986.
4. Cates W: Teenagers and sexual risk taking: The best of times and the worst of times. J Adolesc Health 12:84–94, 1991.
5. Chacko MR, Kozinetz CA, Hill R, et al: Leukocyte esterase dipstick as a rapid screening test for vaginitis and cervicitis. J Pediatr Adolesc Gynecol 9:185–189, 1996.
6. Centers for Disease Control and Prevention: 1993 sexually transmitted diseases treatment guidelines. MMWR 42:1–102, 1993.
7. Centers for Disease Control and Prevention: Policy guidelines for the prevention and management of pelvic inflammatory disease. MMWR 5:1, 1992.
8. Centers for Disease Control and Prevention: Pelvic inflammatory disease: Guidelines for prevention and management. MMWR 40:1–25, 1991.
9. Centers for Disease Control and Prevention: Primary and secondary syphilis—United States, 1981–1990. MMWR 40:314–315, 322–323, 1991.

10. Centers for Disease Control and Prevention: Premarital experience among adolescent women—United States, 1970–1988. MMWR 39:929–932, 1991.
11. Eschenbach DA: Vaginitis including bacterial vaginosis. Curr Opin Obstet Gynecol 6:389–391, 1994.
12. Hillier SL, kiviat NB, Hawes SE, et al: Role of bacterial vaginosis associated microorganisms in endometritis. Am J Obstet Gynecol 175:435–441, 1996.
13. Hutchins CM, Hook EW: Syphilis in adults. Med Clin North Am 74:1389–1416, 1990.
14. Joesoef MR, Schmid GP: Bacterial vaginosis: Review of treatment options and potential clinical indications for therapy. Clin Infect Dis 1(Suppl 20):S72–S79, 1995.
15. Judson FN: Gonorrhea. Med Clin North Am 74:1353–1366, 1990.
16. MacDermott RI: Bacterial vaginosis. Br J Obstet Gynaecol 102:92–94, 1995.
17. Martin DH: Chlamydial infections. Med Clin North Am 74:1367–1387, 1990.
18. McCormack WM Jr, Zinner SH, McCormack WM: The incidence of genitourinary infections in a cohort of healthy women. Sex Transm Dis 21:63–64, 1994.
19. Mertz GJ: Genital herpes simplex virus infections. Med Clin North Am 74:1433–1454, 1990.
20. O'Dowd TC, West RR, Winterburn PJ, Hewlins MJ: Evaluation of a rapid diagnostic test for bacterial vaginosis. Br J Obstet Gynaecol 103:366–370, 1996.
21. Platz Christensen JJ, Larsson PG, Sundstrom E, Wiqvist N: Detection of bacterial vaginosis in wet mount, Papanicolaou stained vaginal smears and in gram stained smears. Acta Obstet Gynecol Scand 74:67–70, 1995.
22. Priestley CJ, Kinghom GR: Bacterial vaginosis. Br J Clin Pract 50:331–334, 1996.
23. Rau FJ, Jones CE, Muram D: Vulvovaginitis in adolescents. In Sanfilippo J, Muram D, Lee P, Dewhurst JC (eds): Pediatric and Adolescent Gynecology. Philadelphia, W.B. Saunders, 1994, pp 187–201.
24. Redondo-Lopez V, Cook RL, Sobel JD: Emerging role of lactobacilli in the control and maintenance of the vaginal bacterial microflora. Rev Infect Dis 2:856–872, 1990.
25. Reife CM: Office gynecology for the primary care physician, Part I: Vaginitis, the Papanicolaou smear, contraception, and postmenopausal estrogen replacement. Med Clin North Am 80:299–319, 1996.
26. Schacter J: Biology of *Chlamydia trachomatis*. In Holmes KK, et al (eds): Sexually Transmitted Diseases, 2nd ed. New York, McGraw-Hill, 1990, pp 167–180.
27. Schmid G: Approach to the patient with genital ulcer disease. Med Clin North Am 74:1556–1572, 1990.
28. Sobel JD: Vaginal infections in adult women. Med Clin North Am 74:1573–1602, 1990.
29. Spaulding C: Bacterial vaginosis. J Fam Pract 41:605–606, 1995.
30. Spinillo A, Capuzzo E, Gulminetti R, Marone P, et al: Prevalence of and risk factors for fungal vaginitis caused by non-*albicans* species. Am J Obstet Gynecol 176:138–141, 1997.
31. Stergachis A, Scholes D, Heidrich FE, et al: Selective screening for *Chlamydia trachomatis* infection in a primary care population of women. Am J Epidemiol 138:143–153, 1993.
32. Sweet RL: Role of bacterial vaginosis in pelvic inflammatory disease. Clin Infect Dis 20(Suppl 2):S271–S275, 1995.
33. Thorpe E, Muram D: STDs in adolescents. In Sanfilippo J, Muram D, Lee P, Dewhurst JC (eds): Pediatric and Adolescent Gynecology. Philadelphia, W.B. Saunders, 1994, pp 336–355.
34. Toomey KE, Barnes RC: Treatment of *Chlamydia trachomatis* genital infection. Rev Infect Dis 12(Suppl 6):5645–5653, 1990.
35. Washington AE, Aral SO, Wolner-Hanssen P, et al: Assessing risk for pelvic inflammatory disease and its sequelae. JAMA 266:2581–2586, 1991.
36. Woods GL: Update on laboratory diagnosis of sexually transmitted diseases. Clin Lab Med 15:665–684, 1995.

CHAPTER 22

Genital Human Papillomavirus Infection

Paritosh Kaul, M.D.

Physicians taking care of adolescent girls frequently encounter genital infections caused by human papillomavirus (HPV). This infection is often associated with abnormal Papanicolaou (Pap) smears. Because genital HPV lesions are sexually transmitted, discovery of such a lesion is an excellent opportunity for the health care provider to offer help, support, and effective health education to the patient. The clinician can use this diagnosis to play an active role in helping the adolescent girl to take charge of her sexual health.

Interest in HPV infection has been increased by its causative role in cervical cancer and its etiologic association with other diseases, including laryngeal papillomatosis, Bowen's disease, and epidermodysplasia verruciformis. It has been recognized as a sexually transmitted disease (STD) and as a possible indicator of sexual abuse in children.

VIRAL CHARACTERISTICS

HPV is a DNA virus that is found most commonly in the skin, lower genital tract, larynx, oral cavity, urethra, bladder, and anal/perianal epithelium. The virus cannot be propagated in tissue culture, and serologic diagnosis is not possible because antibodies to HPV have not been identified. The incubation period for HPV infection varies from 1 to 20 months with an average of 2–3 months. Depending on the type of HPV infection different sites are involved, and specific diseases are produced (Table 1).

EPIDEMIOLOGY

The exact incidence of HPV is unclear at present, but its prevalence among young, sexually active females is high. In a study of 467 female university students using the highly sensitive polymerase chain reaction (PCR) test (see below), the prevalence of HPV was found to be 46%. This figure is much higher than the 11% prevalence found with the ViraPap test. Only 1% of the young women in the study had physical findings, and 9% had a positive history of

TABLE 1. Type of Human Papillomavirus and Site of Disease

Type	Site of Disease
HPV 1, 2, 4	Common skin warts
HPV 4, 6, 11	Anogenital condyloma acuminatum, low-grade squamous intraepithelial lesion of the cervix; laryngeal papillomas; conjunctival lesions
HPV 16, 18, 31, 35, 39, 41–45, 51–56	Anogenital condyloma acuminatum; high-grade squamous intraepithelial lesion of the cervix; anogenital cancers

genital warts. In another study, of 608 young college women, an increased risk of HPV infection was associated with younger age, Hispanic ethnicity, black race, increased number of vaginal-sex partners, high frequencies of vaginal sex and alcohol consumption, and anal sex.

HPV infection is a causative cofactor in cervical cancer. Certain HPV types (16, 18, 31, 33, 35) are regularly found in cervical cancer tissue. However, HPV is not the sole factor, and other associated risk factors for cervical cancer include multiple sexual partners, early coitarche, cigarette smoking, immunosuppression, other genital infections, and in utero exposure to diethylstilbestrol (DES). Women with a high-risk male partner are also at greater risk of developing cervical cancer. Examples include men with multiple sexual partners, men with a history of penile cancer, and men who have had a previous sexual partner with cervical cancer.

Cell-mediated T-cell response plays a role in clinically manifested HPV disease (e.g., warts, Pap smear abnormalities). Spontaneous regression is known to occur in healthy people. The incidence of clinical HPV disease is higher in immunosuppressed patients, including those with human immunodeficiency virus (HIV), renal transplants, and neoplastic syndromes. Prolonged use of steroid medication places adolescents at particular risk of clinical HPV disease Examples include young women with systemic lupus erythematosus (SLE) and chronic inflammatory bowel disease. Adolescents with SLE often present with a huge crop of genital warts, especially during a flare-up of the disease. Treatment in such cases should be aggressive.

DIAGNOSIS

Genital HPV infections may be diagnosed by visual inspection (Fig. 1) and by cytology, histology, and molecular techniques (Table 2). The visualization of condyloma acuminata is usually quite easy, especially with exophytic lesions. However, the lesions may be difficult to visualize when they occur in mucosal folds or are hidden by hair. It is important not to mistake hymenal caruncles for genital warts; use of magnification helps to identify the verrucous nature of HPV lesions. Colposcopic visualization with application of acetic acid, Schiller's iodine, or toluidine blue is superior to examination by the naked eye. False-positive results are associated with colposcopy.

The Pap smear is an integral part of the physical examination of a sexually active female adolescent. HPV infections often are diagnosed by an abnormal Pap smear result. The cytology report often includes koilocytes, which is diagnostic for the virus. Koilocytes are superficial or intermediate squamous cells,

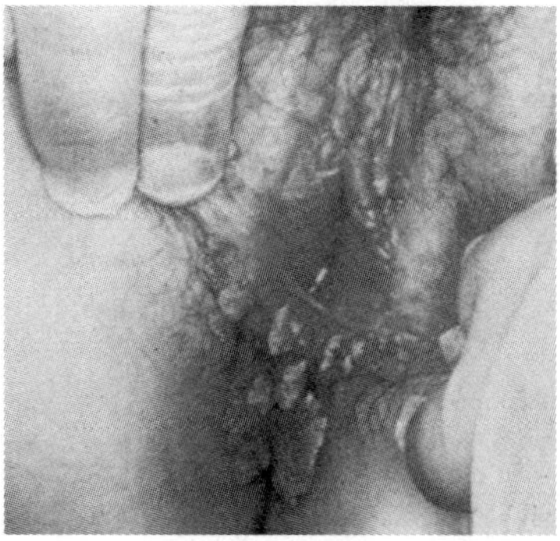

FIGURE 1. Anogenital condyloma acuminatum in an adolescent girl.

which have perinuclear cavitation, irregularly dense cytoplasm, and pyknotic nuclei (Fig. 2). The Pap smear is simply a screening test, however, and has its own limitations. The gold standard for any abnormal cytologic specimen remains tissue biopsy.

Molecular techniques have been developed for detection of subclinical HPV infection. In situ hybridization uses a labeled RNA or DNA probe to detect HPV. The dot-blot technique used in commercial kits (e.g., ViraPap, ViraType) requires collection of an additional specimen that is placed in a collection tube and sent for laboratory analysis. The Southern blot technique has greater sensitivity and specificity than either technique. It uses restriction enzymes, electrophoresis, and DNA probes. Because it is time-consuming and expensive, it is mainly a research tool. PCR is an amplification technique used for research purposes only. It is the most sensitive of all techniques.

MANAGEMENT OF CONDYLOMA ACUMINATUM

Genital warts clear spontaneously in 20–30% of patients. The aim of treatment is local destruction of the lesion. The patient's own host response (if not compromised) causes the lesion to completely heal. Treatment of condyloma acuminatum may be divided into medical and surgical modalities.

Medical Management

Application of 25% podophyllin destroys the lesions, but this tincture must be washed off and reapplied frequently. Podofilox 0.5% (Condylox), a derivative

TABLE 2. Diagnosis of Human Papillomavirus Infection

Method	Comments
Visual inspection	Useful for condylomata acuminata
Colposcopy	Costly and time-consuming; requires special expertise
Papanicolaou smear	Excellent screening test, but has low sensitivity and specificity
Molecular techniques	In situ hybridization Commercially available tests include ViraPap and ViraType Southern blot test: sensitive but costly research tool Polymerase chain reaction: most sensitive; high false-positive rate; research tool

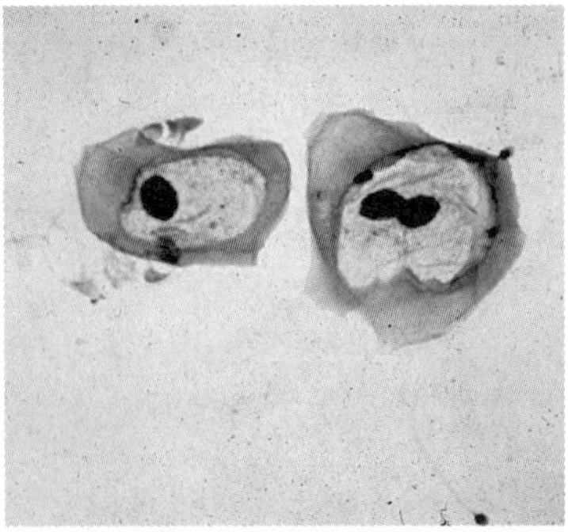

FIGURE 2. Papanicolaou smear of a patient with human papillomavirus infection shows the typical features of koilocytes. (Courtesy of L. G. Koss, M.D.)

of podophyllin, can be self-administered after the first office visit. The total wart area should not be greater than 10 cm^2, and the total amount of solution applied daily must not be greater than 0.5 ml. The solution should be applied externally to the wart with a cotton swab; it does not need to be washed off. Adverse effects include pain, burning, inflammation, and erosion. Its use is contraindicated in pregnancy. Because most young adolescents have difficulty with applying Podofilox, it is preferable to have them come to the office once a week for application by the clinician.

Trichloroacetic acid (TCA) must be applied carefully to the wart. It does not need to be washed off but may cause chemical burns to adjacent normal tissue. The burning sensation may be relieved by application of normal saline, baking soda, or aloe vera gel. TCA should be applied weekly by the clinician.

Imiquimod (Aldara), the newest therapy, is an immune-response modifier capable of stimulating the immune system. It is much less irritating than either podophyllin or TCA and can be safely used by the patient at home. Imiquimod 5% cream should be applied to external genital and perianal warts 3 times/week for up to 16 weeks. The area should be washed after 6–10 hours. Adverse effects include local reactions such as itching, erythema, burning, erosions, ulceration, and pain. The medication may weaken diaphragms and condoms, and no data have been published about its use in patients younger than 18 years. Nevertheless, many providers and patients are pleased with the response to imiquimod, although it takes 3–4 weeks before a visible decrease in warts occurs.

Interferon may be used topically, systemically, or, in refractory cases, intralesionally. It has been used in some centers with variable results. However, it is expensive and associated with adverse reactions, including fever, flulike symptoms, myalgia, and malaise. Its safety in pregnancy has not been established, and effective contraception must be used. Thus, it is a poor choice for adolescent girls.

5-Fluorouracil (5-FU) topical cream has been used successfully in some centers in the treatment of urethral and vaginal condyloma, although it has not been approved by the Food and Drug Administration (FDA) for treatment of warts. It has been used as prophylaxis for recurrence of condyloma after laser therapy, especially in immunocompromised patients. It is applied deeply into the vagina with subsequent application of a tampon to prevent seepage to the outside. Close supervision is required. Serious adverse effects include local reactions such as redness or burning around the vulva. Effective contraception is imperative, and hands must be washed thoroughly after each application.

Bone marrow suppression and gastrointestinal side effects are minimal because of the small amount of absorption. Absorption may increase if the cream is applied to an eroded epithelium. 5-FU generally should be used only by physicians experienced in treating its complications.

Surgical Management

Excision and electrocauterization may be used for local destruction of the condyloma. However, the warts may recur. Cryosurgery is a relatively safe and inexpensive procedure. Although it does not require anesthesia, most patients experience pain. The loop electrosurgical excision procedure (LEEP), which commonly is called large loop excision, is an innovation based on electrocauterization technology. A diathermy wire attached to an electrosurgical unit is used to excise the wart by heat destruction. LEEP requires local anesthesia, but blood loss is minimal. Training and expertise, however, are required.

Carbon dioxide laser has high cure rates with the added advantage of treating vulvar, vaginal, cervical, and perianal lesions concurrently. However, the procedure requires anesthesia and is associated with significant postoperative pain. It is also expensive, and patients need instruction in local vulvar and vaginal care. In addition, bleeding and scarring may occur after the procedure.

EVALUATION AND MANAGEMENT OF PAPANICOLAOU SMEARS

The Pap test is recommended in any adolescent who is sexually active or has been exposed to HPV. It is an excellent screening test but should not be used as a diagnostic tool. Generally, Pap smears with intraepithelial lesions must be assessed by colposcopy and biopsy. Tissue biopsy remains the gold standard for diagnosis of any neoplasia.

It is reassuring that the incidence of invasive cancer in adolescents is relatively low, although the reason is not yet clear. Host factors such as immune response, co-carcinogens (e.g., cigarettes), type of HPV infection, and other biologic properties (e.g., latency, regression, persistence of infection) may explain the low incidence of invasive disease in adolescents.

The technique of Pap smear collection is described in chapter 2. The physician must remember to collect cells from both the endocervix and squamocolumnar junction. The cytopathologist should be provided with the essential history, including last menstrual period, use of hormonal methods of contraception, use of intrauterine devices, previous Pap smear results, and treatments. Pap smears have a false-negative rate of 20–60%, depending on the laboratory.

The Bethesda system, developed in 1988 and further modified in 1991 (Table 3), has become the standard for classification of Pap smears. In addition to giving a cytologic diagnosis, the report comments on specimen adequacy.

Atypical Squamous Cells of Undetermined Significance

Atypical squamous cells of undetermined significance (ASCUS) are the mildest and least specific squamous cell abnormality. The cytologist should

TABLE 3. Aspects of Cervical Cytologic Diagnosis Most Relevant to Adolescents

Specimen adequacy
Satisfactory for evaluation
Satisfactory for evaluation but limited by [reason specified]
Unsatisfactory for evaluation

Descriptive diagnosis

Benign cellular changes
Infection
- *Trichomonas vaginalis*
- Fungal organisms
- Predominance of coccobacilli consistent with shift in vaginal flora
- Bacteria morphologically consistent with *Actinomyces* spp.
- Cellular changes associated with herpes simplex virus
- Other

Reactive changes associated with
- Inflammation
- Atrophy
- Radiation
- Intrauterine devices
- Other

Epithelial cell abnormalities
Squamous cell
1. Atypical squamous cells of undetermined significance (ASCUS) (should be further qualified as to whether reactive or neoplastic process is favored)
2. Low-grade squamous intraepithelial lesion encompassing cellular changes associated with HPV and mild dysplasia/cervical intraepithelial neoplasia grade 1 (CIN 1)
3. High-grade squamous intraepithelial lesion encompassing moderate dysplasia/CIN 2 and severe dysplasia/carcinoma in situ/CIN 3
4. Squamous cell carcinoma

Other malignant neoplasms: specify

Adapted from the the Bethesda System of Classification, 1991.

specify whether an inflammatory or neoplastic process is favored. In adolescents, STDs such as chlamydial infection, cervicitis, or trichomonal vaginitis may cause inflammatory changes resulting in ASCUS. Such infections need to be treated before repeating the Pap smear in 3–6 months. However, if the diagnosis favors a neoplastic process, the follow-up must be as described below for low-grade squamous intraepithelial lesions (LSIL). Two ASCUS smears 3–6 months apart or an ASCUS smear in a high-risk patient (based on HPV typing) should be evaluated like LSIL. For the ASCUS smear that is reactive or unqualified, repeat Pap smears are indicated every 6 months for 2 years or until the adolescent has three consecutive Pap smears that are negative (Fig. 3).

The use of advanced modalities such as HPV DNA-typing, cervicography, and speculography is controversial. These modalities identify patients who are at greater risk, but their low sensitivity and specificity may lead to unnecessary investigations or unjustified reassurance in patients at high risk.

Low-Grade Squamous Intraepithelial Lesion

There are several confounding factors in the management of an adolescent with LSIL on Pap smear. In most patients the LSIL reverts to normal without treatment. A small minority of patients with LSIL progress to malignancy. The most challenging dilemma is that the two groups cannot be differentiated by

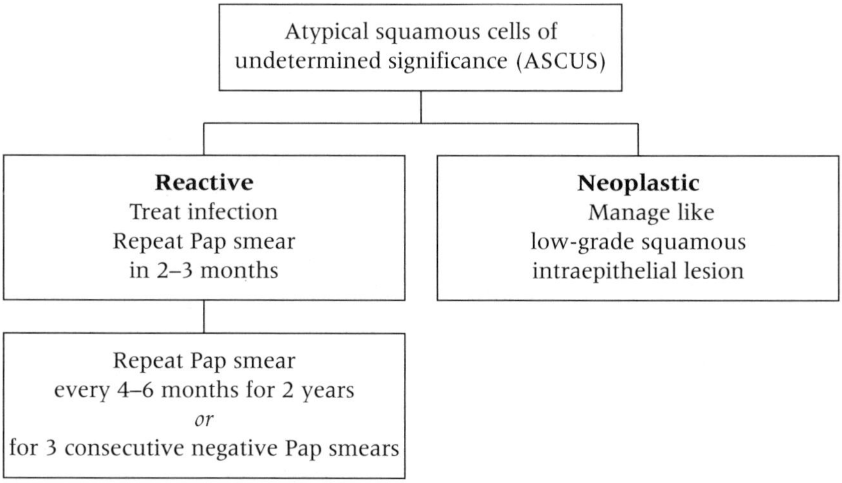

FIGURE 3. Management of atypical squamous cells of undetermined significance (ASCUS).

histopathology. In addition, a few patients with a Pap smear reading of LSIL are found to have a more advanced lesion when evaluated by colposcopy and biopsy.

Once the diagnosis of LSIL is made by Pap smear, the patient should undergo colposcopy along with endocervical curettage and biopsy of the suspicious areas (Fig. 4). In 15% of cases, LSIL has been shown to progress to high-grade lesions. Repeat Pap tests every 4–6 months rather than immediate evaluation with colposcopy and biopsy is also an option, but compliance must be ensured. The most common treatment plan after LSIL is confirmed by surgical biopsy is to excise the lesion by laser, cryosurgery, LEEP, or cone biopsy. Each of these modalities has its advantages and disadvantages. LEEP is the most commonly performed procedure and may produce a thermal artifact that compromises pathologic examination. This technique may not be appropriate

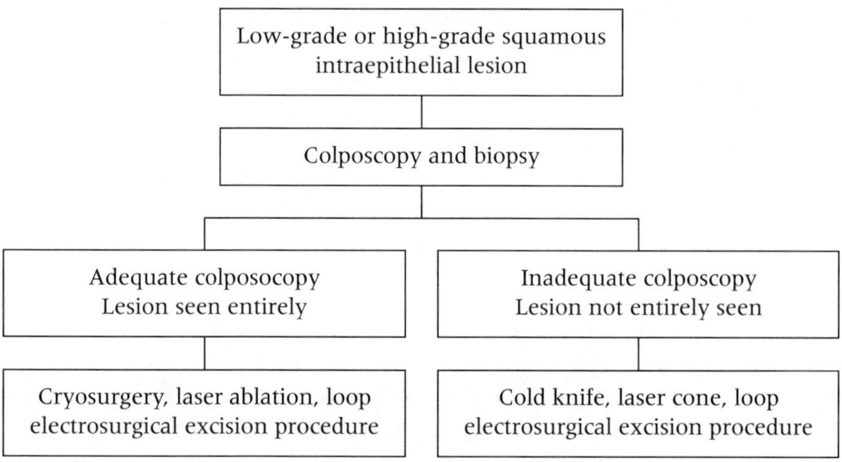

FIGURE 4. Management of squamous intraepithelial lesions.

when the squamocolumnar junction has not been visualized completely. In such cases a cone biopsy is the best option.

High-Grade Squamous Intraepithelial Lesion

High-grade squamous intraepithelial lesions (HSIL) are more frequently encountered in adolescents now than 20 years ago, but they still are relatively uncommon. All Pap tests indicating HSIL must be followed with colposcopy to determine the extent of the lesion. After a negative endocervical curettage, a thorough ablative and/or excisional procedure should be performed, as discussed above.

Follow-up

Careful follow-up is necessary for all adolescents who have undergone the above surgical procedures and should begin at 4 months postoperatively. Patients should have a Pap smear every 4 months for 2 years; if the results are consistently negative, they should have a Pap smear at 6-month intervals for 2 years. Follow-up colposcopy is suggested at yearly intervals.

COUNSELING

Forming an alliance with the adolescent is key to management of HPV infection. The physician can help the patient by effectively communicating information about the disease process. The best approach is to define the problem and the treatment options. Compliance is most likely if the information is given in an age-appropriate and straightforward manner. The adolescent is not a child, but she has not developed the decision-making capabilities of an adult. Therefore, the physician steps in and offers to help her. The young woman needs to be reassured that the warts or the Pap smear abnormality are not cancers and will go away with treatment. She should be educated about the role of the Pap smear and colposcopy in the management of the disease. Spending time with the patient to go over such details ensures compliance and good follow-up and provides a satisfying therapeutic relationship for both the patient and the clinician. This is an excellent opportunity to educate and motivate the patient about STDs and contraception. The management of the male partner of females with HPV or with abnormal Pap smear results is often questioned. Little evidence supports aggressive diagnostic and therapeutic regimens for males.

CONCLUSION

Prevention of HPV in the adolescent population is imperative. The use of newer modalities to detect the presence of the virus, treatment options, and how often to screen patients are still controversial issues. Taking the time to explain and answer questions about the management of the disease ensures the compliance of the patient. The management of genital HPV in adolescents is an opportunity for the health provider to discuss HIV prevention, contraception, and sexuality education.

SUGGESTED READING

1. Bauer HM, Ying Y, Greer CE, et al: Genital human papillomavirus infection in female university students as determined by a PCR-based method. JAMA 265:472, 1991.
2. Broder S: Rapid communication: The Bethesda system for reporting cervical/vaginal cytological diagnoses: Report of the 1991 Bethesda Workshop. JAMA 267:1892, 1992.
3. Diagnostic and Therapeutic Technology Assessment (DATTA): Human papillomavirus DNA testing in the management of cervical neoplasia. JAMA 270:2975, 1993.
4. Gutman LT: Human papillomavirus infections of the genital tract in adolescents. Adoles Med 6:115, 1995.
5. Ho GYF, Bierman R, Beardsley L, et al: Natural history of cervicovaginal papillomavirus infection in young women. N Engl J Med 338:423, 1998.
6. Koss LG: The Papanicolaou test for cervical cancer detection: A triumph and a tragedy. JAMA 261:737, 1989.
7. Kurman RJ, Henson DE, Herbst AL, et al: The 1992 National Cancer Institute Workshop. Interim guidelines for management of abnormal cervical cytology. JAMA 271:1866, 1994.
8. Lorinez AT, Reid R, Jenson AB, et al: Human papillomavirus infection of the cervix: Relative risk associations of 15 common anogenital types. Obstet Gynecol 79:328, 1992.
9. Rosenfeld WD, Rose E, Vermund SH, et al: Follow-up evaluation of cervicovaginal human papillomavirus infection in adolescents. J Pediatr 121:307, 1992.
10. Perlman SE: Pap smears: Screening, interpretation, treatment. Adolesc Med 10:243–254, 1999.

CHAPTER **23**

Pregnancy

Margaret Polaneczky, M.D.
Kim O'Connor, M.S.W.

Despite mild declines over the past decade, pregnancy rates among U.S. adolescents remain the highest in the industrialized world. Each year, approximately 11% of young women aged 15–19 become pregnant. However, among sexually experienced teenagers, the pregancy rate is 22%. The actual number of births to adolescent mothers has remained fairly stable, at approximately 500,000 annually, because of an overall increase in the U.S. teenage population. Overall, 54% of adolescent pregnancies result in birth, 32% are aborted, and 13% end in miscarriage.

Although adolescent pregnancy in general is associated with higher rates of preterm birth and low birth weight, these outcomes are related to sociodemographic factors and lack of adequate prenatal care rather than adolescence itself. If prenatal care and social supports are adequate, pregnancy outcomes need not be worse than in older women, with the possible exception of preeclampsia. However, the social consequences of adolescent childbearing can be substantial. Adolescent mothers face higher rates of long-term poverty and welfare dependence compared with their peers who delay childbearing. Their children tend to have lower cognitive scores, more difficulties in schooling, poorer health, and higher-than-normal rates of future incarceration and adolescent childbearing.

Despite aggressive follow-up, counseling, and provision of contraceptives, clinicians caring for the sexually active adolescent can be guaranteed to encounter pregnancy at some point. Often they are the first health care professional to suspect and identify the pregnancy. Familiarity with the various presentations, diagnosis, and initial evaluation of the pregnant adolescent is therefore essential in dealing with the sexually active adolescent.

DIAGNOSIS OF PREGNANCY

Adolescent providers must maintain continued vigilance for the possibility of pregnancy in their patients, because the signs and symptoms of early pregnancy may be vague, menstrual history less than reliable, and patients reluctant to disclose sexual activity or admit contraceptive noncompliance. A low threshold for performing pregnancy testing is warranted and allows early identification, timely management, and referral of the pregnant adolescent.

Signs and Symptoms of Pregnancy

The most common symptom leading a woman to suspect that she is pregnant is a missed menstrual period. Adolescents should be encouraged to keep track of their menstrual cycles, and the menstrual history should be reviewed carefully at each visit. In taking a menstrual history, it is important to ask both the date of the last menstrual period and whether it was of normal duration and amount. Any account of missed, lighter, shorter, or mistimed menses warrants pregnancy testing. Spotting in early pregnancy around the time of the missed menses, due to invasion of the trophoblast into the decidua (implantation bleed), can be mistaken by the adolescent for a normal menses. It is also important to remember that young women who have not yet menstruated but are sexually active may be at risk for pregnancy, because ovulation occasionally occurs before the first menstrual period.

Menstrual history, however, is not an entirely reliable indicator of pregnancy (Table 1). Only 68% of pregnant adolesents report having missed a menstrual period. Conversely, only about 40% of women reporting a missed period are found to be pregnant. In young adolescents, whose menses may be irregular, this symptom may be even less reliable as a predictor of pregnancy. Other early signs and symptoms of pregnancy include breast tenderness, fatigue, nausea or morning sickness, and frequent urination, all of which may present before the sixth week of gestation. Unfortunately, these symptoms tend to be nonspecific and of variable reliability in predicting pregnancy.

Physical findings presumptive for early pregnancy include softening of the cervix (Goodell's sign), softening of the uterus (Hegar's sign), and a bluish-purple hue in the cervix and vaginal walls due to hyperemia (Chadwick's sign). Although these findings are almost always present at some point during pregnancy, they have been found to be both nonspecific and unreliable in predicting early pregnancy. The palpation of uterine artery pulsations at the vaginal

TABLE 1. The Reliablity of Signs, Symptoms, and Physical Findings in Predicting a Positive Office Pregnancy Test

Symptom/Sign	Sensitivity (%)	Specificity (%)
Delayed menses	68	40
Morning sickness	39	86
Requesting a pregnancy test		36
Any of the following: breast tenderness, morning sickness, fatigue, urinary frequency	50	64
Chadwick's sign (nonblinded)	51	98
Vaginal signs (presumbed combination of Chadwick's, Goodell's, and/or Hegar's signs, blinded)	18	94
Palpable uterine fundus	9	97
Uterine artery pulsations	76	93

From Bastian LA, Piscitelli JT: Is this patient pregnant? Can your reliably rule in or rule out early pregnancy by physical exam? JAMA 278:586–591, 1997, with permission.

fornix may be more reliable than any of these traditional findings, with a sensitivity of 76% and a specificity of 96% in diagnosing pregnancy at 6 weeks or less in blinded studies.

The physical diagnosis of pregnancy is much more reliable with advancing gestational age (Table 2). Enlargement of the uterus can be easily recognized by the experienced examiner by 8 weeks. The uterus becomes palpable abdominally at the pubic symphysis at 11–12 weeks' gestation. Fetal heart tones may be audible with Doppler as early as 10–11 weeks, firmly establishing the diagnosis of pregnancy, but generally they are not reliably heard before 12 weeks' gestation. The uterine souffle often is confused with the fetal heart at this point, but timing of the pulse reveals that it corresponds to the maternal pulse, whereas the fetal heart rate ranges from 120–200 beats per minute. The uterine fundus reaches the umbilicus by 20 weeks' gestation, when fetal heart tones are audible by stethoscope (see Table 2). Fetal movement is also detectable by palpation at this time. From 20–36 weeks' gestation, the fundal height in centimeters corresponds to the gestational age in weeks, and fetal parts may be distinguished as the gestation advances.

Pregnancy Testing

The diagnosis of pregnancy has beeen revolutionized by the development of sensitive and highly specific pregnancy tests. In many ways these tests have replaced physical examination as the cornerstone of early pregnancy diagnosis. All are based on the detection of human chorionic gonadotropin (hCG) in maternal serum or urine.

Levels of Human Chorionic Gonadotropin in Pregnancy

As early as 7 days after ovulation, the implanted trophoblast begins to secrete hCG, a glycoprotein that has a molecular weight of 36,700 daltons and is composed of an alpha and beta subunits. The alpha subunit is almost identical to that of follicle-stimulating hormone (FSH), luteinizing hormone (LH), and thyroid-stimulating hormone (TSH), whereas the beta subunit is specific to hCG. This specificity allows identification of the hCG molecule without cross-reactivity with other hormones.

The placenta is the only normal tissue that secretes hCG in premenopausal females, and most hCG in the maternal circulation is in the form of the intact

TABLE 2. Physical Landmarks in Pregnancy

Landmark	Gestational age (weeks from LMP)
Fetal heart audible by Doppler	10–12
Fundus palpable at pubic symphysis	11–12
Fetal movement detectable ("quickening")	16–20
Fetal heart audible by fetoscope/stethoscope	17–19
Fundus palpable at umbilicus	20
Gestational age in weeks approximates number of cm from pubic symphysis	20–26

LMP = last menstural period.

hCG molecule. However, hCG may be secreted in certain pathologic states, such as choriocarcinoma, embryonal cell carcinoma of the ovary, and neuroendocrine tumors of the lung, adrenal gland, and liver. These diagnoses should be considered when the pregnancy test is positive, but the patient shows no evidence of pregnancy.

Serum Pregnancy Testing by Radioimmunoassay

The most accurate measure of serum hCG levels is a radioimmunoassay (RIA) using highly specific antisera to the beta subunit of hCG. Levels of hCG are measured in international units (IU) per ml, standardized to a powdered preparation of hCG established by the World Health Organization (WHO). Current testing is so sensitive that milli-International units (mIU) are used (Table 3). The current WHO standard preparation is called the *First Reference Preparation* or *1RP* (actually it is the third WHO preparation to date). Providers must know which standard their laboratories use, because hCG levels may vary as much as 50% among various preparations. In addition, levels may vary between laboratories using the same standard preparation. Thus, serial specimens from the same patient should be run at the same laboratory, so that true comparisons can be made over time. RIA can detect hCG levels as low as 2–7 mIU/ml. In general, results < 5 mIU/ml are considered negative.

Levels of hCG, as measured by RIA, rise rapidly after implantation, reaching about 100 mIU/ml in maternal serum by the expected date of the missed menses (Fig. 1). The following facts about hCG levels in normal early pregnancy are critical:

1. Levels of hCG double approximately every 1.7–2 days during the first 8–9 weeks of gestation.
2. A gestational sac is clearly identifiable on vaginal ultrasound at hCG levels of 1,000–2,000 mIU/ml (IRP).

Both ectopic gestations and spontaneous abortions are associated with abnormally low levels of hCG in early gestation as well as with hCG levels that increase at less than normal rates during early gestation. Molar pregnancy and multiple gestations are both associated with higher-than-normal hCG levels. (See abnormal early pregnancy, below.)

After pregnancy termination by delivery or abortion (spontaneous or otherwise), hCG levels decrease gradually (Fig. 2). In general, most first-trimester abortions result in a negative pregnancy test by 40 days after the procedure. However, a pregnancy test may be positive for some weeks afterward and

TABLE 3. Levels of Human Chorionic Gonadotropin (hCG) in Normal Pregnancy

	Weeks from LMP	Beta hCG (mIU/ml)*
Date of missed menses	4	≥ 100
Gestational sac visible on vaginal ultrasound	5 wk ± 2 days	1,398 ± 155
Fetal pole visible on vaginal ultrasound	5 6/7 wk ± 3 days	5,113 ± 298
Fetal heart motion on vaginal ultrasound	6 5/7 wk ± 6 days	17,208 ± 3722

LMP = last menstrual period.

* Beta hCG levels are referenced to the First International Reference Preparation/Third International Standard (3rd IS).

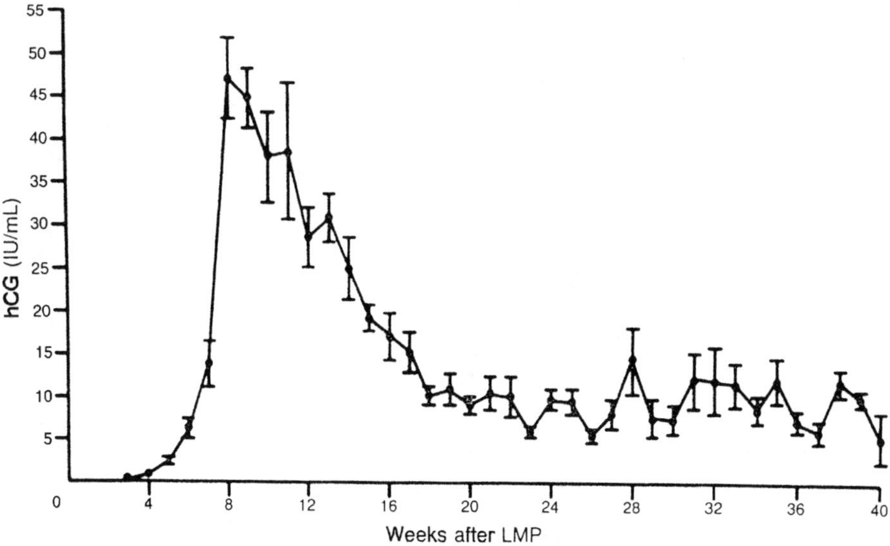

FIGURE 1. Mean serum hCG levels (± SE) throughout normal pregnancy. (From Braunstein GD, Rasor J, Adler D, et al: Serum human chorionic gonadotropin levels throughout normal pregnancy. Am J Obstet Gynecol 126:678, 1976, with permission.)

should not delay the start of hormonal contraception such as depomedroxyprogesterone acetate (DMPA) (see Fig. 2) or Norplant, provided hCG levels are appropriate for the time since pregnancy termination.

Urine Pregnancy Testing

Urine pregnancy tests are based on the identification of hCG metabolites in maternal urine, most of which consist of the "beta-core," a polypeptide fragment of the beta subunit of hCG. These tests are considered "qualitative" for pregnancy; i.e., they can rule pregnancy in or out but cannot reliably predict the level of hCG.

The earlier urine-based pregnancy tests were agglutination inhibition slide tests, which are not recommended for routine office use. The urine pregnancy tests currently used in homes and offices are enzyme-linked immunosorbent assay (ELISA)-type kits based on highly specific monoclonal antibodies to the beta subunit of hCG (standardized to the first reference preparation or third WHO standard). Sensitivities range from 5–25 mIU/ml of hCG. Thus, the urine pregnancy test may be positive as early as 3–4 days after implantation and will be positive by the expected date of the missed menses in almost 100% of normal pregnancies.

Compared with adults, adolescents are more likely to seek pregnancy-testing services rather than do a home-based test. This preference may be due to the cost of the test or embarrassment in purchasing the test kit, among other factors. Practitioners caring for sexually active adolescents should have a reliable, easy-to-use pregnancy test available in their offices (Table 4). If possible, pregnancy tests should be offered on a walk-in basis. In busy practices, pregnancy testing and counseling can be performed by a trained staff member working in

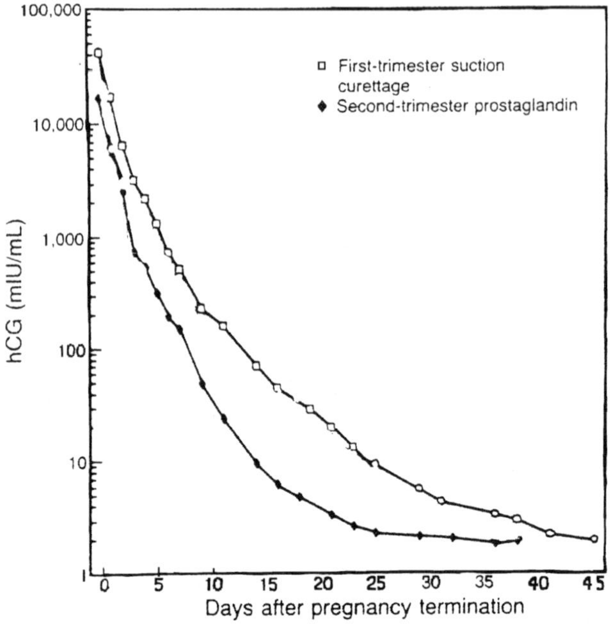

FIGURE 2. Disappearance of hCG (average serum concentrations of hCG) after pregnancy termination. (Adapted from Marrs RP, Kletsky OA, Howard WF, et al: Disappearance of human chorionic gonadotropin and resumption of ovulation following abortion. Am J Obstet Gynecol 126:678, 1976.)

close communication with the clinician. Clear protocols for triage of the patient with a positive test should be used, with identification of points for emergent consultation with the supervising clinician. A pregnancy test triage form can be developed (Fig. 3).

Use of the first morning urine is recommended for all urine pregnancy tests, because it contains the highest concentration of hCG and its metabolites, with levels approximating serum hCG levels. However, this option is not always clinically possible. Clinicians should feel free to use the test on other than first morning urine specimens, with the caveat that a repeat specimen or serum hCG level should be drawn when the urine test is negative but the index of suspicion for pregnancy remains high. Table 5 lists other factors that may affect the performance or interpretation of office-based urine pregnancy tests.

Although most modern test kits have built in negative controls, some manufacturers also offer control samples for periodic quality assurance.

INITIAL EVALUATION OF PREGNANCY

Initial evaluation of the pregnant adolescent includes (1) a careful medical history, with particular attention to the sexual, contraceptive, and menstrual history, and (2) physical examination, including a pelvic exam. The goals of this evaluation are as follows:

1. To confirm the diagnosis of pregnancy
2. To determine the gestational age

TABLE 4. Commonly Used Office-based Pregnancy Tests*

Manufacturer	Name of Test	Specimen Used	Sensitivity mIU hCG/ml†	Comments
Quidel 1-800-874-1517	QucikVue hCG Urine	Urine	25	Positive result: pink-purple line; control: blue line 3 drops sample; results in 3–5 min Control window Store at room temperature
	QuickVue hCG Combo	Urine Serum	20‡ 10‡	Positive result: pink-purple line; 3 drops sample; results in 3–5 min Control window Store at room temperature
	RapidVue	Urine	25	Positive result: pink line; control: blue line Dip strip into urine for 10 sec.; results in 3 min Store at room temperature 2-month shelf life (< most tests); good for high-volume users
Pacific Biotec 1-800-874-1517	Cards QS	Urine	20‡	Postive result: plus sign 3 drops sample; results in 1–3 min Store at room temperature Control window
	Concise Performance Plus hCG	Urine	20‡	Postive result: plus sign 3 drops sample; results in 1–3 min Store at room temperature Control window
Abbott Laboratories 212-518-6000	Test Pack +Plus (hCG Combo)	Urine or serum	25	Postive result: plus sign 3 drops sample; results in 4 min for urine, 7 min for serum Contains both negative control and end-of-assay window (no timer needed) Store in refrigrator overnight; leave at room temperature up to 8 hr daily (shelf life shorter if stored at room temperature, but not a problem for high-volume users)
Hybritech 1-800-854-1957	IconII hCG (urine)	Urine	20	Semiquantitative test Uses spot density compared with positive reference to differentiate hCG levels < 50 mIU from levels > 50 mIU
Wampole	Clearview hCG Duo	Urine or serum	25	5 drops sample; results in 3–5 min Internal control
	Clearview hCGII	Urine	10–25	4 drops sample; results in 5 min Internal control

* All tests are immunoassays based on monoclonal antibodies highly specific for the beta subunit of hCG. They occasionally detect hCG levels even lower than the reported minimal sensitivity; all samples containing ≤ 5 mIU/ml hCG should test negative. The presence of small amounts of blood in the specimen should not alter the results significantly. The cost to providers varies by distributor and quantity purchased but generally ranges from $2–4 per test.

† World Health Organization Third International Standard.

‡ Sensitivities of new products available in early 1998, as reported by the manufacturer. Earlier products (1977) have a sensitivity of 25 mIU for both urine and serum.

Source: Manufacturers' product literature and/or technical support personnel.

The New York Hospital - Cornell University Medical College
Center for Women's Health Care
Obstetrics and Gynecology

Pregnancy Test Visit Patient Assessment

Patient name ______________________________ **DOB** ______________

Pregnancy History

_____Number of previous Pregnancies (Not including present)
_____Number of previous deliveries
_____Number of previous spontaneous abortions
_____Number of previous Ectopic Pregnancies
_____Number of previous elective abortions
_____Number of living children

Last normal menses (LMP)

Date ____________ Late / early / on time (circle one)
Duration __________ (Normal / Abnormal)
Flow ____________ (Normal / Abnormal)
Date of first positive pregnancy test____________

Medical History (check all that apply)

__Hypertension	__Seizure Disorder	__Thyroid Disease
__Heart Disease	__Asthma / Lung Disease	__GI Disease
__Renal Disease	__Lupus	__Other______________

Medications ____

Obstetrical History (Check all that apply)

__Previous Ectopic / Ectopic Risk Factors (Hx. Tubal ligation or reversal, PID)
__Incompetent Cervix / cerclage
__Preterm labor
__Recent hospitalization
__Bleeding
__Abdominal Pain

Previous Prenatal Care this pregnancy

Where________________________Last visit___________Next scheduled appt___________
Does patient have records with her? If do, make a copy today for NYH chart.

Result of Spot Pregnancy Test (circle one) POS NEG

Plan ____

Signature__________________________

Patients with any of the following should be referred immediately for a clinician exam, even if pregnancy test result is negative:History of ectopic, Abdominal pain,Abnormal Bleeding
For patients with significant medical/obstetrical history, consult with the attending regarding how soon the patient needs to be seen.

FIGURE 3. Example of a pregnancy test triage form.

TABLE 5. Factors Affecting Performance of Urine Pregnancy Tests*

1. **Inappropriate timing of specimen.** Inaccurate dates of the last menstrual period can lead to performing the test too soon after the date of conception for a positive result. Repeating the test a few days later is helpful in this situation.
2. **Dilution of urine.** Urine samples taken later in the day, particularly in women with high fluid intake, may have hCG levels below the sensitivity of the test. When possible, patients should be instructed to collect their first morning urine.
3. **Specimen too cold.** Refrigerated specimens are good for up to 48 hours after collection. If necessary, samples can be frozen if testing cannot be done with 48 hours on a refrigerated specimen. However, refrigerated and frozen samples must be returned to room temperature before testing.
4. **Wrong amount of urine used.** Use of too much or too little urine can lead to false-negative results. Some tests are more "forgiving" of this error than others. Follow the instructions strictly.
5. **Reading the result at the wrong time.** Most tests have a fairly strict time window during which the result should be read. Use of a timer is recommended. A few tests (e.g., Abbott) have built in "test done" windows that eliminate the need for a timer. All tests may develop color over time, especially in specimens witht levels of hCG below the reported sensitivity of the test. Such tests should be considered intermediate. Either repeat the test, or confirm with a serum test.
6. **Interfering substances.** Most current tests are not impaired by moderate levels of hemoglobin, glucose, albumin, or other serum proteins or by commonly used medications such as salicylic acid, ethanol, or ampicillin. Thus, although blood-tinged specimens can be used, grossly bloody specimens or specimens with proteinuria above 2+ may lead to false-negative results. If there is any question, either repeat the urine collection or draw a serum hCG.
7. **Visual problems.** Because these tests rely on a faint color reaction, people with red or blue color-blindness are unable to interpret the result. People with visual difficulties may not detect the fine lines seen with lower levels of hCG.
8. **Home-based testing.** In general, home-based urine pregnancy tests have a considerably lower sensitivity and specificity than office-based tests. Most likely this is due to problems with performing the test correctly or to misreading the result of a correctly performed test. Patient management should not be based on the results of a home test alone—a confirmatory specimen in the provider's office is always recommended.
9. **Storage.** Some pregnancy test kits require refrigeration for long-term storage and need to be at room temperature for use (e.g., Abbott +Plus Testpack). Keeping these kits at room temperature all of the time shortens their viability, but this problem does not affect high-volume use. Offices with low testing volumes may best use a kit that can be stored at room temperature. Be sure to read and follow the manufacturer's recommendations for storage. Check the expiration date frequently.

* In all cases, if the suspicion of pregnancy is high and the urine test negative, RIA should be performed on a serum specimen.

3. To identify potential pregnancy complications requiring emergent referral
4. To assess the status of concurrent medical conditions potentially affecting an early pregnancy
5. To educate and counsel the patient about her options for dealing with the pregnancy
6. To make timely referrals for emergent gynecologic care or for abortion, prenatal care, or adoption.

All pregnant adolescents should be referred for management as soon as possible, but patients experiencing any abnormal bleeding or abdominal pain should be referred emergently to rule out the possibility of a life-threatening ectopic gestation. In addition, if there is any question about the viability of the pregnancy, it should be determined as soon as possible. Such information can be critical to the adolescent who is as yet undecided about continuing the pregnancy.

Dating the Pregnancy

By convention, the gestational age is calculated from the first day of the last menstrual period (LMP). This method assumes a 28-day menstrual cycle, with conception occurring on or about day 14 and an average length of term gestation of 266 days. A simple way of estimating the due date is to use *Nagele's Rule:* To the first day of the LMP, add 7 days, subtract 3 months, and add 1 year to obtain the expected date of delivery. Use of a gestational age wheel makes calculation unnecessary, and the computer-savvy clinician can access an online gestational age calculator at *http://www.cpmc.columbia.edu/resources/obgyn-tools/ gestcalc.html.*

It is important to determine not only the date of the LMP but also whether the adolescent is certain of that date. Adolescents who are infrequently sexually active may be more certain of the date of conception than the date of their LMP. Date of conception can be used reliably to predict gestational age. The LMP may be an inaccurate way of predicting gestational age in patients with irregular cycles or recent use of hormonal contraception. In such cases, ultrasound dating may be more reliable. When performed in the first trimester, ultrasound dating is correct within 3–5 days.

Accurate dating of the pregnancy is important in establishing paternity for some adolescents. It is important, therefore, to ask the pregnant adolescent whether she has any concerns about paternity and to address those concerns by giving her an accurate date as soon as possible. For adolescents presenting in the second and third trimesters, accurate dating is not always possible because the margin of error for ultrasound dating is increased later in gestation.

Early Pregnancy Complications

The presence of bleeding and/or abdominal pain or cramping in early pregnancy may indicate spontaneous abortion, ectopic pregnancy, or gestational trophoblastic disease. However, spotting also occurs in approximately 20–25% of normal gestations. Lower abdominal pain and cramping are also common symptoms of normal gestation and often are associated with the presence of a functioning corpus luteum cyst in one or both adnexae. Nonobstetric causes of bleeding (such as cervicitis) or abdominal pain (such as appendicitis) also may occur coincidentally with pregnancy and should be considered.

Spontaneous Abortion

Spontaneous abortion is defined as pregnancy loss before 20 weeks' gestation. Overall, the rate of spontaneous abortion in clinically recognized pregnancies is 15–20%. However, an additional 20% of pregnancies are lost prior to the missed menses and thus are unrecognized clinically as miscarriages. In such cases, the menses is often late and may be heavier than usual.

Most spontaneous abortions occur in the first trimester. Close to 60% are associated with an abnormal chromosomal complement in the gestation, the most common of which is 46XO. Other known causes include uterine or cervical structural abnormalities (i.e., bicornuate uterus, incompetent cervix, uterine fibroids), endocrinologic causes (diabetes, thyroid disease, luteal phase deficiency), autoimmune disorders (systemic lupus erythematosus, anticardiolipin syndrome), teratogen exposure, and infection (e.g., rubella).

Spontaneous abortion is described according to the point along the continuum of pregnancy loss at which the patient presents for evaluation and treatment. Thus it is clinically referred to as either a (1) threatened abortion, (2) inevitable abortion, (3) incomplete abortion, (4) completed abortion, or (5) missed abortion.

Threatened abortion refers to viable pregnancies presenting in the first trimester with bleeding and/or cramping. Pelvic examination reveals the cervix to be long and closed, and ultrasound confirms that the pregnancy is still viable. Expectant management is warranted once viability is confirmed. Some studies suggest that the early fetal heart rate may have prognostic value, with rates less than 90 bpm carrying poor prognosis for successful continuation of the pregnancy. When fetal heart tones may not be confidently confirmed or denied by sonogram, hCG and/or progesterone levels can be used to follow the course of the pregnancy. The possibility of ectopic gestation must always be considered when a patient presents with bleeding and/or abdominal pain, unless an intrauterine gestation can be definitely identified. (See ectopic pregnancy, below.) No specific treatment has been shown to affect the outcome in cases of threatened abortion. However, most clinicians prescribe pelvic and/or bed rest and restricted activity. Use of progesterone has not proved efficacious in the setting of bleeding in an already established pregnancy.

Abortion is considered *inevitable* when the cervical os is open at least a finger's diameter in the setting of bleeding and cramps. When passage of products of gestation has begun, the term *incomplete abortion* is used. At this point, termination of pregnancy by suction curettage is generally performed to prevent further blood loss, to resolve continued cramping, and to reduce the risk of infection. In adolescents, prophylaxis against chlamydial endometritis is generally given because of the high prevalence of asymptomatic chlamydial cervicitis in sexually active teenage girls.

In some cases, there may be a place for expectant rather than surgical management of spontaneous abortion. Determining factors include gestational age of the pregnancy, amount of blood loss, and the patient's desire to avoid surgical intervention as well as the level of support at home and the patient's ability to comply with follow-up. Although expectant management avoids the potential risks of surgical evacuation of the pregnancy, these risks are low. In general, expectant management of inevitable or incomplete abortion is not recommended for adolescents. One exception may be if ultrasound reveals the possible passage of one twin, with continued viability of the remaining twin. In this case, there may be a place for continued observation, depending on the level of bleeding, whether or not two separate sacs and/or placentas are present, and the patient's desire to maintain the pregnancy.

If the cervical os is closed, passage of products is complete, as determined by ultrasound, and bleeding is minimal, the term *completed abortion* is used. Curettage is not required. The term *missed abortion* is used when the true embryo is not viable, the cervical os is closed, and vaginal bleeding occurs. Such patients need suction curettage after dilatation of the cervix.

Corpus Luteum Cysts

Before 7–9 weeks, maintenance of the pregnancy relies on continued production of progesterone by the corpus luteum. The persistent corpus luteum is visible on ultrasound as a cystic structure in the ovary, occasionally as large as 5–6 cm in diameter. Pain from the enlarging corpus luteum is not uncommon and may be confused with an ectopic gestation. Occasionally, hemorrhage into th cyst occurs (hemorrhagic corpus luteum). Management is expectant. The cyst generally resolves early in the second trimester. Avoidance of vigorous sports and intercourse is warranted in the patient who is symptomatic or who has a cyst larger than 5 cm in diameter, because such activitiets may cause rupture of the cyst. Failure of the cyst to resolve by 14 weeks suggests other etiologies. Further management depends n the size of the cyst, whether it is increasing in size, and the presence or absence of associated symptoms.

Gestational Trophoblastic Disease

Gestational trophoblastic disease, or hydatidiform mole, is a relatively common pregnancy complication, occurring in 1:1,000–1,500 pregnancies in the United States annually. A recent review suggests that these rates may be higher among adolescents, particularly in those of Asian descent.[14] Presenting symptoms include bleeding, abdominal pain, and hyperemesis, with the classic physical finding of a large-for-gestation uterus. Among adolescents, excessive vaginal bleeding, occasionally severe enough to warrant transfusion, has been reported to be the most common presenting symptom.

Diagnosis is suggested when the uterus is larger than gestational age (75% of cases) and fetal heart tones are absent. Pelvic sonogram is diagnostic, showing the characteristic sonolucent vesicular material filling the uterine cavity (snowstorm appearance). Levels of hCG are higher than normal, generally above 100,000 mIU/ml.

Treatment is dilatation and suction curettage, a procedure that should be done only by experienced operators because the risk for hemorrhage and uterine perforation are increased compared with normal gestations. Postoperatively, hCG levels must be followed closely until they are less than 2 mlU/ml and then monthly for up to one year as surveillance for recurrent disease. Failure of hCG levels to decline normally or a plateau of hCG levels after evacuation mandates repeat curettage and surveillance for gestational trophoblastic neoplasm and choriocarcinoma. Avoidance of pregnancy in the first postoperative year is recommended, because any increase in hCG levels may confuse or prevent the diagnosis of recurrent or persistent disease. Hormonal methods of contraception are thus the norm. In adolescents, a long-acting hormonal method (i.e., Norplant or DMPA) should be strongly considered.

The recurrence rate of molar pregnancies is generally reported to be between 1% and 2%. However, in adolescents, recurrence rates of 9% have been reported.[11]

Ectopic Pregnancy

Over 100,000 ectopic pregnancies occur annually, accounting for about 2% of all pregnancies. Although the highest rate of ectopic pregnancy occurs among women over 35, adolescents have the highest mortality rate, and the case-fatality rate is five times higher in nonwhite than in white teenagers, most likely because of a tendency to present later in the course of pregnancy.

Risk factors for ectopic pregnancy include history of pelvic inflammatory disease (PID), prior tubal surgery, douching, current intrauterine device (IUD) use, and assisted reproductive technologies. Another important group of adolescents at risk for ectopic gestation are those who become pregnant while using progestin-only methods of contraception, such as Norplant, DMPA, or the mini-pill. The causative factor is the progestin-mediated decrease in tubal motility. The high rates of effectiveness of these methods impart a lower incidence of ectopic pregnancy than in nonusers of contraception. When pregnancy does occur, however, the odds of ectopic pregnancy are markedly increased, as high as 22% in reported series. Thus, current users of progestin-only methods who become pregnant should be presumed to have ectopic pregnancy until proved otherwise.

The classic symptoms of ectopic pregnancy are abdominal pain in the setting of late menses or irregular bleeding. The pain ranges from mild cramps to severe pain resulting in inability to stand erect or walk. Although the pain may be unilateral initially, with progression of the ectopic pregnancy it may become bilateral or diffuse. In cases of rupture or leakage, peritoneal findings and shoulder pain may be present. Occasionally, rectal pain or the urge to defecate results from cul-de-sac irritation. Advanced cases may present with syncope or hypovolemic shock due to blood loss.

Any pregnant adolescent with symptoms suggesting leaking or rupture of an ectopic gestation requires immediate referral for surgical intervention. Fortunately, because of the increasing use of sensitive pregnancy testing, most cases of ectopic pregnancy encountered by the clinician are less acute. A more common presentation consists of irregular bleeding or spotting or no symptoms at all, accompanied by a high index of suspicion due to patient risk factors or smaller-than-expected uterine size for gestational dates. In this case, the mainstay of diagnosis is quantitative hCG levels, transvaginal ultrasound, and, in some cases, serum progesterone levels. In normal early pregnancies, a gestational sac is visible on ultrasound in the uterus at hCG levels of 1,000–2,000 (IRP) (approximately one week after the expected menses), hCG levels should approximately double every 48 hours, and serum progesterone levels are above 25 ng/ml. By correlating these findings with the clinical scenario, algorithms for the diagnosis of suspected ectopic pregnancy have been developed (Fig. 4).

In general, if the hCG level is greater than 2,000 mIU/ml and no pregnancy is identified in the uterus, further evaluation by uterine curettage is indicated. Curettage of the uterus determines whether the diagnosis is a blighted

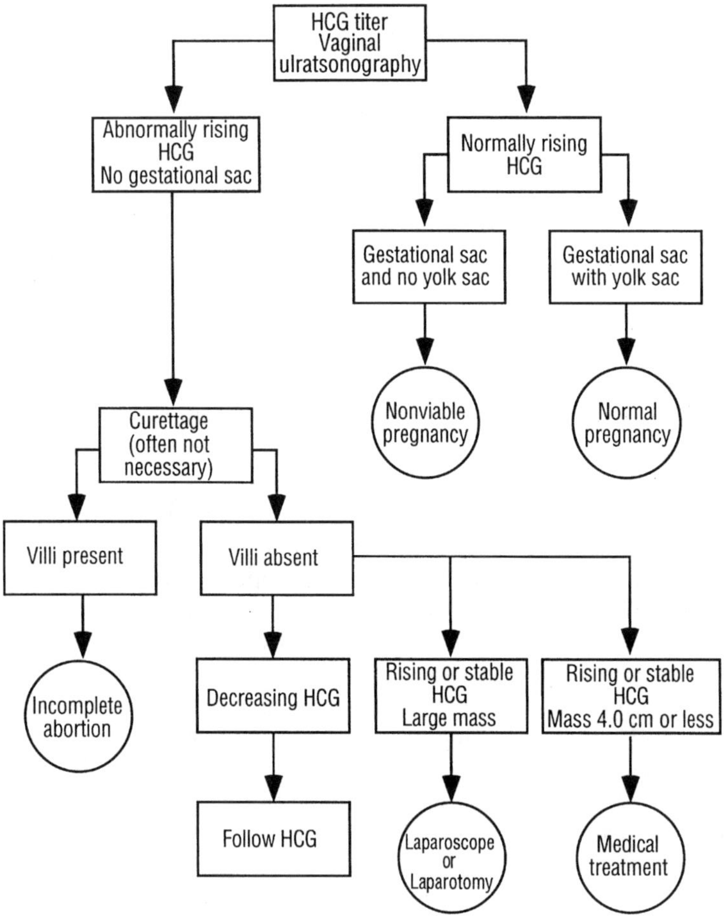

FIGURE 4. Algorithm for the diagnosis and management of suspected ectopic gestations. (From Speroff L, Glass RH, Kase NG: Ectopic pregnancy. In Speroff L, Glass RH, Kase NG (eds): Clinical Gynecologic Endocrinology and Infertility, 5th ed. Baltimore, William & Wilkins, 1994, p 953, with permission.)

intrauterine gestation or an ectopic pregnancy. Lack of villi on curettage or failure of hCG levels to decline after curettage indicates an ectopic gestation. If the hCG level is less than 2,000 mIU/ml and the patient is stable, expectant management with serial hCG levels and sonography can be performed. Levels of hCG are drawn every 48 hours, with repeat sonography at frequent intervals. Failure of hCG levels to rise appropriately indicates an abnormal gestation. Curettage determines whethre the site of the gestation is intrauterine or ectopic. If at any point in the evaluation the patient becomes symptomatic, referral for surgical intervention is indicated.

Surgical treatment is indicated in cases of suspected leaking or ruptured ectopic gestation and if the ectopic gestation is greater than 4 cm in size. Laparoscopy has replaced laparotomy for all but the most acute cases, with preservation of the fallopian tube whenever possible. Treatment depends on the anatomic location of the ectopic pregnancy. Linear salpingostomy with extrusion of the ectopic gestation using hydrodissection is the procedure of choice for ampullary ectopic pregnancies. The tube is left open to heal. Occasionally, fimbrial expression of a distal ectopic ("milking the tube") can be performed, although this procedure is associated with higher rates of postoperative persistent ectopic gestation. Isthmic gestations are treated by segmental tubal resection. Interstitial or cornual gestations require surgical excision of the cornua. Gestations in locations other than the tube are managed accordingly. In all cases of tubal ectopic pregnancy in which the tube is preserved, there is a risk that pregnancy tissue will remain postoperatively. For this reason, hCG levels are followed postoperatively until they are < 5 mIU/ml. Methotrexate therapy is given when levels plateau.

The past decade has seen an increasing use of methotrexate for the medical management of ectopic pregnancy. Criteria for medical management are as follows:

1. Ectopic gestation less than 4 cm diameter
2. No evidence of rupture or leakage
3. hCG levels less than 10,000
4. Ability of the patient to comply with follow-up

Although various regimens have been studied, the most commonly used is a single intramuscular injection of methotrexate in a dose of 50 mg/m^2. Using this regimen, which is rarely associated with side effects, approximately 95% of ectopic pregnancies will resolve. The remainder require either a second dose of methotrexate or surgical intervention because of development of symptoms, persistence of the ectopic gestation, or rupture.

Concerns that adolescents may not be able to comply with medical management of ectopic gestation appear unfounded. A recent review reported comparable success and compliance rates between adolescents and adults.[10] However, the aggressiveness of follow-up and/or interventions to improve compliance among adolescents were not described. It is incumbent on the clinician to maintain contact and to provide aggressive follow-up of the adolescent undergoing medical treatment of ectopic pregnancy.

Septic Abortion

The presence of fever, abdominal pain, and/or bleeding in the setting of early pregnancy suggests septic abortion. The differential diagnosis includes PID (rare in pregnancy), appendicitis, pyelonephritis, and other intraabdominal processes. Referral for immediate treatment, including intravenous antibiotics, hospitalization, and uterine curettage, is indicated.

Determination of Rh Status

In all cases of threatened or spontaneous abortion as well as in ectopic pregnancies, determination of Rh antibody status is mandatory, with prophylactic administration of anti-D gamma globulin (Rhogam) to women at risk for Rh sensitization. Most authorities recommend use of Rhogam in the setting of bleeding at any gestational age in women at risk. Smaller doses of Rhogam are used in first-trimester abortion (50 mg) than typically are given after delivery (300 mg).

Second- and Third-Trimester Pregnancy Complications

Although this chapter focuses on the initial management of the pregnant adolescent, some adolescents manage to evade diagnosis until late in gestation, presenting to the primary care clinician in the late second or third trimester. A brief review of the more emergent presenting symptoms is thus warranted.

Labor

It is unfortunately not entirely uncommon for the pregnant parturient to either deny or avoid the fact of her pregnancy until delivery is imminent, presenting for the first time to the clinician while she is in labor. Unfortunately, the abdominal pain associated with labor is all too often misdiagnosed as impending appendeceal rupture or gastroenteritis by the unsuspecting clinician. Labor pain generally is confined to the lower mid-abdomen in early and false labor but also may be perceived as low back or vaginal pain. As labor progresses, the pain is referred to the entire abdomen. Patient perception of labor pain varies considerably. Signs of imminent delivery may include the passage of a mucus plug ("bloody show"), passage of fluid per vagina (rupture of the membranes), and a feeling of the urge to defecate. Nausea and vomiting, as well as diarrhea, also may occur during labor. In general, a careful abdominal examination reveals the presence of the gravid uterus, and the experienced clinician also may be able to identify fetal parts. Obviously, emergent referral is indicated. Pelvic examination should be deferred if bleeding or rupture of membranes has occurred, unless delivery is believed to be imminent.

Preterm Labor

Preterm labor and delivery are associated with high rates of neonatal morbidity and mortality. Although the cause is unknown, predisposing factors include gonococcal, chlamydial, trichomonal, and bacterial vaginosis; bacteriuria; multiple gestation; uterine fibroids or other uterine anomalies; and a history of preterm delivery. Sociodemographic factors associated with higher rates of preterm delivery in the United States include poverty and black race.

The pain associated with preterm labor may be mild or not noticed at all by the parturient. Although contractions occasionally are palpable by the clinician, examination of the cervix is most important in determining whether the patient is at risk for preterm delivery. The typical cervix is 2–4 cm in length, and cervical dilatation and effacement do not occur until after 36 weeks' gestation in the majority of primiparous patients. Any cervical shortening, effacement, or dilatation before this gestational age requires emergent referral to prevent preterm delivery.

Incompetent Cervix

The incompetent cervix dilates without pain or labor because of pressure from the gravid uterus and its contents. The cervix is unable to support the weight of the advancing pregnancy. Although predisposing factors may include prior second-trimester abortions, uterine anomalies, and history of cone biopsy, some patients have no such history and presumably have an inherent structural abnormality of the cervix.

Patients with incompetent cervix usually present in the mid-to-late second trimester with noticeable cervical shortening and effacement. If cervical dilatation occurs, prolapse of the membranes through the cervix may result, appearing as a fluid-filled balloon in the vagina. This condition often is associated with leakage of amniotic fluid and, if prolonged, rupture of the membranes.

Treatment of the incompetent cervix involves replacement of the membranes and suture of the cervix (cerclage). Prognosis depends on the length and dilation of the cervix, whether rupture of the membranes has occurred, and the presence of coincident intraamniotic infection.

Third-Trimester Bleeding

Bleeding in the late second and third trimesters of pregnancy may be associated with preterm labor, placental abruption (premature placental separation), placenta previa, vasa previa (umbilical vessels presenting in the membranes), incompetent cervix or cervical dilatation, and normal labor. Unless delivery is believed to be imminent, pelvic examination should be deferred because of concerns about placenta previa. Immediate referral should be made. Fetal well-being can be assessed by measuring fetal heart tones using the bell of the stethoscope if Doppler is not immediately available.

Rupture of the Membranes

Membrane rupture may be obvious, characterized by a sudden large gush of straw-colored or pink (blood-tinged) fluid from the vagina. Green or brown fluid suggests passage of meconium by the fetus, a possible sign of fetal distress. Some patients "leak" rather than rupture and note only a small amount of fluid on their underwear or a sensation of feeling wet. During sterile speculum examination, membrane rupture is confirmed by noting (1) pooling of fluid in the vaginal vault; (2) crystallization of the fluid when allowed to dry on a slide and viewed under the microscope ("ferning"); and (3) a dark blue color on testing with nitrazine paper. However, if rupture of the membranes is suspected and delivery is not imminent, pelvic examination should be deferred until referral is made to avoid infection of the fetus with vaginal organisms. This is particularly important in preterm gestations.

Common Medical Conditions Affecting Pregnancy in Adolescents

Adolescents with certain medical conditions are at increased risk for complications during pregnancy. Unplanned pregnancy can be disastrous for either mother or fetus. Clinicians providing care to sexually active adolescents need to be ever vigilant for the possibility of pregnancy in such patients.

Diabetes in pregnancy is associated with an increased risk of congenital abnormalities as well as maternal complications if renal, vascular, or ophthalmic disease is present. Tight glucose control (fasting glucose < 100, postprandial glucose l< 140) is necessary in the first trimester, when organ formation is occurring. Use of hypoglycemic agents is contraindicated because of potential teratogenic effects. Given the narrow time window of organ formation in the fetus, the diagnosis of pregnancy in the noncontrolled diabetic should be considered a medical emergency, and the patient should be referred immediately for prenatal care.

Epilepsy is associated with certain congenital syndromes, due either to direct teratogenic effects of antiseizure medications (e.g., valproic acid, fetal hydantoin syndrome) or to congenital factors that may be associated with seizure disorders in general. Early referral allows adjustment of medication when possible.

Sickle cell anemia and sickle cell trait are associated with urinary tract infections in pregnancy, which may lead to preterm delivery. Pregnancies in adolescents with severe anemia due to sickle cell disease may be complicated by preterm delivery and intrauterine growth retardation. There is a risk of transmission of the disorder to the fetus, depending on the carrier status of the father. Genetic diagnosis is available. Early entrance into prenatal care minimizes complications and allows genetic counseling and testing.

Cardiac disease. Adolescents with congenital or other cardiac disorders, particularly those associated with pulmonary hypertension, may be at increased risk for maternal cardiac compromise due to the increase in plasma volume and other cardiovascular changes associated with pregnancy and delivery. In some patients, pregnancy is contraindicated. Alternatively, others may be led to believe erroneously that pregnancy must be terminated in all cases. Some disorders, such as Marfan's syndrome, are likely to occur in the offspring. These concerns should be addressed early in the pregnancy with the adolescent and her family, and consultation with a maternal-fetal specialist should be sought.

Cancer. Adolescents undergoing chemotherapy or radiation should be referred immediately to a maternal-fetal specialist as soon as pregnancy is diagnosed because of increased risk for congenital anomalies as well as determination of the risk that pregnancy itself may pose to progression of disease and/or options for therapy.

Acne. The use of isotretinoin (Accutane) is considered a contraindication to pregnancy because of high rates of congenital anomalies. Unfortunately, not all adolescents taking this medication are on contraception because of nondisclosure of sexual activity or unplanned sexual activity.

Options Counseling

Most adolescent pregnancies are unplanned. Although some teenagers may suspect that they are pregnant when they present to the clinician, others may be completely surprised by the diagnosis. Some may be brought in for diagnosis by a suspecting parent. For the clinician, the diagnosis and initial evaluation of pregnancy are only the beginning. The clinician has a responsibility to see the pregnant adolescent through what may be a period of uncertainty, confusion, and conflict. This uncertainty may lead to delay in seeking ultimate treatment for the pregnancy, be it abortion or prenatal care.

In counseling the pregnant adolescent about her options related to the pregnancy, the clinician must establish a trusting relationship in which the adolescent understands that she is in a confidential setting and can trust the clinician not to be judgmental. Providing facts specifically related to pregnancy options and decision making is important. Accurate medical information helps to guide the adolescent's decision and should be given in a developmentally appropriate fashion. Information should include an accurate estimate of gestational age as soon as possible, because gestational age sets the time frame in which the decision should be made.

It is important to explore whether the adolescent has thought or talked about the possibility of pregnancy. Many adolescents are embarrassed or ashamed to discuss their sexual feelings and activities, particularly their fantasies and thoughts about pregnancy. Acknowledging these thoughts and emotions can serve to validate and normalize what the adolescent is experiencing. For some adolescents a pregnancy, planned or unplanned, may be an appropriate way to define their social role. Others may see it as a poorly timed, premature event. For some, misconceptions about pregnancy and their ability to have a child may inappropriately influence decision making in what otherwise would be experienced as a poorly timed pregnancy. Such misconceptions need to be addressed. Common concerns include questions about the effects of abortion on future fertility, and misconceptions about the relative risks of abortion compared with pregnancy and childbirth.

That adolescents think and talk about pregnancy does not necessarily mean that the pregnancy is a planned or welcomed event. Many adolescents experience ambivalence about pregnancy. It is important to address the ambivalence directly. It is useful to explore with the adolescent both the positive and negative aspects of pregnancy. What are her positive thoughts and feelings about the pregnancy? What are her negative thoughts and feelings? This strategy names and introduces the adolescent to the myriad emotions that she feels and normalizes and validates their complexity. It also allows the clinician to gather information about the adolescent's life that is directly relevant to the decision she must make. The next step is to take this information and, without interjecting judgment or opinion, help the adolescent to explore the viable options. It is important to mention that three options are available: abortion, adoption, and parenting. Pursue all three and play them out. What does the adolescent think of abortion? What does she think it would be like to have an abortion? Why would she have or not have an abortion? What would it be like to have a baby? Why would she consider having or not having a baby? What are her future goals? What changes would occur in her life if she did or did not have a baby? Does she feel that she could still accomplish these goals? Who could she count on to help her? Why or why not? Can she approach these people to ask for support in the decision process? If so, she should be encouraged to do so.

The clinician should focus on the fact that there is no right or wrong solution. The adolescent's decision must come from within and must be one with which she feels comfortable. This unconditional support is invaluable, because it may well be the only such support that the young person receives.

Referrals

As a clinician, it is important to monitor the ambivalent adolescent's decision process and to assist, when possible, in moving her toward a choice. The adolescent should understand that avoiding a choice is making one, because delays reduce options and may result in poor pregnancy outcomes for those who delay entrance into prenatal care. Once a decision is made, referral should be facilitated by the clinician and/or staff. Facilitation may include assistance with creative strategies for funding of pregnancy terminations, particularly for adolescents who do not seek parental support. The clinician hopefully has developed a network of providers, social workers, and programs that can assist the adolescent in this regard.

If the adolescent decides to continue the pregnancy, the clinician must ensure that she follows through on her scheduled appointment for initiation of prenatal care. Up to 20% of adolescents may delay this appointment for months after the referral is made. Possible barriers to follow-through on the adolescent's part include fear of notifying her parents or guardian, lack of insurance coverage for care, lack of transportation, or difficulties negotiating the health care system, particularly in settings more typically designed for adult patients. Prenatal programs designed specifically for adolescents usually include a significant amount of psychosocial support, prenatal and parenting education, continuity of care, and incentives such as free transportation. Such programs have been shown to reduce significantly adverse perinatal outcomes among adolescent participants. Whenever possible, the pregnant adolescent should be referred to such programs. However, managed care plans may restrict access. The primary care clinician needs to develop and maintain a network of prenatal and gynecologic providers who are experienced and willing to care for the adolescent parturient.

THE NEGATIVE PREGNANCY TEST: AN IMPORTANT OPPORTUNITY FOR INTERVENTION

In general, only 36% of adolescents who request a pregnancy test actually prove to be pregnant. The remaining girls with a negative test constitute a group at extremely high risk for pregnancy. Close to one-half are not using contraception, and the majority hold either positive or ambivalent attitudes toward pregnancy. Up to 15% may actually be attempting pregnancy, and close to 50% believe that their partners want them to become pregnant. The result—60% of adolescents with a negative pregnancy test will become pregnant within the next 18 months.[16]

A negative pregnancy test thus provides an important point of intervention. The intervention needs to be both medical and psychosocial. Such adolescents have a higher rate of multiple partners, and screening for and counseling about sexually transmitted diseases are warranted. Effective contraception is needed; however, the provision of contraceptives alone may not be effective. Thus, the psychosocial factors that may lead the adolescent to choose pregnancy must be explored, as should barriers to effective contraceptive use (see chapter 13). Accomplishing such counseling in the midst of a busy clinical practice is no small feat. Providers working with high-risk populations will want to develop and maintain a network of school and community-based psychologists, social workers, and programs for referral of high-risk adolescents.

DIAGNOSING PREGNANCY IN THE EMERGENCY DEPARTMENT

The pregnant adolescent often presents for the first time in the emergency department, providing an opportunity for early diagnosis and referral. Unfortunately, about one-third will go undiagnosed for a variety of reasons.[13] Pregnant adolescents present to the emergency department with various complaints, not all of which suggest pregnancy. Less than one-half present with a complaint referable to the abdomen or genitourinary tract. Even when such complaints are present, sexual history, menstrual history, and pregnancy testing occasionally are overlooked by the busy clinician. The situation is particularly problematic because less than 10% of pregnant adolescents presenting to the emergency department mention the possibility of pregnancy at the time of initial triage. Only one-third reveal the possibility to the clinician, because they are either unaware of their condition or afraid to admit it. Even when asked, up to 11% deny sexual activity to the clinician. Thus, the emergency provider must have a high index of suspicion for pregnancy in all adolescent girls, regardless of the initial complaint. Retrospective reviews of adult women have found two factors to be highly associated with a positive pregnancy test in the emergency department: a late menstrual period and the patient's own suspicion that she is pregnant. This finding suggests that a menstrual and sexual history should be part of initial triage of all adolescent girls in the reproductive age group. In addition, asking the simple question "Is there any chance that you may be pregnant?," may improve significantly the chances of making the diagnosis in the emergency setting.

SCREENING FOR PREGNANCY BEFORE SURGERY AND RADIOGRAPHY

Teratogenic or abortive effects may result from use of certain anesthetic agents, preoperative medications, and radiation exposure. The best way to identify the pregnant adolescent before anesthesia or radiographic examination and whether pregnancy testing should be mandatory in such situations are controversial issues.

Depending on the institution and the age of the patient, the incidence of pregnancy among presurgical adolescent patients may be as high as 2.4%, and pregnancies have been identified in presurgical patients as young as age 12 in institutions where preoperative pregnancy testing is mandatory.[15] Other hospitals report no pregnancies identified with mandatory testing. This suggests that policies will continue to vary among institutions. At a minimum, a sexual and menstrual history should be taken in all preoperative adolescent patients, and routine pregnancy testing should be considered in institutions with high rates of sexual activity among its adolescents.

The risk to a developing pregnancy of most routinely performed diagnostic radiographs is minimal to none. In general, diagnostic radiographs delivering less than 5 rads are considered safe, and serious risk to the fetus does not occur unless the dose exceeds 10 rads. By comparison, a chest radiograph exposes the fetus to less than 10 millirads of radiation, a pelvic series to less than 50 millirads, and a barium enema to less than 1 rad. Despite the lack of effect of most commonly performed radiologic tests, it is obviously desirable to avoid unnecessary exposure. It seems prudent to screen for pregnancy by determining LMP and asking the adolescent if she suspects that she may be pregnant before diagnostic radiographs are taken.

Radiation therapy, on the other hand, poses significant risk to a developing pregnancy. In addition to pregnancy screening, adequate contraception minimizes the risk of exposing an unrecognized pregnancy to teratogenic radiation.

FOLIC ACID

Because most adolescent pregnancies are unplanned, the need for folic acid should be addressed in all sexually active adolescents. The United States Public Health Service recommends that all women of childbearing age consume 400 μg/day. This recommendation is based on research studies among women whose pregnancies were at high risk for neural tube defects (namely, women who had a previous child born with a neural tube defect). These studies showed that daily folic acid consumption before and during pregnancy led to a 71% reduction in the incidence of neural tube defects.

The daily recommended dose of folic acid can be obtained from the following dietary sources:

- ½ cup cooked dried peas, beans, or lentils
- ½ cup dry roasted peanuts, soybeans, sunflower seeds, or sesame kernels
- 1 packet of instant fortified oatmeal
- 1 medium avocado
- 1 cup fresh or frozen orange juice
- 1 cup dark, leafy green lettuce
- ½ cup cooked fresh asparagus, brussel sprouts, okra, spinach, or turnip greens (be careful: overcooking of these foods may destroy the folic acid)

Taking a daily multivitamin with 0.4 mg (400 μg) is the best way to ensure adequate doses of folic acid. Most multivitamins contain this amount.

CONCLUSION

Every clinician caring for adolescent girls will confront the diagnosis of pregnancy and its sequelae. The adolescent patient may or may not be aware of her pregnancy, and her family often is unaware of her condition. The primary care provider can make a positive difference in the outcome of the pregnancy and the psychological health of the girl and her family by handling the situation with knowledge and sensitivity. Providing information about pregnancy options and helping adolescents with decision making while being supportive and nonjudgmental are difficult and time-consuming tasks, but they are essential to ensure a healthy outcome.

ACKNOWLEDGMENT

This chapter was originally published by the authors in *Pediatric Clinics of North America*, Vol. 46, No. 4, pp 649–670, 1999, and was modified by the authors for inclusion here.

REFERENCES AND SUGGESTED READING

1. Centers for Disease Control and Prevention: State-specific birth rates for teenagers, United States, 1990–1996. MMWR 46:837–842, 1997.
2. Henshaw S: Teenage abortion and pregnancy statistics by state, 1992. Fam Plan Perspect 29:115–122, 1997.
3. Yordan EE, Yordan RA: An overview of adolescent pregnancy. J Pediatr Adolesc Gynecol 9:111–118, 1996.
4. Bastian LA, Piscitelli JT: Is this patient pregnant? Can you reliably rule in or rule out early pregnancy by physical exam? JAMA 278:586–591, 1997.
5. Lobo R, Mishell DR, Davajan V: Endocrinology of pregnancy. In Mishell's Textbook of Infertility, Contraception and Reproductive Endocrinology, 4th ed. Boston, Blackwell Science, 1997, pp 185–190.
6. Fossum GT, Davajan V, Kletsky OA: Early detection of pregnancy with transvaginal ultrasound. Fertil Steril 49:788–791, 1988.
7. Hatcher RA, et al: Pregnancy testing and management of early pregnancy. In Contraceptive Technology, 16th ed. New York, Irvington, 1994, pp 453–471.
8. Wilcox AJ, Weinberg CR, O'Connor JF, et al: Incidence of early loss of pregnancy. New Engl J Med 319:189–194, 1988.
9. Speroff L, Glass RH, Kase NG: Ectopic pregnancy. In Clinical Gynecologic Endocrinology and Infertility, 5th ed. Baltimore, Williams & Wilkins, 1994, pp 947–967.
10. McCord ML, Muram D, Lipscomb GH, et al: Methotrexate therapy for ectopic pregnancy in adolescents. J Pediatr Adolesc Gynecol 9:71–73, 1996.
11. Bayatpur MM, Reyes J: Gestational trophoblastic disease among adolescents. Adolesc Gynecol 6:220–222, 1993.
12. Stephenson JN: Pregnancy testing and counseling. Pediatr Clin North Am 36:681–695, 1989.
13. Causey AL, Serago K, Wahl NG, Voelker CL: Pregnant adolescents in the emergency department: Diagnosed and not diagnosed. Am J Emerg Med 15:125–129, 1997.
14. Ramoska EA, Sacchett AD, Nepp M: Reliability of patient history in determining the possibility of pregnancy. Ann Emerg Med 18:48–50, 1989.
15. Malviya S, D'Errico C, Reynolds P, et al: Should pregnancy testing be routine in adolescent patients prior to surgery? Anesth Analg 83:854–858, 1996.
16. Kempen PM, Norton P, Vu H: A risk index for pregnancy during anesthesia. J Clin Anesth 9:194–199, 1997.
17. Zabin LS, Sedivy V, Emerson MR: Subsequent risk of childbearing among adolescents with a negative pregnancy test. Fam Plann Perspect 26:212–217, 1994.

CHAPTER 24

Abortion

Melanie A. Gold, D.O.

Each year, one million American adolescent girls become pregnant, and 85% of their pregnancies are unintended. Many chose abortion as a way to resolve the pregnancy. The incidence of abortion is reported in three ways:

1. The abortion *percentage* is the total number of abortions obtained by women in different demographic categories (e.g., age, marital status, race, parity) and expressed as the percentage of all abortions performed that year.
2. The abortion *rate* for any given year is calculated by the total number of abortions per 1,000 women in the population.
3. The abortion *ratio* is expressed as the number of abortions compared with the total number of live births in any given period.

Young women between the ages of 11 and 19 account for 20% of all abortions; women aged 20–24 years account for another 32%.[1] Girls under 15 years of age account for fewer than 1% of all abortions. Older adolescents and young adult women have the highest abortion rates, whereas younger adolescents and women over 35 have the lowest rates.

In 1992, 112 pregnancies occurred per 1,000 U.S. women aged 15–19 years; of these, 61 ended in births, 36 in abortion, and 15 in miscarriage. Rates of pregnancy, birth, and abortion are 2–3 times higher in African-American adolescents than in white adolescents.[2] Among all adolescents 15–19 years of age, the birth rate rose 12 points between 1987 and 1991 but decreased somewhat in the latter half of the 1990s.

Abortion ratios are highest for adolescents under 19 years of age and for women aged 40 years or older. Among adolescents, the abortion ratio is highest for those younger than 15 (more pregnancies end in abortion) and lowest for 19-year-old women (more pregnancies end in live births). In the 1990s, the abortion ratio decreased for women aged 15–19 years.

Over one-half of the reported legal abortions are obtained at 8 weeks or less of gestation. Most women (88%) obtain abortions during the first 12 weeks of pregnancy. However, adolescents younger than 19 are more likely than older women to obtain abortions later in pregnancy (Table 1). Fewer than 1% of all abortions occur after 21 weeks' gestation, and almost all of these are completed before 23 weeks. Seventy-eight percent of all women obtaining abortions are unmarried, and 43% have no living children.[1] The majority (99%) of

TABLE 1. Reported Legal Abortions by Weeks of Gestation and Age, United States, 1996

	All Women		Women ≥ 20 yr old		Women < 20 yr old	
Gestation	*Number*	%	*Number*	%	*Number*	%
8 wk or less	347,024	55	289,414	57	57,310	45
9–10 wk	142,828	22	111,846	24	30,982	24
11–12 wk	62,248	11	51,557	23	17,691	14
13–16 wk	38,061	6	27,329	10	10,732	8
16–20 wk	27,942	4	19,783	5	8,159	6
≥ 21 wk	10,094	2	6,735	1	3,359	3
TOTAL	635,197	100	506,664	100	128,233	100

Adapted from Centers for Disease Control and Prevention: Abortion surveillance—United States, 1996. MMWR 48:1–42, 1999.

legal abortions are performed by curettage; fewer than 1% are performed by intrauterine injection of saline or prostaglandin. One-half of all abortions occur among women who do not use any form of contraception. Adolescents are less likely to use effective contraception than older women, particularly within the first 6 months after coitarche (see chapter 13).

ATTITUDES TOWARD ABORTION

Adolescents' attitudes toward abortion are correlated with a number of demographic variables. The most consistent and strongest correlate is with religious identification and participation. Affiliation with Catholic or fundamentalist churches that espouse antiabortion ideology is associated with increased opposition to abortion. Likewise, frequent attendance at religious services, which is a proxy for religiosity, has been found to be associated with increased opposition to abortion. Socioeconomic status also has been correlated with abortion attitudes. People from poor socioeconomic backgrounds are less likely to support pro-choice attitudes than those from middle- and upper-class backgrounds. In addition, the higher the level of education, the more likely a person is to approve of abortion. Lastly, family-related beliefs are strongly correlated with abortion attitudes. People with more traditional or conservative views, such as opposition to premarital sex or divorce, are more likely to oppose abortion. A study by Gondor found that college students' decisions about abortions for girls under 18 are based predominantly on personal values (96%) and the influences of parents (50%), friends (45%), family members (33%), and religious beliefs (36%).[3] Fewer college students acknowledged the influence of health care providers (18%), media (18%), or teachers (14%).

A study of the abortion attitudes of adolescent males found that 13% of 15–19-year-old males approved of abortion under all 8 of the hypothetical situations presented to them, whereas 14% disapproved in every case.[4] Eighty-five to 90% approved of abortion when the pregnancy endangered the woman's health or was the result of a rape. The young men were more accepting of abortions for health reasons than for social or economic reasons. Males living in wealthier social environments were twice as likely as their poorer counterparts to approve of abortion. Respondents who placed greater importance on religion were more likely to disapprove of abortion.

Despite the demonstrated safety of legal abortion and more than 30 years of experience with the procedure, adolescents still believe that abortion is unsafe. In a study conducted in 1975, 20% of adolescents thought that legal first-trimester abortion was unsafe and 13% thought that having an abortion would make them sterile.[5] A study conducted in 1996 found that 32% of adolescent girls thought that abortion was unsafe.[6] Almost three-quarters (72%) of these inner-city adolescents believed that having an abortion might impair future fertility. A 1992 focus-group study of adolescents from across the U.S. revealed that young people have inaccurate knowledge about abortion and the laws governing it.[7] The adolescents expressed erroneous beliefs based on anecdotal evidence about abortion and portrayed the procedure as medically dangerous and emotionally damaging. One participant had "heard" that having three or more abortions could lead to sterility, and other adolescents suggested that even one abortion could cause infertility. Despite the degree of geographic diversity of the sample, the adolescents' views were surprisingly homogeneous. Four major themes arose from the focus groups:

1. Negative attitudes toward abortion were balanced by support for choice. Although most adolescents were personally opposed to abortion, they supported continued legality of abortion and felt that women should have the ability to make a choice.

2. They had negative attitudes toward mandatory parental notification and consent laws.

3 Most expressed incorrect beliefs that abortion is medically dangerous and predominantly illegal, despite the reality of extremely low mortality and morbidity rates and the passage of laws legalizing abortion in the 1970s.

4. The primary sources of adolescents' attitudes toward abortion were from anti-abortion views, conservative morality, and religion.

BARRIERS TO ABORTION

There are numerous barriers to abortion. Examples include distance from facilities providing abortion, gestation limitations, costs, and harassment.[8] Among women who obtained outpatient abortions, 16% traveled 50–100 miles from their homes, and 8% traveled more than 100 miles to the abortion facility. Travel distance is a particular barrier for adolescents, who often do not have their own means of transportation or the funds to take public transportation to a far-away town. As gestational weeks increase, fewer providers are available to perform abortions. Although 98% of providers will perform abortions at 8 weeks of gestation, only 48% will perform abortions at 13 weeks and only 13% will provide abortion services at 21 weeks. This trend forms a particular barrier for adolescents, who often delay seeking abortions. Most abortion facilities set both upper and lower gestational age limits for performing abortions. The most common lower gestational age limit is 6 weeks from the last menstrual period because surgical abortion at an earlier point was perceived to increase the likelihood of complications and because the small size of the embryo makes it difficult to be sure that the pregnancy has been terminated. With the availability of medical abortion methods and manual vacuum aspiration techniques, pregnancies can be safely terminated before 6 weeks' gestation.

Appointment availability and cost are other potential barriers. One-half of outpatient facilities estimate that more than 4 days elapsed from the time a woman contacts the facility until she can obtain her abortion; more than 13% say that more than 1 week elapsed. Difficulty obtaining an abortion can further delay the procedure and thus increase the cost. The large majority of abortions are paid for directly by the patient rather than by insurance. One-third of all women do not have insurance, and even fewer adolescents are insured. Many insurance companies do not include abortion service coverage, and, except in states such as New York and California, medical assistance does not cover fees for abortion-related services. Most states prohibit the use of public medical assistance funds to cover the cost of the abortion procedure; thus, low-income adolescents and young women may have limited access to abortion services. Finally, even women whose insurance covers abortion services may not have met the required deductible, or they may not want to use their insurance because of concerns about confidentiality and stigma. The average cost of a first-trimester abortion with local anesthesia in an outpatient facility is $300–$400, excluding other expenses such as travel, time missed from work, and additional medical services such as ultrasonography.[8] The cost increases sharply with gestations longer than 12 weeks. The average charge for an abortion at 16 weeks is approximately $600; at 20 weeks the average charge is over $1000. The majority of abortions are performed in outpatient facilities, but when they are performed in a hospital, the charges are six times higher. Costs are significantly higher if a patient wishes general anesthesia.

Another barrier facing young women seeking abortion services is harassment by antiabortion protesters. Violence aimed at abortion facilities and providers creates several barriers. Patients are fearful of walking through crowds of antiabortion picketers outside abortion facilities, and abortion providers are fearful of violence aimed at themselves and their families. In the U.S., there is a physician shortage—84% of the counties have no abortion providers. The reasons for inadequate abortion providers are a combination of poor access to abortion training and fear of antiabortion violence. Many obstetric/gynecologic residencies have not required training in first- or second-trimester abortion techniques, and several generations of obstetrician/ gynecologists lack adequate experience or training in abortion procedures. However, in January 1996 the Accreditation Council for Graduate Medical Education (ACGME) required obstetric/gynecologic residencies to train their residents in abortion techniques unless students have moral or religious objections. Abortion providers see harassment and other expressions of antiabortion sentiment as major problems that affect their ability to perform abortion, and many physicians who otherwise might perform abortions fail to do so because of fear of community backlash and targeting of their general obstetric practices by antiabortion groups.

Fear about the impact of an abortion on future fertility and concern about increased cancer risks, particularly breast and ovarian cancer, are also patient barriers to abortion. Antiabortion propaganda has widely disseminated the myth that having an abortion will damage a woman's future fertility. The link between history of an abortion and higher prevalence of breast cancer is still debated in the medical literature. Many women are unaware of the significant health risks associated with pregnancy and delivery in contrast to the lower morbidity and mortality rates associated with a first-trimester abortion.

Waiting periods are yet another barrier facing women who seek an abortion. Many states enforce a mandatory 24-hour waiting period. Such laws require that a woman must wait a minimum of 24 hours from the time she is counseled about having an abortion before she can undergo the procedure. Other states have shorter delays of 1–8 hours. These laws impose added impediments to obtaining abortion for adolescent and young women who live a far distance from an abortion facility or do not have their own means of transportation.[9] Every health care provider of sexually active adolescents should be aware of state laws regarding mandatory waiting periods.

Adolescents under the age of majority (18 years) face unique barriers to obtaining an abortion. Many states restrict a minor's access to abortion by requiring single or dual parental notification and/or consent. Over one-half of the states in the U.S. mandate some kind of parental involvement in a minor's abortion decision. Only two states, Connecticut and Maine, and the District of Columbia have laws that affirm a minor's ability to obtain an abortion on her own consent. Parental notification laws require medical personnel to notify a minor's parents of her intention to obtain an abortion, whereas parental consent laws require medical personnel to obtain written permission from one or both parents before performing the abortion. Laws vary greatly from state to state and change frequently. Table 2 shows the current laws regarding minor parental consent and notification.

As of 1995, 26 states had laws mandating at least one parent's involvement in a girl's abortion decision.[10] In 16 of these states, a girl must have the consent of one or both parents; in the other 10, one or both parents must be notified of the girl's plan to obtain an abortion. All states with parental notification or consent laws must provide an alternative court-bypass system in which a judge can authorize the abortion if he or she determines that the minor is mature enough to make the decision by herself. If the judge finds the girl too immature to make the decision, the judge can still authorize the abortion if he or she deems that it is in the girl's best interest. Some states allow a physician to waive parental involvement, and some allow professional counseling instead of parental involvement. Although the court-bypass system appears to be a reasonable alternative, few adolescents know about it or are resourceful enough to negotiate the judicial system without adult assistance. The adolescent who uses judicial bypass must not only face a judge but also work her way through a confusing legal system and repeatedly answer potentially judgmental questions by strangers. Generally, it is the youngest, poorest, and least educated adolescents who are the least able to use judicial bypass; thus, they are most likely to end up either becoming teen parents or turning to illegal, unsafe abortions.

Restrictive laws such as parental notification or consent often create delays in seeking prompt medical care; consequently, even if an adolescent does ultimately obtain an abortion, she may delay seeking care until after the 8th week of gestation, thus incurring a higher risk of complications and higher costs.[11] In Minnesota parental notification laws have been found to be associated with a

TABLE 2. Parental Involvement in a Minor's Abortion Decision Laws by State, 1997

State	Parent Consent	Parent Notification
Alabama	X	
Arkansas		X, dual parent notification
Delaware		X, notice to grandparent or mental health professional
Georgia		X
Idaho		X, dual parent notification, no judicial bypass
Indiana	X	
Iowa		X, notice to grandparent
Kansas		X
Kentucky	X	
Louisiana	X	
Maryland		X, physician may waive
Massachusetts	X	
Michigan	X	
Minnesota		X, dual parent notification
Mississippi	X	
Missouri	X	
Montana		X
Nebraska		X
North Carolina	X, may be given by grandparent	
North Dakota	X, dual parent consent	
Ohio		X, notice to grandparent, stepparent, adult sibling
Pennsylvania	X	
Rhode Island	X	
South Carolina	X, may be given by grandparent	
South Dakota		X
Utah		X, dual parent notification, no judicial bypass
Virginia		X
West Virginia		X, second physician may waive
Wisconsin	X, by another adult over age 25	
Wyoming	X	

No parent involvement laws: Alaska, Arizona, California, Colorado, Florida, Hawaii, Illinois, Nevada, New Hampshire, New Jersey, New Mexico, New York, Oklahoma, Oregon, Tennessee, Texas, Vermont, Washington

Minor consent laws affirming minor's ability to consent to abortion: Connecticut, District of Columbia, Maine

Adapted from Frost JJ: Family Planning Clinic Services in the United States, 1994, Family Planning Perspectives 28:98, 1996; The Alan Guttmacher Institute: The lawmakers grapple with parent's role in teen access to reproductive health care, Issues in Brief, Washington, DC, 1995; and Donovan P: State Reproductive Health Monitor, issue of September 1997.

decrease in pregnancies, but minors also were found to have a greater proportion of abortions in the second trimester as compared with earlier abortions after institution of the laws.[12] In Massachusetts, parental notification laws had a minimal effect on the numbers of births and abortions but were associated with a significant increase in the number of out-of-state abortions.[13] In Mississippi, after institution of a parental consent requirement in 1993, the ratio of minors to adults who sought abortion in the state declined by 13%, a decrease offset by a 32% increase in the ratio of minors to adults who obtained abortions out of state. There was also a 28% drop in out-of-state minors who came to Mississippi for abortions. Current legislation for a "Teen Endangerment Act" was passed by the U.S. House of Representatives and awaits Senate vote. The legislation would criminalize anyone—including ministers, grandparents, and siblings—for helping a teenager cross state lines to obtain an abortion. This poses a further barrier for teenagers seeking abortions. After institution of the parental consent requirement, the ratio of minors to adults who obtained abortions after 12 weeks' gestation increased by 19%. Thus, parental consent laws do not seem to decrease abortions in minors but do increase out-of-state abortions and delay abortion services, thus increasing the risk of complications.[14]

The presumed purpose of parental notification and consent laws is to improve parent–child communication about abortion decision making. Abortion providers encourage adolescents to discuss with parents or other important family members their plans to obtain an abortion, and 61% of adolescents discuss their abortion decision with parents even without state requirements to do so.[11] The younger the adolescent, the more likely she is to have discussed her abortion plans with her mother. Adolescents who choose not to inform their parents about their abortion decision often do so because of a family history of substance abuse or emotional, physical, or sexual abuse. For such adolescents, forcibly involving the parents may result in further abuse or deterioration of the parent–child relationship. Rather than inform parents, some adolescents resort to unsafe, illegal abortions or attempt to perform the abortion themselves. In doing so they risk serious injury or death and, in some states, criminal charges.

ABORTION METHODS

First Trimester

A pregnancy of shorter duration than 13 weeks since the last menstrual period is considered the first trimester. The standard method for abortion is a surgical technique called vacuum aspiration or suction curettage. This method is performed most frequently in an outpatient setting—a doctor's office or clinic. Generally, a local anesthetic is used in the form of a paracervical block to numb the cervix; however, some women prefer general anesthesia, although its use increases the risks of the abortion procedure.

Second Trimester

Terminating a pregnancy after the 13th week is a more complicated procedure because of the larger fetus and the greater blood supply to the placenta and uterus. There are two main methods of abortion in the second trimester: dilatation and evacuation (D&E) and induction methods in which labor is artificially induced by instilling medication into the uterus. Although many second-trimester abortions are performed in an outpatient setting, both methods are occasionally performed in a hospital, particularly after the 20th week. More than one-third of all abortions after 12 weeks are obtained by adolescent girls.

MEDICAL METHODS

In the 1990s, two medical modalities of inducing therapeutic abortion have emerged. One method entails oral administration of an antiprogesterone (mifepristone [RU486]), followed by administration of a prostaglandin, usually misoprostol, by either the vaginal or oral route. The other method involves an injection of methotrexate, a cytotoxic, folic acid antagonist, followed by administration of a prostaglandin (misoprostol) by either the oral or vaginal route. Both regimens have been shown to be 90– 95% effective and are safe for termination of pregnancies up to 7 weeks' gestation.[15–17] Although not currently approved by the Food and Drug Administration (FDA) for use as an abortifacient, methotrexate has had FDA approval for other uses for decades. Mifepristone is used widely in several European countries and is currently under investigation by the FDA for use in first-trimester abortions. Mifepristone in combination with a prostaglandin has been used by almost 200,000 women in Europe for early termination of pregnancy. Mifepristone blocks the action of progesterone, which is necessary to sustain the pregnancy. Mifepristone softens and opens the cervix, thins the uterine lining, and primes the uterus to respond to the prostaglandin with contractions.

The mifepristone-misoprostol method can be used successfully up to 49 days from the beginning of the last menstrual period. Ultrasonography is frequently used to confirm gestational size because efficacy decreases after 7 weeks of pregnancy. Three visits are required for the mifepristone regimen. At the first visit the woman receives a medical history, physical exam, and lab tests to rule out anemia and thrombocytopenia and to detect Rh factor. Informed consent is obtained, and if the woman is eligible, she takes 600 mg of mifepristone orally. Two days later an ultrasound is performed to determine if the pregnancy is still intact because a small percentage of women abort with mifepristone alone. If the woman is still pregnant, she takes 800 μg of misoprostol in the form of two tablets by mouth or intravaginally and is observed in the clinic for 4 hours.

Sixty-six percent of women have an abortion within 4 hours of taking the misoprostol, and 80–88% have an abortion within 24 hours. Twelve days after the misoprostol is taken, the woman is examined to ensure that the pregnancy has aborted. Within 14 days of treatment, 95–97% of women have a complete abortion. Two to 4% of women have an incomplete abortion, and 1% have an ongoing pregnancy. If the medical abortion is not complete by the 14th day, the woman is strongly advised to obtain a surgical abortion. Mifepristone has few side effects. The most common side effects are due to prostaglandin and include vaginal bleeding, cramping, nausea, vomiting, and diarrhea. The average number of days of bleeding is 8–9 compared with the shorter duration of 5 days with a surgical abortion. Women may see passage of fetal tissue, which to some is distressing.

For the methotrexate regimen, after the woman receives a medical history, physical exam, and lab tests confirming pregnancy, blood type, and Rh type, an injection of 50 mg/m^2 of methotrexate is administered intramuscularly, often in the deltoid or gluteus muscle. Five to 7 days after the injection, 800 μg of misoprostol is given either orally or intravaginally. With this regimen 90–95% of women abort within 2 weeks. The duration of bleeding after a methotrexate-misoprostol abortion is longer than after a mifepristone-misoprostol abortion and can last up to 4–6 weeks.

SURGICAL ABORTION METHODS

Menstrual Extraction

The term *menstrual extraction* designates the evacuation of the contents of the uterus or extraction of the endometrial lining before the diagnosis of pregnancy is established by laboratory test or physical examination. This procedure is conducted early in pregnancy (4–6 weeks' gestational age) and entails inserting a soft, small-bore catheter, called a Karmen cannula, through the cervical os into the uterus, attaching it to a 60-ml syringe, and manually aspirating the uterine contents. The procedure was used more commonly before the development of sensitive pregnancy tests and was called menstrual regulation because it removes the endometrial lining before a missed menses. The procedure had fallen out of favor because many women had unnecessary menstrual extractions when they were not pregnant. However, with current highly sensitive urine pregnancy testing, patients can be selected more appropriately. Concern about missed or incomplete abortion and retained tissue has caused many physicians to refrain from offering early surgical abortion. However, research indicates that vacuum aspiration is safe and effective before 6 weeks' gestation when a protocol including highly sensitive urine hCG assays, high-resolution pre- and postoperative ultrasonography and careful on-site tissue inspection is followed.

Aspiration and Curettage

More than 99% of abortions performed at 12 weeks or less of gestation are performed by suction aspiration followed by curettage.[1] The standard D&C or suction aspiration method is performed in two stages. Dilatation is performed either mechanically or with osmotic dilators. After administration of local anesthesia or after the woman is asleep under general anesthesia, the cervix is dilated over several minutes by inserting and removing rods or dilators of progressively larger diameters. The more gradual method of dilating the cervix is to insert sterile, absorbent short-fiber rods made of synthetic material or seaweed. The rods are left in the cervix over several hours to overnight. The rods slowly absorb moisture from the cervix and enlarge the cervical os, allowing greater dilatation than with mechanical methods. Because the osmotic dilators expand slowly, they allow more dilatation with reduced likelihood of tearing the cervix.

When osmotic dilators are used, they generally require two visits to the clinic or office for completion of the abortion procedure. After the cervix is dilated by mechanical or osmotic methods, the physician inserts a cannula that is attached to an aspiration machine. The mild suction of the machine empties the contents of the uterus as the cannula is gently rotated. Then the walls of the uterus are checked for residual fragments or remnants with a curette. The entire procedure takes about 10 minutes. Some women experience menstrual-type cramping during the procedure and often experience menstrual-like bleeding for several days after the procedure.

Dilatation and Evacuation

After 12 weeks' gestation, the most frequently used procedure is curettage, which usually is reported as dilatation and evacuation (D&E). The D&E procedure is an expansion of the vacuum aspiration procedure. However, the cervix requires far greater dilatation to allow passage of the fetal tissue. The cervix is generally dilated with osmotic dilators, which may take a few hours to two days to dilate the cervical os completely. Full os dilatation is crucial to avoid cervical laceration or tearing. After dilatation, the physician uses a large-bore cannula similar to that used in the first-trimester vacuum aspiration procedure to suction out the contents of conception. The tissue forceps are used to grasp and remove fetal parts that are too large to be suctioned. Once the uterus is emptied, the uterine walls are checked with a curette to determine that the abortion is complete and that no fetal or placental tissue remains. The procedure can take up to 30 minutes to complete and frequently is performed under general anesthesia.

Amnioinfusion

Fewer than 2% of all abortions in the U.S. are performed by the instillation method, and nearly all of them are performed in the hospital. Approximately one-half of intrauterine instillations involve saline and are performed at 16 weeks' gestation or greater. The physician anesthetizes the skin of the abdomen with local anesthetic and passes a needle into the amniotic sac in the uterus. Medications are injected or instilled into the amniotic sac to induce contractions. Medications include prostaglandin, urea, saline, or a combination regimen. Sometimes prostaglandin gel is also used intravaginally to assist in ripening and softening of the cervix. After several hours of induced labor, the patient expels the fetus vaginally.

Mechanical Stimulation and Hysterotomy

Mechanical stimulation is one of the oldest abortion techniques. A catheter or bougie is inserted into the cervical os to stimulate an abortion. The method is still used in Japan in combination with other methods, such as laminaria and resorcinol, but it is rarely used in the U.S. Hysterotomy, a procedure in which the fetus is surgically incised for manual removal, is rarely performed because of the high morbidity rate.

Intact Dilatation and Extraction

The controversial and widely publicized "partial birth abortion" procedure is an inflammatory term not recognized by the medical community and does not refer to a specific, medically defined method of abortion. The terminology of the proposed bill banning the procedure refers to an intact dilation and extraction (D&X) procedure. The D&X is a variation of a D&E in which the cervix is dilated and the fetus is removed intact by breach delivery after partial evacuation of intracranial contents to allow delivery of the head. This procedure is generally performed after 19 weeks' gestation but may be indicated at any time after 16 weeks. It has been argued that the intact D&X procedure is safer for the pregnant woman than a D&E. The danger of the proposed bill banning the procedure is its vague terminology, which could be applied to all forms of D&E, which is currently the most common abortion method used in the second trimester. The American College of Obstetricians and Gynecologists (ACOG) has opposed the bill.

COMPLICATIONS

Generally, the earlier an abortion is performed, the less complicated and safer it is. The safest time to have a surgical abortion is between 6 and 10 weeks from the last menstrual period. Of women who obtain abortions before 13 weeks' gestation, 2.5% have a minor complication that can be handled in an outpatient facility; fewer than 0.5% require hospitalization or surgical intervention. Complication rates are higher for abortions between 13 and 24 weeks. General anesthesia is an added risk factor for complications. Other factors that affect complication rates are the skill and training of the provider, the type of anesthesia, the woman's overall health, and the abortion method.

A vasovagal response during or immediately after completion of the abortion procedure is not uncommon. Women may experience diaphoresis, bradycardia, and hypotension, but symptoms usually respond quickly to reverse Trendelenburg position and oral fluids.

A missed abortion occurs when the abortion procedure does not terminate the pregnancy. Missed abortion occurs in less than 0.5% of cases and is more common when the abortion procedure is conducted less than 6 weeks from the last menstrual period. The treatment for missed abortion is to repeat the procedure.

Another possible complication from surgical abortion is accumulation of blood clots in the uterus, which requires another suction procedure for removal. Retention of blood clots occurs in less than 1% of cases, whereas retained tissue, called an incomplete abortion, occurs in less than 0.5% of cases. When tissue remains in the uterus, repeat suctioning is also required.

In less than 3% of cases an infection occurs after the procedure. The majority of postabortal pathogens are preexisting sexually transmitted organisms, such as *Neisseria gonorrhoeae* and *Chlamydia trachomatis*, rather than skin pathogens that have contaminated surgical instruments. All adolescents should be screened for asymptomatic cervical infection with sexually transmitted organisms before abortion and, if necessary, treated. Postabortal infections respond well to current broad-spectrum antibiotics.

In less than 1% of cases, a tear of the cervix may require suturing. Cervical tears or lacerations occur less commonly when cervical dilatation is achieved with osmotic dilators. Perforation of the uterus with associated bowel injury occurs in less than 0.5% of cases. Intervention depends on the extent of the injury. Minor or small perforations of the uterus alone may heal without surgical intervention, whereas larger tears or injury to bowel, bladder, or ureters require surgery and, in rare cases, hysterectomy.

Postabortal syndrome (uterine hypotonia) occurs in less than 1% of cases. It is caused by excessive bleeding into the uterus because the uterus fails to contract normally. In rare cases, uterine hypotonia requires blood transfusion. Cervical stenosis may result from excessive cervical dilatation or cervical trauma and usually presents as postabortion amenorrhea. Cervical stenosis is treated with cervical dilatation using a uterine sound or small Pratt dilator.

Signs of postabortion complications include severe pain; chills or a temperature of 100.4°F or greater; bleeding that is heavier than a normal period or soaks through more than one sanitary napkin pad an hour; passage of clots that are larger than a quarter; foul-smelling discharge or drainage; and continuing symptoms of pregnancy. Complications from amnioinfusion are related to difficulties in accurate placement of the instillation needle, adverse physiologic reaction to maternal absorption of the instillate, incomplete emptying of the uterus, and uterine trauma from uncontrolled contractions.

SAFETY AND RISKS

Abortion is one of the most common surgical procedures performed in the United States; it is also one of the safest. Induced abortion has one-half the mortality risk of a tonsillectomy and one one-hundredth the mortality risk of an appendectomy. The risk of death from pregnancy and childbirth is 16 times greater than the risk of death from abortion. Not surprisingly, general anesthesia makes the abortion procedure significantly riskier. There is a 2–4-fold greater risk of death associated with general anesthesia than with local anesthesia.[18] General anesthesia also doubles the risk of uterine perforation and cervical laceration compared with local anesthesia. The risk of hemorrhage requiring blood transfusion and intraabdominal hemorrhage requiring surgery is also more common when abortion is performed under general as opposed to local anesthesia. However, patients whose abortions are performed under local anesthesia are more likely to have mild complications such as postoperative fever.[19] Eighteen possible abortion-related deaths were reported in the U.S. in 1990, of which 10 proved to be abortion-related (five were associated with legal abortion and five with spontaneous abortion).[1]

PSYCHOLOGICAL IMPACT

Severe psychological or psychiatric disturbances after abortion occur in a minority of women and usually consist of depression and/or anxiety. Psychosis is rare (reported in only 0.003% of cases).[20] The most common emotional response after an abortion is relief. Psychological distress tends to be greatest before rather than after an abortion. Anxiety, depression, anger, guilt, and shame are significantly less 6 months after the abortion compared with the preabortion period. Women at the highest risk for postabortion adjustment problems are single or nulliparous, have a history of serious emotional problems or conflictual relationships with sexual partners, lack social support for their decision, or have strong ambivalence toward abortions.[21] Women with negative religious or cultural attitudes toward abortion also are more likely to experience increased conflict than women with positive attitudes.

PRACTICAL MEASURES FOR THE PRIMARY CARE PROVIDER

Preabortion Visit

Pregnancy is diagnosed by a positive human chorionic gonadotropin (hCG) level in urine or serum, enlargement of the uterus on bimanual examination, and visualization of a gestational sac or fetus by ultrasound. When pregnancy is diagnosed by the primary care provider, the adolescent should be counseled about pregnancy options. It is common for an adolescent to be unsure of her decision about pregnancy outcome. It is often helpful to refer her to a social worker or counselor to review in depth her circumstances and feelings surrounding different choices. The health care provider should review the three pregnancy options: termination, continuation, and keeping the infant or placing it in adoption services after delivery. If the patient chooses to continue her pregnancy and if the primary care provider does not provide prenatal care, the patient should be referred as soon as possible to an obstetrician for prenatal care and screening for sexually transmitted infections (STIs). However, if the patient is unsure or considering an abortion, preabortion screening for STIs should be performed. In addition, wet mount to rule out bacterial vaginosis should be done. If an annual Papanicolaou smear has not been collected, one should be done so that results are available at the postabortion visit.

Depending on the date of the last menstrual period and uterine size by palpation, the physician should counsel the patient about what to expect from the abortion procedure and select the best site for referral. If the patient is obese or the uterine size is unclear, it is often helpful to obtain an ultrasound to confirm gestation age before referral for an abortion. For patients with medical assistance, the cost of an ultrasound obtained as part of an abortion is not covered by medical assistance. However, if the patient is sent for an ultrasound to confirm gestational size before deciding on abortion vs. prenatal care, medical assistance covers the cost. The purposes of preabortion counseling are to reduce anxiety, to provide information about the abortion procedure, and to screen for underlying psychopathology that may contribute to poor emotional outcome. Additional goals should be to help the young woman understand and cope with her feelings and to help prevent future unintended pregnancies. Table 3 is an example of a postabortion instruction sheet that may be given to patients before they undergo abortion.

TABLE 3. Postabortion Instructions for Patients

What to do:
Rest
Eat good food
Drink plenty of fluids
Check your temperature twice daily for 1 week, then once daily for 1 week

What to expect:
Bleeding similar to a normal period lasting no longer than 3 weeks
Mild cramping similar to menstrual cramps

For 2 weeks after the abortion *do not*:
Take tub baths (showers are okay)
Use tampons (use sanitary pads only)
Douche
Have sexual intercourse
Go swimming
Participate in strenuous activity, such as heavy lifting or running

Call the place where you had your abortion if you have any of the following:
Temperature more than 100.4°F for more than 8 hours
Bleeding that is heavier than a normal period
Bleeding for more than 4 weeks
Passing large blood clots
Severe cramps
Severe, persistent abdominal pain
Feeling faint or dizzy

Office Postabortion Follow-Up

Many patients prefer to have their postabortion follow-up visit with their usual primary care provider. When the abortion procedure is uneventful and the patient experiences no interim complications (e.g., excessive bleeding or clotting, pain, fever), it is appropriate and even advisable for the postabortion check-up to be performed by the primary care provider. The postabortion check up is best scheduled within 2–3 weeks after the procedure. The main purposes of the check-up are to ensure that the abortion was successful (e.g., the patient is no longer pregnant), that there are no intercurrent infections, that the patient has recovered both emotionally and physically from the procedure, and that she has chosen a contraceptive plan for the future.

The postabortion check-up begins with an interim history, including severity and duration of pain and need for analgesia, bleeding severity and duration, clot size, history of fever, experience of sexual intercourse since the procedure, and, if applicable, type of contraception used. The physical exam should include examination of the breasts for masses, tenderness, and galactorrhea; abdominal exam for masses and tenderness; and a gynecologic exam. A speculum exam should include examination of the vagina for any abnormal discharge and visualization of the external cervical os for closure. A wet mount examination of vaginal discharge is helpful to rule out bacterial vaginosis or other infections that can occur after instrumentation of the cervix and destruction of normal lactobacilli by antiseptic swabbing of the vagina before the abortion. A bimanual exam should be done to confirm that the uterus is small, firm, and nontender and that it has involuted and returned to its usual intrapelvic position. A highly sensitive pregnancy test that detects 50 mIU hCG or less will remain positive for up to 4 weeks after the procedure and thus cannot be used at the 2-week follow-up as confirmation that the abortion was successful. A less sensitive pregnancy test, such as a slide agglutination-antibody test, which detects 1,000 mIU or more of hCG, can confirm successful termination of pregnancy, or the patient can return in 2–3 weeks for a standard urine hCG test as long as her uterus is small and firm on bimanual exam.

Postabortion Contraception

Because ovulation may occur as early as 2–3 weeks after the abortion, it is important to begin discussing contraceptive choices at the preabortion counseling visit and to ensure that the young woman has ample information about available contraceptive methods from which to choose a postabortal contraceptive plan. Condom use always should be recommended, and concomitant use of a spermicide should be advised if no other hormonal or barrier method is selected. Oral contraceptive pills can be started the day of or the day after a first-trimester abortion procedure. However, if the abortion is obtained in the second trimester, it is often recommended to delay initiation of oral contraceptives for 3–6 weeks to decrease the risk of hypercoagulability and thromboembolism. Depo-Provera is a frequently chosen method and can be administered on the day of procedure. However, it is important to counsel the patient to expect menstrual alterations, which may be difficult to distinguish from bleeding from retained products. If a patient has medical contraindications to estrogens and wishes to use an oral method, progestin-only pills can be started on the day of both a first- or second-trimester abortion.

A diaphragm is infrequently used by adolescents or young women, but if it is the chosen method of contraception, it must be refitted 1 month after an abortion performed in the second trimester. Diaphragms do not require refitting after a first-trimester abortion. Intrauterine devices (IUDs) are infrequently recommended for use by young women, but if this method is deemed appropriate, the IUD can be inserted at 2 weeks after a first-trimester abortion or 4 weeks after a second-trimester abortion. Because many adolescents and young women choose to be abstinent after an abortion and may have unanticipated unprotected intercourse, it is important to discuss the availability of emergency contraceptive pills (ECPs). All patients should be given information about ECPs after their abortion. In addition to failed abstinence, condoms break, pills are forgotten, diaphragms slip, and subsequent Depo-Provera shots are missed.

CONCLUSION

Primary care providers for sexually active female adolescents should be knowledgeable about the abortion-related laws in their state. Abortion is safest when performed early by well-trained and experienced providers. Patients who are counseled fully about the procedure and receive thorough contraceptive counseling after their abortion can decrease the risk of future unintended pregnancies.

National Abortion Federation (NAF), 1755 Massachusetts Avenue NW, Suite 600, Washington, DC 20036, phone (202) 667–5881, toll-free hotline 1-800-772-9100, www.prochoice.org.

REFERENCES AND SUGGESTED READING

1. Centers for Disease Control and Prevention: Abortion surveillance—United States, 1992. MMWR 48:1–42, 1999.
2. Henshaw SK: Teenage abortion and pregnancy statistics by state, 1992. Fam Plann Perspect 29:115–122, 1997.
3. Gondor M, Cavanaugh RM, Henneberger PK, et al: Young adult's knowledge, attitudes, and behavior about abortions in young women. J Pediatr Adolesc Gynecol 9:21–26, 1996.
4. Marsiglio W, Shehan CI: Adolescent males' abortion attitudes: Data from a national survey. Fam Plann Perspect 25:162–169, 1993.
5. Reichelt P, Werley H: Contraception, abortion, and venereal disease: Teenagers' knowledge and the effects of education. Fam Plann Perspect 7:83–88, 1975.
6. Gold MA, Coupey SC: Attitudes of inner-city female adolescents towards medical and surgical abortion. J Pediatr Adolesc Gynecol 11:127–131, 1998.
7. Stone R, Waszak C: Adolescent knowledge and attitudes about abortion. Fam Plann Perspect 24:52–57, 1992.
8. Henshaw SK: Factors hindering access to abortion services. Fam Plann Perspect 27:54–59, 87, 1995.
9. Althaus FA, Henshaw SK: The effects of mandatory delays on abortion patients and providers. Fam Plann Perspect 26:228–231, 233, 1994.
10. Alan Guttmacher Institute: Issues in Brief: Lawmakers grapple with parents' role in teen access to reproductive health care. November 1995, pp 1–6.
11. Henshaw SK, Kost K: Parental involvement in minor's abortion decisions. Fam Plann Perspect 24:196, 1992.
12. Rogers JL, Boruch RF, Stoms GB, DeMoya D: The impact of the Minnesota Parental Notification Law on abortion and birth. Am J Public Health 81:294–298, 1991.
13. Cartoof VG, Klerman LV: Parental consent for abortion: Impact of the Massachusetts law. Am J Public Health 76:397–400, 1986.
14. Henshaw SK: The impact of requirements for parental consent on minor's abortions in Mississippi. Fam Plann Perspect 27:120–122, 1995.
15. Henshaw RC, Naji SA, Russell IT, et al: A comparison of medical abortion (using mifepristone and gemeprost) and surgical vacuum aspiration: Efficacy and early medical sequelae. Hum Reprod 9:2167–2172, 1994.
16. Creinin MD, Darney DP: Methotrexate and misoprostol for early abortion. Contraception 48:339–348, 1993.
17. Hausknecht R: Methotrexate and misoprostol to terminate early pregnancy. N Engl J Med 333:537–540, 1995.
18. Peterson HB, Grimes DA, Cates W Jr, et al: Comparative risk of death from induced abortion at ≤ 12 weeks' gestation performed with local versus general anesthesia. Am J Obstet Gynecol 141:763–768, 1981.
19. Grimes DA, Schultz KF, Cates W Jr, et al: Local versus general anesthesia: Which is safer for performing suction curettage abortions? Am J Obstet Gynecol 135:1030, 1979.
20. Zoles G, Blacker CV: The psychological complications of therapeutic abortion. Br J Psychiatry 160:742–749, 1992.
21. Payne EC, Kravitz AR, Notman MT, Anderson JV: Outcome following therapeutic abortion. Arch Gen Psychiatry 33:725–733, 1976.
22. Pavl M, Lichtenberg ES, Borgetta L, et al: A Clinician's Guide to Medical and Surgical Abortion. Philadelphia, Churchill-Livingstone, 1999.
23. Hern WM: Abortion Practice. Boulder, CO, Alpenglo Graphics, 1990.
24. American Academy of Pediatrics Committee Statement: The adolescent's right to confidential care when considering abortion. Pediatrics 97:746–751, 1996.
25. Cartoof VG: Adolescent abortion: Correlates and consequences. Adolesc Med 3:283–298, 1992.

CHAPTER 25

Lesbian Adolescents

Caitlin C. Ryan, A.C.S.W.
Donna Futterman, M.D.

Lesbian adolescents experience the same health and mental health concerns as their heterosexual peers, with the addition of challenges related to having a stigmatized identity. Although lesbian adolescents represent all racial and ethnic groups, socioeconomic levels and backgrounds, they are generally invisible. Fear of rejection, humiliation, and discrimination prevents many from disclosing their sexual identity to providers, parents, peers, and adults who normally provide support for adolescents. Most lesbian adolescents are reluctant to disclose their sexual identity or share confusion about their sexual orientation with providers, particularly during an initial interview. Providers can build rapport by not assuming that all youth are heterosexual and by creating a nonjudgmental, supportive environment in which adolescents feel safe to disclose health problems and concerns.

IDENTITY DEVELOPMENT

Parents or providers may assume that same-sex behavior equals same-sex identity. Regardless of their sexual identity, however, many adolescents may experiment with same-sex behavior. In addition, adolescents may self-identify as lesbian or gay without having been sexually active. Sexual identity develops over a period of time. Most early models of homosexual identity development were based on the experiences of middle and upper-middle class white gay men.[1] Nearly all models recognize the impact of stigma, which affects the formation and expression of homosexual identity, involves increasing acceptance of identity, and includes disclosure to nongay persons. These models generally include the following stages: (1) awareness of same-sex feelings; (2) identity confusion (and cognitive dissonance), with gradual reframing of negative myths and misconceptions; (3) self-identification as lesbian or gay; and (4) integration of sexual identity into all aspects of life. More recent models explore the impact of gender, race, and ethnicity on sexual orientation.[2] Such models contend that factors such as legal and economic realities, racial/ethnic group, geographic area, family, and support systems determine the extent to which disclosure may be possible; thus, widespread disclosure should not be construed as the only measure of identity integration, as earlier models suggest.

Development of sexual identity in racial and ethnic minority youth is more complex and is shaped by several factors, including attitudes, values, and beliefs about sexuality, gender, and sex roles; responsibilities for childbearing; religious values; degree of acculturation into mainstream society; and the importance of family and ethnic communities in providing acceptance and support.[3,4] Identifying as openly gay may jeopardize acceptance by family and ethnic community, while racism in mainstream society and the predominantly white lesbian/gay community devalues core aspects of self. As a result, lesbians and gay males of color are generally less visible than their white counterparts and must balance the needs and demands of separate communities and allegiances while facing additional stressors and challenges in consolidating sexual, racial, and ethnic identities.

The cognitive and emotional isolation that lesbian and gay youth experienced in past decades may make it even more difficult to understand same-sex feelings and attractions. Increasing access to information and wider availability of support services for lesbian and gay youth have contributed to greater self-awareness of sexual identity at younger ages. Studies of adolescent sexual orientation show that the age of "coming out" or self-identification as lesbian or gay has been steadily dropping (Table 1).[5] These findings precipitated further research that shows that awareness of sexual attraction in heterosexual and homosexual youth occurs at a mean age of 10, with attraction marking the first event in a developmental sequence (of attraction, fantasy, and behavior).[6] As a result, providers will be more likely to care for self-identified lesbian and bisexual youth than during previous decades when sexual identity consolidation was more likely to occur at a later age and providers were less aware of their patients' sexual identity.

Impact of Stigma

A primary task of identity development for lesbian adolescents is learning to manage a stigmatized identity. Although the vast majority of lesbian adolescents grow up to lead healthy, productive lives, the challenge of transforming a stigmatized identity into a positive one represents a significant developmental crisis, regardless of age. Negative attitudes about homosexuality, myths, and misperceptions are internalized from early childhood. As a child or young adolescent begins to acknowledge and label same-sex feelings and attractions, internal conflict, cognitive dissonance, identity confusion, and even self-loathing

TABLE 1. Average Age at Which Event Occurs

	Adults (Retrospective Studies)		**Adolescents (Prospective Studies)**	
Behavior/Identity	*Males*	*Females*	*Males*	*Females*
First awareness of same-sex attraction	13	14–16	9	10
First same-sex experience	15	20	13–14	14–15
Self-identification as lesbian or gay	19–21	21–23	14–16	15–16

may result. Adolescents may repress, deny, or attempt to change such feelings through a range of coping behaviors, including heterosexual activity, use of alcohol and drugs, pregnancy, and displacement activities, such as extensive immersion in sports, school, or extracurricular activities. Internalized as self-hate and low self-esteem, stigma can have social, behavioral, and health-related consequences and increase risk for unprotected sex, sexually transmitted infections (STIs), human immunodeficiency virus (HIV), substance abuse, psychological distress, and suicide.

Support for adolescents who are struggling with issues related to emerging sexual identity is essential. Providers should explain the difference between identity and behavior: some individuals may identify as lesbian or gay without being sexually active, just as others may be sexually active with same-sex partners without identifying as lesbian or gay. Moreover, some adolescents may become sexually active to repress or confirm same-sex feelings and identity. Providers should explain that adolescents have options other than becoming sexually active to learn about their sexual identity and suggest alternatives, such as educational materials and support groups. Adolescents who may be experiencing same-sex feelings and attractions need reassurance and support that such feelings are common and do not necessarily indicate homosexual identity. Sexual identity evolves over time, and attempts to force resolution do not accelerate the process. For youth who may be lesbian, access to accurate information and positive role models helps to reframe negative stereotypes and provides options for developing positive career and personal goals for a satisfying, productive life. Providers should make referrals to support groups* for lesbian, gay, and bisexual youth, which are increasingly available in urban areas and smaller cities, and to knowledgeable counselors when appropriate.

Parents, too, need accurate information and an opportunity to understand and grieve the loss of a child's heterosexual identity with its attendant hopes and dreams of marriage, grandchildren, social acceptance, and career. Like adolescents and young adults who struggle with an emerging sexual identity, parents and families experience a parallel "coming out" process and are affected by the stigma associated with homosexuality. Acceptance takes time, and realization of the extensive resources and support available in the lesbian/gay community, including successful lesbian/gay role models, career, long-term relationships, and parenting options, helps parents to adjust to what, for most, is initially disturbing news. Referral to Parents, Families and Friends of Lesbians and Gays (P-FLAG)†—a national organization with chapters in many urban communities that provides education, information, and support for parents and families of lesbians, gay men, and bisexuals—helps many parents learn to cope and ultimately accept their adolescent's sexual identity. Referral to knowledgeable family therapists who understand the dynamics of coming out is also helpful. Providers should be aware that not all parents eventually accept an adolescent's lesbian

* For information about local support services for lesbian, gay, bisexual, and transgender youth, contact the National Youth Advocacy Coalition at 202-319-7596, www.nyacyouth.org.

† For information about local P-FLAG chapters, contact the national office at 202-638-4200, e-mail PFLAG@aol.com or web address, http://www.pflag.org.

or gay identity, and coming out may precipitate negative repercussions, including violence and expulsion from the home. Thus, adolescents often need guidance and counseling to help determine the best timing and circumstances in which to disclose their sexual identity to families and others whose reactions will affect the adolescent's emotional and physical well-being.

PRIMARY CARE

An initial work-up provides an opportunity for the provider and adolescent to share key information and begin to build rapport and trust. These interactions are especially important since they form the basis for future provider–client relationships and help-seeking behaviors. Sensitivity to sexual identity, in particular, will encourage disclosure and help to establish appropriate communication patterns for a lifetime of care. The goal with any adolescent whose sexual orientation is unknown is to facilitate, not force, disclosure. Health and risk behaviors are best assessed in the context of an adolescent's life, including family, school, interests, peers, interests, activities, coping style, and behaviors. An excellent assessment tool for adolescent interviews is the HEADS questionnaire, developed by staff of Children's Hospital of Los Angeles, which has been adapted for use with youth who may be lesbian, gay, or bisexual (Table 2).[7,8] In addition, Table 3 provides a general guide to primary care for lesbian adolescents.

Providers should ensure that both the adolescent and parent(s) understand that information they share will not be disclosed, except in serious situations such as those involving suicidal feelings or sexual abuse. When confidentiality is openly discussed, adolescents are more willing to seek care for sensitive health concerns. Assurances about confidentiality are particularly important for lesbian youth, who may experience rejection, discrimination, loss of critical relationships (e.g., family and close friends), and ejection from their homes if confidentiality related to their sexual identity is breached.

Reproductive Health, Sexually Transmitted Infections, and Parenting

Because lesbian youth may have internalized distorted perceptions about their psychology and health needs and risks, education should be provided about sexual health. Studies of health behaviors, particularly among older lesbians, show lack of routine gynecologic care. In a national lesbian health survey, for example, 23% of 17–24-year-old lesbians and 5% of lesbians over age 55 had never received a Pap smear.[9] Fear of ridicule or lack of understanding among providers, including misconceptions that gynecologic care is relevant only for heterosexual females, inhibits lesbians from obtaining routine screening and ongoing care. Others may become alienated and reluctant to seek care as a result of intense pressure from providers who, failing to realize that they were treating lesbian patients, tried to determine their method of birth control. Providers should explain the need for routine gynecologic check-ups for lesbian adolescents and provide guidance on reproductive health. Because lesbian adolescents who are sexually active may have sex with

TABLE 2. Adolescent Risk Profile Interview (HEADS Assessment)

H	**Home**		Where do you live? Who do you live with? How much time do you spend at home? What do you and your family argue about? Can you go to your parents with problems? Have you ever run away from home?
E	**Education**		What grade are you in? What grades are you getting? Have they changed? Have you ever failed any classes or been kept back a grade? Do you ever cut classes? Have you ever been teased or attacked in sachool?* Do you work after school or on weekends? What are your career/vocational goals?*
A	**Activities**		What do you do for fun? What activities do you do during and after school? Are you active in sports? Do you exercise? Who do you do fun things with? Who are your friends? Who do you go to with problems? What do you do on weekends? Evenings?
		If appropriate:	Does anyone in your home/family know you are lesbian/gay/bisexual? Why/why not?* Do any of your friends know you're gay?* Do you have any gay friends? Are they your age, older?* Do you go anywhere to meet other gay people?* Do you go to gay bars or clubs?* What do you know about local social and recreational organizations for lesbians and gay men?*
D	**Drugs**		Do you drink coffee or tea? Do you smoke cigarettes? Have you ever smoked one? Have you ever tried alcohol? When? What kind and how often? Do any of your friends drink or use drugs? What drugs have you tried? Have you ever injected steroids or drugs? When? How often do you use them? How do you get money to pay for drugs?* Are drugs used or available in places where you hang out?*
S	**Sexual activity/ identity**		Have you ever had sex unwillingly? How many sexual partners have you had? How old were you when you first had sex? How old was your partner?* Have you ever had sex with men? Women? Both? Do you think you might be lesbian, gay, or bisexual?* Do you think you need to have sex to find out if you're lesbian, gay, or bisexual?* Do you want to become pregnant?* Have you ever been pregnant? Have you ever had an infection as a result of having sex? Do you use condoms and/or another form of contraception for STD and HIV prevention? Have you ever traded sex for money, drugs, clothes, or a place to stay? Have you ever been tested for HIV? Do you think it would be a good idea to be tested?

Table continued on following page.

TABLE 2. Adolescent Risk Profile Interview (HEADS Assessment) *(Continued)*

S	**Suicide/depression**	How do you feel today on a scale of 0–10? (0 = very sad, 10 = very happy) Have you ever felt less than a 5? How long did that feeling last?* What made you feel that way? Does thinking you may be lesbian, gay, or bisexual make you feel that way?* Did you ever think about hurting yourself, that life wasn't worth living, or hope that when you went to sleep you wouldn't wake up?

• Adapted for use with adolescents who may be lesbian, gay, or questioning their sexual identity. From Goldenring JM, Cohen EH: Getting into an adolescent's H.E.A.D.S. Contemp Pediatr 5:75–90, 1988. Adapted in Ryan CC, Futterman D: Lesbian and Gay Youth: Care and Counseling. Adoles Med 2:207–374, 1997, with permission.

male partners, screening should include possible pregnancy and STIs, including trichomonas, gonorrhea, chlamydia, and syphilis. HIV counseling should be provided and voluntary testing offered. Lesbians who have unprotected sex with bisexual males or gay male friends may be at increased risk for HIV infection. Although risk for STIs is substantially lower for lesbians who have sex only with other females, some sexually transmitted diseases can be transmitted between women, including HPV, bacterial vaginosis, and trichomonas. Herpes and chlamydia also have been reported in lesbians who have had only female sexual partners, and although extremely rare, at least two cases of HIV infection are reported to have been transmitted between female partners. By providing health guidance that includes same-sex and opposite-sex practices, providers can ensure that all youth receive appropriate prevention messages, whether or not sexual orientation is known.

Unfortunately, health promotion and prevention literature often fails to mention lesbians, gay males, or bisexuals, so many lesbian or gay youth—who already have internalized misconceptions about their health needs and risks—do not apply the message to themselves. It is not uncommon, for example, for lesbian youth to assume that they cannot become pregnant; as a result, they may not realize that they should use birth control methods, including condoms. Lesbian youth also may have questions about parenting. Increasingly, more lesbians are choosing to parent through donor insemination and conception as well as foster care and adoption. As public acceptance of lesbians and gay men has grown, sanctions and stressors associated with being a lesbian or gay parent have decreased. More lesbians are choosing to have children, as single mothers or part of a same-sex couple. For lesbian adolescents, pregnancy may be a choice, an attempt to hide their sexual identity, or the result of failure to use contraceptives with male partners. Providers should ensure that lesbian adolescents understand their risk for pregnancy as a result of unprotected intercourse, while providing birth control information and health guidance on STIs and HIV.

Rape and Trauma

Lesbian youth are at risk for antigay violence, including rape and assault. Victimization is a common experience, particularly for youth who are stereotypically lesbian or gay, and ethnic minority youth are more frequent victims.

TABLE 3. Primary Care for Lesbian Adolescents

Physical examination

1. Height and weight with percentiles
2. Blood pressure and pulse
3. Eyes, ears, nose, mouth, teeth, and gums
4. Thyroid
5. Lymph nodes
6. Breasts
7. Heart, lungs, and abdomen
8. Back/spine
9. Tanner staging of pubertal development
   Breasts and pubic hair pattern
10. Anogenital exam/inspection
    - *Anal exam, if indicated*
    - Pelvic exam, if symptomatic, sexually experienced, or > 18 years old (speculum and bimanual)
11. Skin
12. Neurologic and mental status exam

Patient education

1. Breast self-exam
2. Genital exam (internal and external)
3. Menstrual history
4. Guidance (parenting, injury prevention, diet and fitness, adolescent development, and healthy lifestyles)

Laboratory screening

1. Hemoglobin or hematocrit (sickle cell screen, if indicated; consider complete blood count for youth with chronic illness, such as HIV infection)
2. Urinalysis
3. Liver function tests (SGOT, SGPT) for substance-using adolescents
4. Cholesterol screening, if indicated by obseity, other history
5. Pregnancy-related tests
   - Serum hCG, if indicated by history or or clinical exam
   - Rubella serology before pregnancy

Immunizations

1. Diphtheria/tetanus
2. Measles, mumps, and rubella
3. Hepatitis A, hepatitis B (prescreen homeless and HIV-positive youth for exposure to hepatitis B with HepBsAg, cAb, sAb)
4. Influenza yearly for chronic illness (including HIV) and homeless youth
5. Varicella, if not immune

Tuberculosis evaluation

1. Skin testing
2. Baseline chest x-ray if anergic or PPD-positive
3. Facilitating completion of evaluation

Sexual identity

1. Behavior
   - Same-sex and opposite-sex patterns
   - Age of coitarche and age of partners
   - Consensual and nonconsensual acts
   - Types of sexual experience
     Outercourse
       a. Kissing
       b. Massage and petting
       c. Masturbation
     Intercourse
       a. Vaginal-penile
       b. Oral-genital, oral-anal
       c. Anal-genital
   - Condom use (settings and partner type)
   - Concurrent substance use
   - Survival sex
2. Disclosure of sexual orientation
   - Family
   - Friends/partner(s)/roommates
   - Classmates/coworkers
   - Teachers/supervisors/counselors
   - Role of health care provider

Sexually transmitted diseases

1. Screening
   - Gonorrhea (triple site: genital, oral, anal)
   - Chlamydia (cervical or urine screen)
   - Vaginal wet mount (candidal infection, vaginosis, trichomoniasis), if indicated by history or exam
   - Hepatitis B prevaccination screen: hepBsAg, cAb, sAb (consider hepatitis C serology if HBV-positive or partner has HCV)
   - HIV antibody (consent and confidentiality)
   - Human papillomavirus/dysplasia
       a. Cervical Papanicolaou (Pap) smear
       b. *Consider anal Pap and anoscopy if perianal warts present*
   - Syphilis
2. Treatment issues
   - Adherence
   - Test of cure
   - Partner issues
3. Prevention
   - Risk reduction skills

Reproductive health

1. Contraception
2. Pregnancy decision making
3. Parenting skills

Vision testing and audiometry

Referral for dental care

Other referrals

From Ryan C, Futterman D: Lesbian and Gay Youth: Care and Counseling. New York, Columbia University Press, 1998, with permission.

Surveys of bias-related experiences among lesbian and gay adults show that during their lifetime more than one-half have experienced some kind of violence because of their sexual orientation.[10] Typically, depression, anxiety, fear, low self-esteem, and self-blame follow victimization; posttraumatic stress disorder is a more serious complication. Witnessing pervasive antigay victimization and harassment increases anxiety and fear of discovery among closeted youth and has a sobering effect on key developmental tasks such as career development and life choices.

Antigay victimization heightens vulnerability and often intensifies negative feelings about sexual orientation, causing the adolescent and others to perceive the act as punishment for being gay. Reactions may be heightened or minimized depending on an individual's stage of coming out or degree of self-acceptance. Family and peer support are important resources for recovering from trauma. Among youth who have not disclosed their sexual identity, parents may react with anger and "blame the victim" if the adolescent's sexual orientation is disclosed as a result of an assault or rape. Referral to a knowledgeable mental health provider is especially important for adolescents who may internalize the bias nature of their attack. Recovery from victimization and antigay violence is facilitated by: having a strong support system, access to supportive counseling, positive coping skills, access to lesbian/gay community resources and perceiving the attack as an act of prejudice rather than personal failure.

Childhood sexual abuse, which has not been found to occur with any greater frequency in lesbians than in heterosexual women,[11] also has a range of psychological and behavioral consequences that increase risk for further victimization and health concerns, including depression, posttraumatic stress disorder, substance abuse, suicidal ideation, and behavioral risk for HIV infection. Victims also experience sexual identity confusion, which further confounds and prolongs identity consolidation.

Substance Use

Alcohol and drug use are common among adolescents; however, information about the prevalence of substance use in lesbian and gay youth is limited. Some studies of urban gay youth show higher rates of alcohol and drug use, while others do not. Lesbian and gay youth use alcohol and drugs for many of the same reasons as heterosexuals—to experiment and assert independence, to relieve tension and increase self-esteem, and to self-medicate for underlying depression or mood disorder. For lesbian adolescents, vulnerability may be enhanced by social stigma and the need to hide or deny their sexual orientation. Nevertheless, careful screening for substance use is important, particularly for sexually active adolescents, because substance abuse increases risk for STIs and HIV.

Human Immunodeficiency Virus and AIDS

Even though new treatments offer promising options for prolonging life and decreasing AIDS-related disorders, relatively few adolescents currently receive care for HIV disease, and most do not know they are infected. Limited availability of HIV counseling and testing blocks access to HIV-related care for many youth. Without knowledge of one's HIV status, early intervention and aggressive therapy are not possible. Guidelines are available for providing routine counseling and offering HIV testing to adolescents in primary care settings,[12] and all sexually active youth should routinely receive HIV counseling and be offered testing (with informed consent). New testing options, such as oral test kits, facilitate testing in a variety of settings without having to draw or store blood. Regardless of HIV status, all sexually active youth should receive ongoing HIV education and prevention information, including a demonstration of condom use and help in developing a risk reduction plan that includes practical, achievable goals.[12]

A primary concern in working with adolescents with HIV infection is helping them adjust to their HIV status. Access to support services and psychosocial care is especially important for adolescents who have a range of needs that change with the stage and course of disease. Overall goals for primary care include (1) determining the stage of HIV disease and health status; (2) providing ongoing health maintenance for HIV and primary care needs; (3) monitoring immune function and viral load; (4) providing access to state-of-the-art treatment; (5) providing education about HIV and risk reduction; (6) identifying and addressing psychosocial needs; and (7) providing access to appropriate clinical trials. Because treatment and care must consider an adolescent's developmental stage and cognitive capacity, providers need to develop an individualized treatment plan that includes these considerations. Guidance is available for discussing new treatment options with adolescents.[12,13]

Mental Health Care

Although no differences in psychological adjustment have been seen in studies of lesbians and gay males and their heterosexual peers, adolescents and adults who are struggling with sexual identity may experience a range of psychological reactions during the process of coming out (becoming aware of and integrating their sexual identity). Once the crisis has passed, psychological distress clears and symptoms associated with coming out resolve. Although coming out is a normal stage of sexual identity development, lesbian and gay youth are at risk for misdiagnosis and inappropriate treatment during this period and require support from their primary care provider. Referral to a knowledgeable counselor or mental health practitioner is also helpful.

Lesbians and gay males who have integrated a positive identity show better psychological adjustment, greater satisfaction and lower rates of depression or stress than gay people in conflict with their identity. However, providers should be aware that identity development takes place over time, and integrating a positive identity requires access to supportive peers and adults, accurate information, and connection to a community where acceptance and validation are provided. As with other aspects of their identity, adolescents integrate or consolidate their sexual identity gradually by exploring the congruency of feelings, behavior, and self-perception, and through interactions with others.

During the process of coming out, adolescents are especially vulnerable. Providers may encounter parents or even some adolescents who seek treatment that attempts to change their sexual orientation. Experts in adolescent medicine caution against such attempts, which raise many ethical concerns, often contribute to negative self-esteem and mental health problems, and are generally unsuccessful over time. According to the American Academy of Pediatrics' Statement on Homosexuality and Adolescence, "Therapy directed specifically at changing sexual orientation is contraindicated, since it can provoke guilt and anxiety while having little or no potential for achieving changes in sexual orientation."[14] Moreover, the American Psychiatric Association (APA) states that "there is no published scientific evidence supporting the efficacy of 'reparative therapy' [also known as conversion therapy] to change one's sexual orientation."[15] Furthermore, the APA "opposes any psychiatric treatment, such as 'reparative' or 'conversion' therapy which is based upon the assumption that homosexuality per se is a mental disorder or based upon a prior assumption that the patient should change his/her homosexual orientation."

Even though the APA removed homosexuality from its list of mental disorders more than 20 years ago, some practitioners still attempt to change an individual's sexual orientation, and in recent years, such efforts appear to have intensified. Providers should caution parents against referring the adolescent for "reparative therapy" and instead, seek treatment from a mental health practitioner who will help the adolescent manage fears and confusion, while providing support for identity development. In making referrals, providers should assess carefully the agency's or practitioner's attitudes, experience, treatment philosophy or bias, and knowledge of the needs of lesbian, gay, and bisexual adolescents.

Lesbian and gay youth also report significant stress associated with school and related activities and high levels of stress associated with the stigma of homosexuality. In one of the few studies of gay-related stress, the most stressful events reported by gay and bisexual male adolescents included coming out to others, having their sexual orientation discovered by others, and being ridiculed because of their sexual identity. Many youth describe harassment, verbal and physical abuse, and negative attitudes of teachers and peers. However, some adolescents are more affected by the cumulative effects of stigma and stress as a result of earlier negative life experiences or heightened internal vulnerability. Accurate assessment for depression and suicidal ideation are especially important. Depression, somatic complaints, and suicidal ideation, in particular, are associated with emotional conflict and stress and may be indicators of internal stress in youth who are struggling with undisclosed sexual identity issues.

Although high rates of suicidal ideation and behavior have been reported in many previous studies of lesbians and gay males, these studies have been criticized for not using representative samples. A recent probability study of adolescent risk behaviors among high school students in Massachusetts showed that lesbian and bisexual youth and those who reported same-sex experiences were more than 3.5 times as likely as heterosexual youth to have attempted suicide during the past 12 months.[17] These youth were also more than four times as likely as their heterosexual peers to have skipped school during the

TABLE 4. Suicide Risk and Victimization—Massachusetts Youth Risk Behavior Survey, 1997[17]

Reported Behaviors	Lesbian/Gay/Bisexual* Students	Other Students
Attempted suicide in the past year	41/4%	11.5%
Skipped school in the past month because they felt unsafe en route or at school	16.5%	3.4%
Was threatened/injured with a weapon at school in the past year	25.3%	3.6%

* Includes both lesbian and bisexual students and female students who reported same-sex experiences.

past month because they felt unsafe and more than seven times as likely to have been threatened or injured with a weapon at school during the past year (Table 4).

These findings underscore the need for including a mental health assessment in a routine medical work-up and carefully assessing all youth who present with depressed mood. The assessment should include the adolescent's emotional state, family and environmental circumstances, history of suicidality, motivation, impulsivity, and suicidal behavior among peers. Adolescents who have attempted suicide in the past are at much greater risk for attempting and completing suicide. Providers should ask whether the youth has developed a plan for committing suicide, which signals a much more serious intent. Youth who are actively suicidal should be placed in a safe environment. Those who express suicidal thoughts or feelings should be referred for counseling with provider follow-up within the next few days. Although data about risk for suicide among lesbian youth are limited, in one of the few studies of lesbian and gay adolescents lesbians were more than twice as likely to have attempted suicide and to have used more lethal means. In another survey, lesbian youth were at higher risk than other age groups, and attempts occurred twice as often in victims of child sexual abuse, rape, and antigay violence.

ANTICIPATORY GUIDANCE

Providers routinely offer anticipatory guidance to adolescents and parents but may feel uncomfortable or uncertain in counseling nonheterosexual youth. In addition to routine topic areas of health and nutrition, safety and risk-taking, sexuality, adolescent development, relationships, school activities and future plans, providers can help lesbian adolescents and their parents to cope more effectively by discussing the following concerns.

Identity

Providers should ask lesbian adolescents what it means to be a lesbian, explore their myths and misconceptions, and provide accurate information and referrals to appropriate community services. Lack of accurate information and positive role models, including supportive heterosexual adults, is a significant problem for lesbian youths. Support and acceptance help to reframe negative internalized perceptions and to enhance self-esteem, which is essential for lesbian and gay youth.

Disclosure

Adolescents need guidance about when and how to disclose their sexual identity to parents, friends, and others in their social network. They should be counseled to think about the consequences of disclosure and to take their time in sharing information that has many repercussions, including rejection, abuse, and ejection from their homes. Adolescents need time and support, including referral to a youth support group and knowledgeable counselor, to explore the best option for disclosing their sexual identity.

Sexual Behavior and Prevention

As with all youth, lesbian teens should be cautioned about the risks of STIs, HIV, and possible pregnancy and counseled to use condoms and reduce risky behaviors in terms that specifically discuss the risk for lesbian adolescents. Providers should explore and address any misconceptions lesbian youth may have; for example, lesbian adolescents may think that having sex with a male partner or becoming pregnant ensures their heterosexuality. Adolescents should understand clearly that they have options other than sexual activity to learn about being lesbian or gay. Examples include referrals to support groups, reading books about lesbian and gay youth, and access to lesbian, gay, and bisexual community ties. This is particularly important since adolescents are at high risk for HIV infection; in fact, one-quarter of all HIV-infected persons are under age 22.

Substance Use

Adolescents should be counseled about substance use and the risk of chemical dependency. Use of alcohol and drugs to manage low self-esteem and isolation, shame, and internalized homophobia can increase risk of addiction. Moreover, the lack of supportive, age-appropriate activities for lesbian and gay youth restricts opportunities for socialization. In rural communities and small towns, for example, bars may be the only place for lesbians and gay males to socialize. Lesbians who are victims of antigay violence and sexual abuse are at increased risk for substance abuse and should receive appropriate counseling and referrals.

Mental Health

Providers should offer counseling about stressors that affect gay youth such as fear of discovery, shame, and isolation. Adolescents should understand that no psychological differences have been seen in studies of lesbians and gay males and their heterosexual peers. However, depression and thoughts about suicide have been reported by lesbian and gay youth, particularly those who have been sexually abused or who are having problems with family, school, or peers. Adolescents should be encouraged to share these feelings with their provider if they occur or persist.

Discrimination

Providers should discuss the potential risks of discrimination and antigay violence and encourage lesbian and gay youth to socialize in groups and to seek appropriate counseling and follow-up care if they are victimized. Violence has many emotional and somatic effects, including self-blame and heightened vulnerability, that increase risk for other health and mental health problems. Referral to support groups helps to build self-esteem and provides a buffer against stigma and discrimination while building self-esteem and positive coping skills.

Social Support

Providers should assess the adolescent's support system, including peers and adults. Social support plays an important role in self-acceptance and social development. Many lesbian and gay youth report losing friends after they come out to them. Providers should explore both negative and positive experiences and identify potentially vulnerable youth for appropriate referrals.

Access to Lesbian/Gay Communities

Access to lesbian/gay communities provides access to accurate information, support, and resources, including opportunities for exposing misconceptions and stereotypes and learning the broad range of diversity and occupational and career choices that are possible as lesbian and gay adults. In many urban communities, support groups and social and recreational services are available for lesbian and gay youth to reduce isolation and provide access to supervised, safe environments where they can socialize without fear of ridicule, harassment, or abuse.

Career Plans

Career planning is an important developmental task for all youth, but it is particularly difficult for lesbian and gay adolescents who lack positive models for occupational and vocational choices. Negative stereotypes about appropriate behavior and vocational options further limit choices. Providers can assist by exploring career or vocational plans and helping youth to understand that their sexual orientation should not limit their life options.

CONCLUSION

Although providers initially may not be aware of adolescents who are lesbian or bisexual, these youth are highly attuned to behaviors that signal acceptance or rejection and make decisions about disclosing their identity based on a provider's openness and perceived potential for being nonjudgmental. Because many lesbian youth internalize myths and misconceptions about what it means to be lesbian or gay and because they struggle with the health and behavioral effects of stigma, they are at increased risk for many physical and mental health concerns that are preventable and can be ameliorated with appropriate assessment and guidance. Appropriate care for lesbian adolescents does not require special skills or extensive training. Awareness that all youth are not heterosexual, sensitivity in conducting routine interviews, and understanding the stressors that affect lesbian and gay youth enable providers to provide quality care for this medically underserved and often invisible population.

REFERENCES

1. Troiden RR: Homosexual identity development. J Adolesc Health 9:105–113, 1988.
2. McCarn S, Fassinger RE: Re-visioning sexual minority identity formation: A new model of lesbian identity and its implications for counseling and research. Counsel Psychol 24:508–534, 1996.
3. Morales ES: Ethnic minority families and minority gays and lesbians. In Bozett FW, Sussman MB (eds): Homosexuality and Family Relations. Binghamton, NY, Harrington Park Press, 1990.
4. Greene B: Ethnic minority lesbians and gay men: Mental health treatment issues. J Consult Clin Psychol 62:243–251, 1994.
5. Herdt G, Boxer A: Children of Horizons, 2nd ed. Boston, Beacon Press, 1996.
6. McClintock M, Herdt G: Rethinking puberty: The development of sexual attraction. Curr Direct Psychol Sci 5:178–183, 1996.
7. Goldenring JM, Cohen EH: Getting into an adolescent's H.E.A.D.S. Contemp Pediatr 5:75–90, 1988.
8. Ryan CC, Futterman D: Lesbian and gay youth: Care and counseling. Adoles Med 8:207–374, 1997.
9. Bradford J, Ryan C: The national lesbian health survey: Final report. Washington, DC, National Lesbian and Gay Health Foundation, 1987.
10. Badgett L, Donnelly C, Kibbe J: Pervasive patterns of discrimination against lesbians and gay men: Evidence from surveys in the United States. Washington, DC, National Lesbian and Gay Task Force, 1992.
11. Bradford J, Ryan C, Rothblum ED: The national lesbian health care survey: Implications for mental health care. J Consult Clin Psychol 62:228–242, 1994.
12. Ryan CC, Futterman D: Lesbian and Gay Youth: Care and Counseling. New York, Columbia University Press, 1998.
13. Hoffman ND, Futterman D, Myerson A: Treatment issues for HIV-positive adolescents. AIDS Clin Care 11:1–23, 1999.
14. American Academy of Pediatrics: Homosexuality and adolescence. Pediatrics 92:631–634, 1993.
15. American Psychiatric Association: Gay and lesbian issues: Fact sheet. Washington, DC, American Psychiatric Association, 1994.
16. American Psychiatric Association: Position statement on psychiatric treatment and sexual orientation. Washington, DC, American Psychiatric Association, 1998.
17. Goodenow C, Abels M, Netherland J: Lesbian and bisexual adolescent girls: Risk behaviors and stressors. Presented at the American Psychological Association conference, Boston, 1999.

CHAPTER 26

Sexual Assault, Rape, and Sexual Abuse

Kathy Silverman, D.O.

Incidents of sexual assault, rape, and sexual abuse involving adolescent girls and young women are quite common (Tables 1 and 2). Exposure to disease and physical and psychological trauma associated with forced sexual encounters are frequent causes of both acute and chronic dysfunction. The ability of the clinician not only to respond appropriately to the acute issues related to sexual assault but also to recognize and address the more insidious and long-term sequelae of rape or molestation is crucial to the preservation of the physical and mental health of adolescent victims. An appropriate response requires that the clinician be aware of the historical, physical, and evidentiary components of a rape evaluation. In addition, he or she must be cognizant of the long-term sequelae of sexual assault and alert to the often subtle clues that a girl may have had an untoward and traumatizing past sexual experience. Sexual assault evaluations require careful interviewing techniques and sensitivity to the psychological needs of the assaulted young woman.

EPIDEMIOLOGY AND RISK FACTORS

The Uniform Crime Report of the United States Department of Justice documented that nearly 100,000 rapes of women were reported in 1996.[1] This number does not include statutory rape or other sex offenses, nor does it take into consideration that rape is known to be a vastly underreported crime. The National Crime Victims Research and Treatment Center estimates that nearly 700,000 women are raped each year in the United States and that 60% of these victims are teenagers.[2] Rape is mainly a crime against young women, with more than 50% of assaults involving victims below the age of 18 years.[3]

Unlike adult women, adolescent victims of sexual assault frequently know their assailant. Date and acquaintance rape are much more common in this age group, often beginning as a mutually agreeable interaction and escalating to a forced or coerced sexual encounter.[4] In many such situations drugs or alcohol is involved. Some studies have shown that girls who are victims of

TABLE 1. Legal Definitions

First-degree sexual assault

Sexual penetration of a part of a person's body by an object into the genital, oral, or anal openings, which occurs when there is

1. force or coercion, or
2. mental or physical inability to communicate unwillingness to engage in such an act.

Second-degree sexual assault

Sexual contact without penetration that could include intentional touching of a person's sexual or intimate parts or the intentional touching of the victim's clothing covering these intimate parts when there is

1. force or coercion, or
2. mental or physical inability to communicate unwillingness to engage in such an act.

Third-degree sexual assault

Sexual penetration by a person 18 years or older of a person under the age of consent.

Adapted from American Academy of Pediatrics, Committee on Adolescence: Sexual assault and the adolescent. Pediatrics 94:761–765, 1994.

sexual assaults are involved in more risk-taking behaviors than girls who are not victimized.[5,6] Factors associated with rape in the adolescent age group are listed in Table 3.

REPORTING

Many victims of sexual assault seek medical services before contacting the police. Health care providers must be familiar with the laws in their state, which may either mandate reporting or preclude reporting without the per-

TABLE 2. Medical Definitions

Rape

A sexual assault in which the penis of the assailant is placed into the genitalia of the victim, either without consent or by threat or coercion.

Acquaintance rape

Rape in which the assailant and victim know each other.

Date rape

Sexual assault is perpetrated by an individual whom the victim voluntarily accompanied on a date.

Sexual assault

Any contact of an offender with the genitalia of a nonconsenting victim.

Sexual molestation

Noncoital sexual activity between a child and an adolescent or an adult, which may include viewing, genital or breast fondling, or oral–genital contact.

Statutory rape

Having sex with a person under statutory age. The offense may be with or without the victim's consent, and ignorance of the victim's age is usually no defense.

Sexual abuse

Sexual acts performed against a minor by a parent, guardian, relative, or acquaintance.

Sodomy

Generally referred to as oral and anal copulation.

Adapted from American Academy of Pediatrics, Committee on Adolescence: Sexual assault and the adolescent. Pediatrics 94:761–765, 1994; Black's Law Dictionary, 6th ed. St. Paul, MN, Black, Henry West Publishing, 1990.

TABLE 3. Factors Associated with Adolescent Rape Victims

Alcohol and drug use	Staying out very late
Interactions with strangers in unsupervised settings	Physical, emotional, or mental limitations
Accepting rides from strangers	Homelessness
Interactions with older males	

Adapted from Holmes MM: Rape management. Contemp Pediatr 15:62–79, 1998.

mission of the victim. In some states, laws requiring parental notification of the sexual assault of a minor may supersede considerations of confidentiality.

When reporting is not mandated, clinicians may wish to encourage such reporting at the time of the assault. The opportunity always exists for the adolescent, at some later date, to change her decision and not pursue legal action. In addition, financial assistance from State Crime Victims Compensation Boards almost always is contingent upon the crime having been reported.

CLINICAL EVALUATION

History

Clinical assessment should be done in a setting that maximizes privacy, and a female assistant should be present if the examining clinician is male. Neither parents nor police should be present. A separate interview may be done with parents and police at a different time. A detailed account of the assault as well as a complete medical and psychosocial history should be obtained (Appendix A). The description of the assault should include the date, time, and place of the attack; description of the assailant; who was involved, if known; specific sexual acts; violent acts; and the weapon, if one was used. It also should note what the victim did after the assault that may have altered evidence (e.g., if the victim changed her clothes, showered, douched, wiped the genital area, inserted or removed a tampon, brushed her teeth, urinated, or had a bowel movement). Special interviewing techniques have been published for use with young children and may be appropriate to use with very young or mentally handicapped adolescents.[7] In some cases, particularly those involving children and the mentally handicapped, videotaping the interview may be helpful in assisting later prosecution.

Physical Examination

Rape victims are trauma victims and require immediate identification and treatment of serious or life-threatening injuries. After the initial assessment, the victim of a sexual assault should undergo a complete physical examination, including an age-appropriate genital examination. If the patient seeks care within 72 hours of the assault, evidence may be obtained that will assist with subsequent prosecution (Tables 4 and 5). Beyond 72 hours, the yield from an evidentiary examination is negligible.[8] Rape crisis centers and most emergency rooms have "rape kits" and protocols to aid in the collection of evidence and in the treatment and referral of rape victims. It is essential that

TABLE 4. Medical Specimens

1. Gonorrhea cultures from oropharyngeal, anal, endocervical (postmenarcheal girls), and vaginal (premenarcheal girls) areas if indicated by history. Nonculture tests should not be used.
2. Chlamydia cultures from endocervical (postmenarcheal girls), vaginal (premenarcheal girls), and rectal areas if indicated by history. If a test other than culture is used, a second test based on a different diagnostic technique must be used to verify positive results.
3. Syphilis screen
4. Hepatitis B screen
5. Pregnancy test for pubertal girls
6. HIV antibody test
7. Wet mount to look for *Trichomonas vaginalis,* bacterial vaginosis, and sperm.

(Only conduct a speculum examination on premenarcheal girls if major trauma is suspected. Use a pediatric speculum. Sedation is usually required. Only saline should be used if lubrication is needed for speculum insertion.)

Adapted from Hampton H: Care of the woman who has been raped. N Engl J Med 332:234–237, 1995.

the victim's physical and emotional well-being take precedence over evidence and data collection and that she be allowed a sense of control throughout the examination.

Documentation of the examination should include vital signs and height and weight. A description of the victim's general appearance (e.g., damaged clothing), behavior, and emotional state should be included in the report. The genital examination should describe the labia majora and minora, perihymenal region, hymen, posterior fourchette, fossa navicularis, clitoris, and the periintroital vaginal tissue.[9] If a speculum examination is done, the vaginal mucosa and cervix should be described. In cases of sodomy, the buttocks, perianal, and anal areas should be described.

TABLE 5. Forensic Specimens

Forensic specimens are obtained to identify blood, hair, skin, and semen from the assailant. Contamination of specimens must be avoided. All specimens must be properly labeled, sealed, and delivered to law enforcement officials.

1. Clothing worn during the assault should be scanned with a Wood's lamp to detect semen.
2. The victim should disrobe over a clean sheet or piece of paper, and her clothes as well as any foreign materials should be collected and placed into a paper bag.
3. Fingernail scrapings should be obtained.
4. Dried secretions (semen, blood, saliva) should be collected with a saline-moistened swab.
5. Saliva sample of the victim should be taken.
6. Blood sample of the victim for ABO type should be taken.
7. Alcohol and toxicology samples of the victim (serum and urine) should be obtained.
8. Hair samples from both pubic and scalp areas of the victim should be taken.
9. Debris combed from the victim's pubic hair should be collected.
10. Oral, vaginal, and anal samples should be collected with sterile cotton swabs.
11. Vaginal aspirate should be collected by pipette to look for sperm.

Adapted from Neinstein L: Adolescent Health Care: A Practical Guide, 3rd ed. Baltimore, MD, Williams & Wilkins, 1996, pp 1143–1172.

All areas of trauma should be diagramed and described. Photographs with patient identification included (a hand-held sign with the patient's name will suffice) should be taken whenever possible. A colposcope, hand-held magnifying lens, or application of toluidine blue helps to visualize injuries and, at times, colposcopic photography is available.

MANAGEMENT

The urgent care of the adolescent victim of sexual assault includes identifying and treating any injuries that may be present; evaluation and prophylaxis for sexually transmitted diseases (STDs); assessment of the need for emergency contraception; counseling regarding possible exposure to human immunodeficiency virus (HIV), including advice regarding HIV prophylaxis and immediate and subsequent testing; an appraisal of the adolescent's psychological response to the assault; and, as addressed previously, decisions regarding the collection of evidence and reporting to the police or protective authorities. In addition, before discharge from the acute situation, an attempt should be made to make definitive arrangements for subsequent counseling and medical care.

As sexual assault often involves force or violence, the adolescent should be examined for any evidence of trauma that may require either immediate treatment or documentation for subsequent prosecution. Bruises, abrasions, bite marks, and lacerations are common in both genital and nongenital areas. Lacerations must be differentiated from deeper stab wounds. In addition to a general appraisal for trauma, specific attention should be paid to the identification of genital injury. Often there is no evidence of genital injury; however, hymenal tears, genital lacerations, or abrasions may be present and require attention and documentation. Virginal adolescents may have particular concerns regarding hymenal integrity, and such concerns should be addressed. Infrequently, an assault results in major trauma to the genital or anal area, which demands immediate gynecologic or surgical intervention.

The sexual assault victim also needs evaluation and prophylaxis for STDs. Even in the absence of acute findings, the adolescent should receive prophylaxis for *Chlamydia trachomatis, Neisseria gonorrhoeae, Trichomonas vaginalis,* bacterial vaginosis, and hepatitis B if antibody-negative.[10] Specific regimens for prophylaxis have been published by the Centers for Disease Control and Prevention (CDC) (Table 6).[10]

If the victim was not protected by effective contraception and is not pregnant, emergency contraception should be offered. A number of different combinations of oral contraceptive pills may be used for this purpose (Table 7). Because these regimens often cause nausea, an antiemetic may be taken 1 hour prior to each dose. The patient should be alerted to the possibility that her next menstrual period may be early or late and that emergency contraception may fail. A pregnancy test should be performed 2 weeks after the assault if menses has not occurred.[11] If a teenager does become pregnant as a result of a rape, she should receive options counseling regarding her decision to terminate or carry the pregnancy.

Although transmission of HIV through an isolated sexual assault is rare, the adolescent victim and her family may be concerned about this possibility. The

TABLE 6. STD Prophylaxis

- Postexposure hepatitis B vaccine for those who have not been previously immunized or infected. Administer at initial visit, and at 1–2 and 4–6 months after the first dose.
- Serologic test for syphilis
- Empiric therapy for gonorrhea, trichomonas, bacterial vaginosis, and chlamydia. Recommended regimen:
  Ceftriaxone, 125 mg IM, in a single dose for gonorrhea
  plus
  Metronidazole, 2 gm orally, in a single dose for trichomonas and bacterial vaginosis
  plus
  Azithromycin, 1 gm orally, in a single dose,
  or
  Doxycycline, 100 mg twice daily for 7 days, for chlamydia
- HIV: Test for antibody. Routine prophylactic treatment is not recommended; however, if the assailant is known to be HIV-positive, prophylactic multiagent treatment should be offered after counseling.
- Injuries (major trauma, lacerations, burns, abrasions)
  Tetanus booster (dT), 0.5 ml IM, if more than 5 years since last booster.
- Follow-up:
  Serologic tests for syphilis and HIV should be repeated at 6, 12, and 24 weeks after the assault if the previous results were negative. For pregnant or allergic patients, refer to the CDC Guidelines for alternative regimens.

Adapted from Centers for Disease Control and Prevention: 1998 Guidelines for Treatment of Sexually Transmitted Diseases. MMWR 47(RR-1), 1997.

benefit of prophylactic therapy for sexually transmitted HIV infection is not known. Postexposure therapy with zidovudine has been associated with a decreased risk of HIV transmission in health care workers who had a percutaneous exposure to HIV-infected blood. Clinicians who offer rape victims prophylaxis against HIV infection should take into account the potential risks and benefits of such therapy, the likelihood of exposure, and the time that has lapsed since the assault.[12] If the victim desires preventive therapy, she should be informed of the possible adverse effects of the medication, the unknown efficacy, and the need for strict adherence to the dosing regimen and close follow-up care. In addition, she should be informed that prophylaxis is most likely to work best if started immediately after the assault. According the the CDC, if

TABLE 7. Suggested Regimens for Emergency Contraception

Ovral
  2 tablets orally (within 72 hours after assault), and
  2 tablets orally 12 hours after the first dose.

Lo/Ovral, Levlen, Nordette
  4 tablets orally (within 72 hours after assault), and
  4 tablets 12 hours after the first dose.

Triphasil or Tri-Levlen
  4 yellow tables (within 72 hours of the assault), and
  4 yellow tablets 12 hours after the first dose.

Levonorgestrel (progestin-only)
  1 tablet (0.75 mg) orally (within 72 hours after assault), and
  1 tablet (0.75 mg) orally 12 hours after the first dose.

therapy is initiated, it should be given according the to guidelines for occupational mucus membrane exposure. It should be noted that HIV postexposure prophylaxis is expensive and that because of its unproven efficacy, many health insurance companies will not reimburse for the cost. Before prescribing, baseline testing should be done to evaluate for preexisting HIV infection.

The adolescent rape victim may suffer acute and severe psychological trauma. In many ways the assault has a far greater impact on the psyche than upon the genitalia. Feelings of guilt, humiliation, and depression may overwhelm the young woman. Besides any long-term psychological considerations, there may be an immediate need to protect her against self-destructive thoughts and acts. When the girl appears to be at risk for suicide or terribly frightened of returning to her home, school, or neighborhood, a brief hospitalization may be indicated.

The anxiety of the moment prevents many rape victims from remembering their treatments or instructions. All treatments and advice given to the adolescent should be explained thoroughly and, when possible, committed to writing. If family members are involved and concerned, they should participate in hearing explanations of complex medication regimens so that they can help to reinforce adherence. Patient education materials specific to the needs of the adolescent victim complement information offered during the acute encounter. In addition, the patient should be supplied with a telephone number to call if she has any questions or concerns. Before discharge, arrangements should be made for medical follow-up and referral to counseling professionals with expertise in working with rape victims.

ACQUAINTANCE AND DATE RAPE

National data indicate that each year an excess of 100,000 females, aged 12 years and over, are victims of rape or attempted rape, and in approximately 50% of cases the victims know their assailant.[11] Victims of acquaintance rape often feel that by knowing their assailant, they in some way contributed to the rape.

Girls and young women express ambivalent opinions about forced sex. In one study of adolescents, 32% of girls thought that a forced sexual encounter was all right if a couple had been dating for a long time; 31% believed it was all right if the woman initially agreed to have sex but then changed her mind; and 27% thought it was all right if she "led him on."[13] In the same study, 54% of the adolescent boys thought forced sex is justified if the woman had said yes and then changed her mind, and 40% thought forced sex was all right if the man spent a lot of money on the date. Another study of high school students showed that a significant number of both males and females thought that forced sex was acceptable in the following circumstances: she says yes and then says no; she has led him on; she gets him sexually excited; she gets drunk or high and passes out; she has had sex with some of his friends; they have had sex before; he buys her dinner and pays for her movie; or she is wearing sexy clothing.[4] These studies indicate that gender biases regarding male prerogatives and rape myths, including the belief that rape victims bring it upon themselves, are commonly held stereotypes among adolescents.

TABLE 8. Tips for Avoiding Date Rape Drugs

- Do not share drinks.
- Do not accept a drink from a punch bowl.
- Do not accept a drink that you have not seen poured.
- Do not leave your drink unattended and then go back and drink from it.
- Do not drink anything that has an unusual taste or appearance.
- Do not mix alcohol and drugs; the result can be lethal.

Often the use of alcohol or drugs is implicated in date and acquaintance rape. Alcohol use and drinking to intoxication are frequent occurrences in adolescent social interactions. When intoxication becomes a part of the dating situation, it may have one of several adverse effects, such as reducing the girl's ability to resist a sexual assault, decreasing the inhibitions of both parties, increasing aggressive behavior, or facilitating the misinterpretation of sexual intentions.

The use of "date rape drugs" is an emerging problem. In particular, two substances, flunitrazepam (Rohypnol™) and gammahydroxybutyrate (GHB) have been implicated.[14] Both are odorless and tasteless and hence easily used to adulterate a beverage without arousing suspicion. Suggestions to assist young women in protecting themselves against "date rape drugs" are found in Table 8. Anticipatory guidance for adolescent dating should include some specific suggestions (Table 9).

PSYCHOLOGICAL CONCERNS

In the weeks and months after a sexual assault, victims often complain of insomnia, difficulty concentrating, depression, and somatic symptoms (Table 10). In addition to these complaints, which may be expressed by women of any age, there are some concerns that, although not specific to adolescents, are encountered more commonly in this younger age group. Adolescent girls often express feelings of guilt, shame, and self-blame as well as concerns about the loss of virginity.

Posttraumatic stress disorder (PTSD) is yet another frequent consequence. Symptoms of PTSD may persist for weeks or months and involve reliving the event, avoidance of experiences that were previously enjoyed, avoidance of situations that are reminiscent of the assault, and autonomic symptoms of anxiety, including palpitations, chest pain, and diaphoresis. PTSD more commonly follows instances of rape by a stranger in which there has been violence, in

TABLE 9. Anticipatory Guidance for Dating

- Let your date know what your limits are.
- Be aware of situations in which you do not feel in control or are uncomfortable, and get out of them as quickly as possible.
- Try group dating if you do not feel comfortable with your date, or arrange to meet in a public place.
- Do not date people who do not respect you.
- A girl has the right to say no at any time.

Adapted from American College of Obstetricians and Gynecologists, Committee on Adolescent Health Care: ACOG Committee Opinion: Adolescent Acquaintance Rape, No. 122, 1993.

TABLE 10. Prevalence of Psychological Symptoms Following Rape

Behavior	Percent
Denial	54
Phobias	46
Psychosomatic complaints	44
Insomnia	31
Depression	27
School problems	15
Attempted suicide	10

Adapted from Felice M, Grant J, Reynolds B, et al: Follow-up observations of adolescent rape victims. Clin Pediatr 17:311–315, 1978.

which a weapon was used, or in which serious injury has been sustained.[15] Both individual and group counseling may be helpful. Recovery for an adolescent is often dependent on family support, and assistance to the family may be necessary to enable them to provide this support. It should be noted that young women suffering from PTSD subsequent to a rape often seek medical attention for a variety of somatic complaints. The clinician should appreciate that psychological distress often manifests as somatic symptoms. It also may be quite difficult for a girl to raise concerns about her mental health and to disclose the rape event. The opportunity to identify and address PTSD as a result of sexual assault should not be missed.

SCREENING FOR PREVIOUS SEXUAL ASSAULT

Questions about sexual activity should be incorporated routinely into the health care encounter with an adolescent. This questioning should include inquiries into whether she has ever been subject to forced, involuntary, or coerced sexual acts (Table 11). Many young women have experienced unwanted sexual episodes, which may range from touching to repetitive rape. Many victims do not seek medical care at the time of an assault, nor are they likely to volunteer information about such traumatic episodes unless they are specifically questioned. Even when specifically questioned, the victim often needs several visits and the establishment of a trusting relationship with the clinician before she will disclose her assault experience. The routine incorporation of questions about unwanted sexual activity lets the patient know that her clinician is receptive to a discussion of rape or abuse. If she acknowledges recent abuse, she requires an evaluation similar to that noted previously for an acute

TABLE 11. Screening Questions for Sexual Assault

- How old were you when you first had sex?
- Was having sex something that you wanted to do?
- Have you ever been forced to have sex, or have you ever been raped?
- Has anyone ever touched you in a way that made you feel uncomfortable?
- Did you ever have sex when you were under the influence of drugs or alcohol?
- Has anyone ever tried to make you have sex when you did not want to?
- Have you been in an abusive relationship?
- How old are the people you date or with whom you have had sex?

sexual assault. Even if the sexual assault occurred weeks, months, or years before, the adolescent still may be a candidate for counseling because of ongoing psychological sequelae.

CONCLUSION

Underreporting and regional variances make it difficult to quantify the number of women victimized by sexual assault in the United States each year. The number is clearly in excess of 100,000, with a majority being adolescents. The clinician caring for girls and young women no doubt will encounter, at one time or another, a patient who either presents for care because of a rape or is suffering the consequences of a previous assault. Therefore, health care providers taking care of adolescents should be familiar with not only the nuances of gathering a sexual assault history and collecting evidence for a potential prosecution but also the requisites for providing acute treatment, including prophylaxis against sexually transmitted diseases and pregnancy and the need to address the psychological trauma associated with an assault. In addition, the clinician needs to be alert to the somatic symptoms, which, at times, are the only indicator that a young woman has been victimized in the past. The potential long-term consequences of rape, including posttraumatic stress disorder, mandate an appropriate and sensitive response to girls and young women who have been victimized whenever and wherever they present for care.

REFERENCES

1. Federal Bureau of Investigation: Uniform Crime Reports: Crime in the United States: 1997. Washington, DC, Government Printing Office, 1997.
2. Crime Victims Research and Treatment Center: Rape in America. Charleston, SC, Medical University of South Carolina, 1992.
3. Schafran LH: Topics for our times: Rape is a major public health issue. Am J Public Health 86:15–16, 1996.
4. Davis TC, Peck GQ, Storment JM: Acquaintance rape and the high school student. J Adolesc Health 14:220–224, 1993.
5. Piepert JK, Domalgalski LR: Epidemiology of adolescent sexual assault. Obstet Gynecol 84:867–871, 1994.
6. Shreir LA, Pierce JD, Emans SJ, DuRant RH: Gender differences in risk behaviors associated with forced or pressured sex. Arch Pediatr Adolesc Med 152:57–63, 1998.
7. Yuille JC, Hunter R, Joffe R, Zaarn J: Interviewing children in sexual abuse cases. In Goodman G, Bottoms B (eds): Child Victims: Child Witnesses; Understanding and Improving Children's Testimony; Clinical, Developmental and Legal Implications. New York, Guilford Press, 1993.
8. Crane E, Gershel J: Clinical Manual of Emergency Pediatrics, 3rd ed. St. Louis, McGraw-Hill, 1997.
9. Neinstein L: Adolescent Health Care: A Practical Guide, 3rd ed. Baltimore, MD, Williams & Wilkins, 1996.
10. Centers for Disease Control and Prevention: 1998 Guidelines for Treatment of Sexually Transmitted Diseases. MMWR 47(RR-1), 1997.
11. American Academy of Pediatrics, Committee on Adolescence: Sexual assault and the adolescent. Pediatrics 94:761–765, 1994.
12. Post-sexual exposure prophylaxis: A round table discussion. AIDS Clinical Care 10:9–12, 1998.
13. Parrot A: Acquaintance rape among adolescents: Identifying risk groups and intervention strategies. J Soc Work Hum Sexuality 8:47–61, 1989.
14. Schwartz RH, Weaver AB: Rohypnol, the date rape drug. Clin Pediatr 37:321–322, 1998.
15. American Medical Association, Council on Scientific Affairs: Violence against women. JAMA 267:3184–3189, 1992.

APPENDIX A

Rape Protocol/Data Sheet

Emergency department

Consent for treatment
Date and time of entry into the emergency room, time evaluated, and if discharged, time of discharge
Name of evaluator(s)
Name of translator if one was used
Mode of arrival to the emergency room (ambulance, police, driven by family or friend)

Identifying information

Victim's name, address, telephone number, date of birth, social security number
Alleged perpetrator's name, address, telephone number, race, and age, if known
Name of person giving the history if other than the victim

History

Chief complaint of the victim, in the victim's own words.
Description of the assault: date, time, and place of the assault. Has assault occurred within the last 72 hours?

Specific sexual acts

Vaginal, oral, or anal contact with penis, fingers, mouth, or object.
Masturbation of the victim by the assailant or masturbation of the assailant by the victim.
Did ejaculation occur? If it did, then where did the assailant ejaculate?
Was there fondling, kissing, licking? If yes, describe at what part of the body.
Was contraception used? If so, what kind?

Violence

Was a weapon used? If so, what kind and how was it used?
Was force used? If so, what kind?
Were threats used? If so, what were they?
Describe injuries sustained during the sexual assault and any preexisting injuries.

Physical complaints

Bleeding, pain, discharge

Activities following the assault

Douching, wiping, showering, changing clothes, brushing teeth, brushing hair, inserting or removing a tampon, urinating, bowel movement

Substance use

Was there voluntary use of drugs or alcohol?
Was the victim's mental status in any way impaired?
Was a "date rape drug" used?

Ongoing abuse

Does the victim know the assailant, and is there the potential for ongoing abuse?

Behavioral complaints

Suicidal ideation, depression, anxiety, phobia, fear, sleep disturbance, anorexia, sexual acting out, decline in academic performance, inability to concentrate.

Medical history before event

Illnesses, surgeries, injuries, previous assaults

Allergies

Immunizations

Tetanus booster, hepatitis B vaccine

Review of systems

Include a thorough gynecological history: menarche, date of last menstrual period, contraception, previous sexual experience, last sexual encounter, STDs (include dates and treatments), pregnancies, previous HIV testing and results, use of tampons, douching, previous sexual abuse or assault.

Also include a psychiatric history: suicide attempts, mental illness, therapy, admissions, medications.

Social history

Household members (names, ages, relationship to victim)
Educational level of victim and any developmental delay
Substance abuse (type, last use, frequency)

Physical examination

General description: include condition of clothing worn (e.g., torn, blood-stained), behavior, and emotional state.

Vital signs, height, weight, race

Complete physical examination (patient should be undressed and in a gown)

Careful inspection of skin and mucus membranes

Describe, diagram, photograph all areas of trauma (patient's name should appear in the photograph).

Oral examination

Look for trauma and culture if indicated by history.

Genital examination

External: describe sexual maturity rating (Tanner stage), perineum, labia majora and minora, periurethral tissue, posterior fourchette, fossa navicularis.

Describe, diagram, and photograph findings (areas of trauma and where semen and debris were found). Use colposcopic photography if available.

Speculum examination

Vaginal mucosa, cervix, secretions, evidence of STDs, trauma

Bimanual examination

Uterus, adnexae, cervix, tenderness, any palpable abnormalities. Describe position of the patient during the genital examination (lithotomy, knee to chest, frog leg, supine) and any instrumentation used (speculum, colposcope).

Rectal examination

External: describe surrounding skin and buttocks (skin tags, fissures, hemorrhoids, abrasions, lacerations, hematomas).

Internal: digital exam: tone, masses, guaiac test. If major trauma is suspected a sigmoidoscopy can be done.

Describe, diagram, and photograph findings (areas of trauma and where semen and debris were found). Use colposcopic photography if available.

Laboratory testing

Lab and forensic data collected (see Tables 5 and 6)
Pregnancy test
Toxicology screens of blood and urine if indicated by history

Management

STD prophylaxis/treatment (see Table 6)
Pregnancy prophylaxis (see Table 7) if indicated
HIV counseling, testing (and prophylaxis if desired)
Immunizations (hepatitis B, tetanus booster) if indicated
Report to police: date, time, precinct, person taking report, person collecting forensic evidence
Report to social services, if indicated: date, time, person taking report, case number
Disposition of rape kit and forensic evidence: all specimens labeled, evidence packaged, sealed, signed, and delivered to law enforcement officials, who must sign to receive it.

Follow-up

7–14 days: repeat STD tests and pregnancy test.
Hepatitis B vaccine. If not already immune, give the first shot at initial visit, the second shot 1 month later, and the third shot 6 months later.
Repeat syphilis test, HIV test, and hepatitis test at 6, 12, and 24 weeks if previous tests were negative.
Psychological assessment initially and referral for counseling for patient and family.

Adapted from Neinstein L: Adolescent Health Care: A Practical Guide, 3rd ed. Baltimore, MD, Williams & Wilkins, 1996; American Academy of Pediatrics, Committee on Adolescence: Sexual assault and the adolescent. Pediatrics 94:761–7654, 1998.

Index

Entries in **boldface type** indicate complete chapters.